Family Caregiving Across the Lifespan

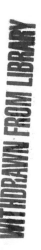

FAMILY CAREGIVER APPLICATIONS SERIES

Series Editors

David E. Biegel, *Case Western Reserve University*
Richard Schulz, *University of Pittsburgh*

Advisory Board Members

Volumes in This Series:

Family Caregiver Applications Series
Volume 4

Family Caregiving Across the Lifespan

Eva Kahana
David E. Biegel
May L. Wykle

Published in cooperation with the
Center for Practice Innovations,
Mandel School of Applied Social Sciences
Case Western Reserve University

SAGE Publications
International Educational and Professional Publisher
Thousand Oaks   London   New Delhi

For information address:

SAGE Publications, Inc.
2455 Teller Road
Thousand Oaks, California 91320

SAGE Publications Ltd.
6 Bonhill Street
London EC2A 4PU
United Kingdom

SAGE Publications India Pvt. Ltd.
M-32 Market
Greater Kailash I
New Delhi 110 048 India

Printed in the United States of America

Library of Congress Cataloging-in-Publication Data

Main entry under title:

Family caregiving across the lifespan / edited by Eva Kahana, David E.
    Biegel, May L. Wykle.
        p. cm. — (Family caregiver applications series; v. 4)
    "Published in cooperation with the Center for Practice Innovations,
    Mandel School of Applied Social Sciences, Case Western Reserve
    University."
    Includes bibliographical references and index.
    ISBN 0-8039-4430-6. — ISBN 0-8039- 4431-4 (pbk.)
    1. Chronically ill—Care. 2. Caregivers. I. Kahana, Eva.
    II. Biegel, David E. III. Wykle, May L. IV. Series.
    RC108.F357 1994
    362.1'0425—dc20   93-43663

94 95 96 97   10 9 8 7 6 5 4 3 2 1

Sage Production Editor: Diane S. Foster

This book is dedicated to the younger and older
members of our families who have made us
appreciate the uplifts as well as the burdens
of caregiving in chronic illness

Contents

Acknowledgments

The idea for this volume grew out of an interdisciplinary conference, entitled "Family Caregiving Across the Lifespan," that was cosponsored by the Mandel School of Applied Social Sciences and the University Center of Aging and Health, Case Western Reserve University. The conference, which was funded in part by the George Gund Foundation, was cochaired by Drs. Kathleen J. Farkas and May L. Wykle and was held at Case Western Reserve University in the fall of 1990. Seven of the chapters in this volume are revisions and expansions of papers that were presented at that conference, and the remaining seven chapters are papers invited by the editors on topics that address the overall themes of the volume.

This project would not have been possible without the expertise, commitment, and dedication of the contributors to this volume. They portrayed good humor and patience throughout the process of completing this manuscript.

The development of this volume benefited from the combined assistance of a number of individuals. Judy Simpson, senior program officer at the George Gund Foundation, helped secure the financial resources necessary to make this project a reality. Marquita Flemming, editor at Sage Publications, provided continued support and encouragement for our work. We are deeply grateful to Tammy Lorkovich and Neale Chumbler from the Department of Sociology and to Patricia Kilrain, Altaf Husain, and Kris Keffer from the Mandel School of Applied Social Sciences, who provided assistance with the preparation of this manuscript. We also appreciate the efforts of Linda Wykoff, who assisted in editing the manuscript.

Series Editor's Foreword

Most of us think of caregiving in relation to frail and disabled elderly persons. A prototypical case is the elderly wife caring for her husband with Alzheimer's disease, or the middle-aged daughter caring for her mother who no longer is able to navigate through life on her own. This book dispels this narrow view of caregiving and shows us that caregiving occurs at all ages and for a broad range of health conditions. Disability, dependence, and the need for help from those around us have no age limits.

Expanding the caregiving paradigm is the central theme of this book. The editors of this volume have brought together leading researchers from numerous disciplines including sociology, psychology, nursing, public health, and social work to broaden our view of caregiving at several levels. The conceptual framework for caregiving is enlarged to include the broader social system within which individual caregivers operate. The temporal context for caregiving is expanded to include chronic illnesses that occur throughout the life course, such as AIDS, cancer, and heart disease, and caregiving tasks and challenges are examined from a normative life course perspective.

Finding coherence in so much diversity is an accomplishment unachievable by any individual. It is therefore no accident that this volume has three editors. Eva Kahana brings to this effort her extensive experience in the sociology of aging and her understanding of life course development. David Biegel has been a major contributor to research on the interface between individual caregivers and formal support systems, and May Wykle long has been recognized as a national expert on cultural variations in the caregiving experience. Working closely together, this

team has created a volume that expands the discourse on caregiving to
many new domains and defines the caregiving research agenda for the
years ahead.

Richard Schulz
Series Coeditor

Introduction

OVERVIEW OF THE VOLUME

Social scientists as well as human service professionals long have been fascinated by the human interactions involved in providing assistance and caring for family members with chronic illness. The study of caregiving has assumed an important role in family studies and among scholars involved in the study of stress and coping. In the practice arena, the family context of chronic illness comprises a major underpinning of the field of family medicine, a growing specialty in primary care. Human service professionals ranging from social workers to nurses and clinical psychologists have developed therapeutic interventions to address needs of families caring for persons with chronic illness. Increasing public debate and media attention also have been directed at long-term care options and financing of home care, including innovative adjuncts to family caregiving such as hospice and respite care.

Several converging social trends have resulted in the increasing importance of studies of caregiving across the life span and across diverse health problems. The social significance and potential burden of caring for family members with chronic illness represent a normative demand on families (Zarit, Pearlin, & Schaie, 1993). Increased life expectancy has resulted in greater prevalence of Alzheimer's disease and other chronic illnesses associated with late life. Advances in medical technology, coupled with DRG financing of hospital stays, also have resulted in increasing use of home care rather than acute hospitalization for cancer and other illnesses requiring relatively high-technology care. In addition, the growing epidemic of the Acquired Immune Deficiency Syndrome (AIDS) has posed challenges for caregiving to a much younger group than those who in the past typically were cared for in traditional family settings. The deinstitutionalization of persons with mental illness has produced greater requirements for home care and other informal services for individuals with mental illness and developmental disabilities. Recent advances in entitlements and legal protection of individuals who are physically challenged also have opened up new horizons for functioning and empowerment for this group, bringing with these new horizons greater needs for support by informal and formal caregivers.

One result of this growing interest in caregiving has been a large increase in the caregiving literature in recent years. For example, between 1987 and 1991, there was a 41% increase in the number of journal articles concerning caregiving abstracted in *Psychological Abstracts,* a 200% increase in caregiving articles abstracted in *Sociological Abstracts,* and an increase of 307% in caregiving articles abstracted in *Medline* while the total number of articles abstracted in these databases increased by only 9% or less per database.

The response to this proliferation of caregiving literature has led to debate among scholars about the merits of further investment of scientific resources in the study of caregiving with the belief by some that we do not need further studies to document or describe caregiver stress (Zarit & Toseland, 1989). It has been argued that caregiving may be an overstudied phenomenon that is not likely to lead to many new insights about the social world or illness or the psychosocial interior of the family.

Upon closer scrutiny of the caregiving literature, however, it becomes clear that only one small corner of this complex paradigm has received most of the attention by researchers: burdens of caregivers of physically frail elders or elders with Alzheimer's disease. At the same time, much less is known about the nature, components, antecedents, and sequelae of caregiving involving other age groups and diverse illness situations. Previous reviews of caregiving research have identified a number of significant limitations in both conceptualization and method of caregiving research. Conceptual limitations relate to a general lack of theoretical grounding and a narrow perspective typically limited to focus on ill effects on designated family caregivers of patients suffering from a specific disease. The need for examination of the caregiving experience *across* as well as *within* particular illnesses has been particularly stressed (Biegel, Sales, & Schulz, 1991). In terms of methodological limitations, the literature is characterized by cross-sectional studies that lack comparison groups and shared instruments and that usually are based on convenience samples of caregivers, often comprising clinical populations.

Recently there has been a call to broaden the conceptual framework of caregiving research to include a wider range of variables that affect caregiving (Chiriboga, Weiler, & Neilson, 1988-1989; Pearlin, Mullan, Semple, & Skaff, 1990). Pearlin and colleagues' work in particular, which George (1990) calls a tour de force, also emphasizes the need for further examinations of the process and context of caregiving. Significant gaps in knowledge exist in regard to the contextual perspectives in caregiving (Burton & Sorensen, 1993). Caregiving generally has been explored in terms of individual care providers without regard to the broader social system within which caregiving interactions are embedded.

This volume aims to consider the broad spectrum of chronic illnesses that necessitate family caregiving throughout the lifespan and to discuss responses to these challenges by both caregiving families and caregiving systems. In doing so, we hope to move the caregiving paradigm beyond the narrow orientation to understanding that arises when the focus is only on specific ailments, such as Alzheimer's disease; on specific age groups, such as the very old or very young; or on specific individuals (i.e., the caregiver dyad—caregiver and/or care receiver). This book is predicated on the belief that much can be learned about caregiving by understanding its broader social and temporal contexts. At the same time, the study of caregiving also is seen as a valuable avenue for exploring broader theoretical concerns of behavioral and social sciences, including human development, social exchange, and the impact of chronic stress on psychological well-being.

The interplay between broader society and the personal caregiving context of individuals generally has been considered in terms of formal and informal caregiving systems. However, ecological approaches to caregiving permit us to consider new and previously neglected areas of that interface. Thus, for example, definitions of the family can be broadened to include non-kin significant others such as partners and even community volunteers caring for AIDS patients (Brennan & Moore, this volume). The physician's role as an important part of the caregiving context may be explored (Medalie, this volume). Furthermore, society's role may be analyzed as it directly affects needs and options of both caregivers and care receivers (Aldous, this volume). Society can influence relationships between caregivers and care receivers by the stigma attached to certain health problems such as AIDS or Alzheimer's disease. To the extent that these conditions are stigmatized, those afflicted will have diminished access to both formal and informal caregivers, and caregivers may experience greater burden. Laws recently enacted through the Americans with Disabilities Act serve to provide greater access as well as protection against discrimination for persons with disabilities, thereby easing burdens of caregivers and opening up options for independent living for persons with physical or mental impairments.

Addressing limitations inherent in the extant literature poses difficult challenges to scholars in the field. Nevertheless, each limitation also translates into need for further work in this field and contradicts the view that caregiving is an overresearched field. This book represents one effort in the direction of clarifying and extending conceptual approaches in caregiving research. It is thus predicated on the view that clarification of concepts must precede significant advances in research.

The expanded caregiver paradigm (Kahana, Kahana, Johnson, Hammond, & Kercher, this volume) addresses several of the most basic questions relevant to caregiving—the who, when, what, how, and why of caregiving. First, who are the important agents of caregiving? This question might be characterized as the spatial axis of caregiving. The definition of the caregiver as an individual or as a group, as part of a formal or informal system reflects one of the central themes in caregiving research and a central determinant of relevant processes and outcomes of caregiving.

Specifically, contributions to this book serve to expand the caregiving paradigm by broadening the focus of inquiry to include both members of the caregiving dyad and significant nonfamily caregivers. In addition, the social context in which caregiving is embedded is addressed by focus on the family and the broader social system. In contrast to studies of caregiving that focus only on singular actors in the caregiving paradigm, such as the major family caregiver, an entire section of this volume is devoted to discussions of the interface between informal and formal caregivers and society at large as they provide the context to family caregiving.

A second central question addresses when caregiving is likely to involve different challenges and elicit different responses for both the caregivers and the care receivers. The paradigm is expanded temporally through consideration of age and life stage of both the caregiver and the care receiver. Thus, caregiving may be placed in a life course perspective in which both age- and stage-specific and more universal dimensions and consequences of caregiving may be identified (Birkel, 1991). The effects of chronic illness on families, including the challenges posed by caregiving, may best be understood if placed in the context of normal developmental tasks faced by individual members of the family and the family unit (Rustad, 1990). Although a life course perspective represents the most common application of the temporal perspective, considerations of temporal dimensions also may include stages of illness, family life stage, and historical and cohort influences. Several of the contributors to this volume assume a developmental approach to understanding family caregiving, whereas others focus on unique characteristics and consequences of caregiving during a specific life stage.

The third central question relevant to the caregiving paradigm asks about the what and how of caregiving. What actually constitutes the process of caregiving? What transactions take place in the course of caregiving exchanges, and what are the consequences of caregiving transactions? Expanding the caregiving paradigm along a transactional axis involves recognizing that caregiving is part of a broad range of responses that individuals may make in the context of family and interpersonal relationships. Specifically, with regard to perceived needs of others, responses may range from provision of assistance to indifference and neglect and even harm-inducing or abusive behaviors (Birkel, 1991). The emergent social support literature with its recent focus on both care withholding and supportive behaviors provides a useful conceptual framework for understanding the transactions or processes involved in alternative caregiving relationships.

The value of providing support to caregivers has been underscored in the work of Zarit, Reever, and Bach-Peterson in their research on caregivers of patients with dementia (1980). Beyond specifying the types of social provisions involved in caregiving there is great need and much room for elaborating on the question of *what* types of processes or transactions occur. Several of the chapters in this volume represent progress in addressing caregiving processes. In particular the work of Given and Given highlights the transactions involved in helping family members cope with the multiple challenges of living with cancer.

The question of what are the outcomes or consequences of giving care for the caregiver represents the major concern of prior caregiving research. In addition to addressing processes of caregiving, an expanded caregiving paradigm also involves a broader view of the consequences of caregiving. Rather than limiting considerations of caregiving outcomes only to explanation of negative consequences for caregivers, the expanded paradigm explored in this volume also addresses potential benefits of caregiving. The positive values or potential benefits of caregiving have been noted by Horowitz (1985). Such benefits have been conceptualized as representing "uplifts" that may counteract the stresses posed through "hassles" of caregiving (Kinney & Stephens, 1989). Satisfaction with caregiving roles also has been reported by family caregivers to stroke patients (Silliman, Earp, Fletcher, & Wagner, 1988). In this volume, the chapter by Young and Kahana looks at dyadic outcomes that range from adverse sequelae for both caregivers and care receivers, to situations in which one party benefits while the other suffers, and finally to mutually beneficial outcomes for caregivers and care receivers.

In addition to questions related to the who, when, how, and what of caregiving, a relatively neglected but important background consideration involves the why of caregiving. What are the motivational bases for getting involved in the provision of costly assistance to others? The term *caregiving* suggests a positive or nurturant response to perceived or real needs of others. It thus reflects a willingness to acknowledge unmet needs and respond to them in a manner helpful to those in need albeit at a cost to the provider of assistance (Birkel, 1991). Students of caregiving have been particularly concerned with understanding these costs to the caregiver with caregiving paradigms largely directed toward understanding the stressful impact of caregiving and the psychosocial and physical impacts of care provision (Zarit & Toseland, 1989).

Are there unique decisions involved in coming to the aid of others despite potentially high costs to the caregiver? Some students of caregiving argue that rather than involving a unique set of interactions caregiving may represent a more intensive form of a prior pattern of help giving in families (Walker & Pratt, 1991). Others point to the powerful influence of decisions to become caregivers. An innovative and comprehensive conceptualization of the why of family caregiving in a developmental context is provided in this volume in Midlarsky's contribution.

This book also represents a response to the need for breaking down disciplinary barriers and narrow, age-limited orientations to understanding caregiving. Caregiving has been a subject of inquiry among sociologists, social workers, psychologists, and nurses. Each of these disciplines approaches issues of caregiving with its own set of conceptual frameworks, methodological preferences, and terminology. Often these disciplinary frameworks come to comprise barriers to communication and even barriers to motivation to understand progress in other fields.

As different age groups and different disciplinary groups increasingly compete for research and (even clinical) funding dollars, incentives are created for exaggerating differences and deemphasizing similarities in caregiving issues across the life span. Yet true scientific understanding can be derived only if we appreciate both commonalities and differences in challenges posed by, and adaptations made in response to, the needs of persons with chronic illness.

Consideration of caregiving issues across a wide variety of ages, life and family stages, and illness situations allows for better understanding both of general processes involved in caregiving and of unique aspects of caregiving situations. Furthermore, dissemination of extant knowledge across the lifespan can diminish duplication studies and lead to a more cumulative knowledge base.

ORGANIZATION AND CONTENT OF THE VOLUME

As indicated above, despite the large and increasing number of publications pertaining to family caregiving in recent years, there are many remaining gaps in knowledge. No single volume can provide a comprehensive analysis of family caregiving. The focus of this interdisciplinary volume is to address conceptual issues in caregiving. Thus, the caregiving paradigm is expanded in time and space by focusing on caregiving in the context of the family life cycle. Unique adaptive tasks and common challenges faced by caregivers to such populations as chronically ill children, mentally ill young adults, adult AIDS patients, and chronically ill elders are discussed.

The volume is divided into three parts. Part I, "Paradigms for Caregiving," presents four chapters that address the caregiving paradigm and the relationship of family caregiving research to family life studies. In Chapter 1, Kahana, Kahana, Johnson, Hammond, and Kercher attempt to integrate alternative conceptual approaches to caregiving through exploration of developmental, dyadic, and system-based perspectives. The chapter offers an interdisciplinary perspective that incorporates developmental psychological approaches to understanding challenges to personality development of individual caregivers and care receivers. It uses sociological perspectives to help understand caregiving families at different points in the life cycle. Kahana and colleagues present multidimensional views of the temporal aspects of caregiving through both an examination of the life stages of individual caregivers and care receivers and a discussion of family life cycle stages. The social context of caregiving is discussed through a focus on caregiving groups or systems ranging from the family to society at large.

Continuing the theme of family life cycles, in Chapter 2 Aldous provides an in-depth discussion of the family life cycle literature and, in so doing, places caregiving research within the context of the broader literature on families. She discusses social and economic changes in society that have impacted on families and draws implications of these changes for family caregiving. Five stages of family life are discussed: formation, child rearing, child leaving home, middle years, and final years. For each stage of the lifespan, Aldous compares and contrasts important issues and caregiving activities facing families and places our understanding of caregiving in a broader societal perspective. Gaps in the caregiving literature are noted, especially the unevenness of caregiving research, with the caregiving literature about young families being particularly sparse.

In Chapter 3 Midlarsky bridges two related literatures with common themes, altruism and caregiving, that are seldom discussed in the same context. She focuses on altruism as a major theoretical framework relevant to interpersonal motivations or orientations underlying helping behavior in general and caregiving in particular. The development of altruism throughout the life span is explored, particularly as it relates to caregiving in chronic illness situations. In undertaking this task, Midlarsky places particularistic aspects of caregiving research in the more global theoretical context of helping and motives for helping. The chapter addresses the issue of why people help despite the often high personal costs of caregiving and calls attention to relevant related concepts, such as nurturance, that traditionally are not considered in the caregiving literature. The chapter also reviews evidence from developmental and social psychology that can inform our conceptualization of caregiving.

In the fourth and final chapter in Part I, Litwak, Jessop, and Moulton present an original theory of caregiving that melds life-course considerations with a task-specific theory of social support. The chapter's focus on the relationship between informal and formal care helps set the stage for later examinations of this topic, which are featured in Part III of this volume. In this chapter, Litwak and colleagues expand Litwak's task-specific theory, which originally was developed in work with the elderly, and then they apply it to different stages of the lifespan from early childhood through old age. The chapter discusses the interrelationship of informal and formal caregiving and the life-course factors that affect one's choosing of a formal resource over an informal one. Such factors include physical maturation; incest and privacy norms;

parenting norms; gender role reversal; parent/child role reversals; and grandparent, female, sibling, and spousal overloads. The authors discuss the fact that the pressures for using formal organizations to substitute for informal ones are very different at different stages of the lifespan. The chapter discusses the need (a) for more research to empirically establish at which stage of the life course there will be more pressure to use formal services and (b) for research that is needed to examine which stresses at each life stage are the most important in affecting use of services.

Part II, "Illness and Life Stage: Challenges for Caregiving," contains six empirical chapters that continue discussion of conceptual aspects of caregiving, ranging from the expansion of the caregiving paradigm, caregiving processes and tasks, to the positive aspects of caregiving. The chapters encompass caregiving with children, young adults, the middle-aged, and the elderly. A range of chronic illnesses is discussed as well, including AIDS, mental illness, cancer, and heart disease.

Chapter 5 addresses a care-receiving population that has received less attention than others, namely, caregiving with young children. Patterson and Leonard present a longitudinal, qualitative study of families caring for medically fragile children. The framework for caregiving includes the full family system: the sibling as well as the marital unit. Distinctions of caregiving impact are based on gender roles of mothers and fathers. The chapter identifies critical themes of strains related to home care of children with chronic illness: losses (privacy and spontaneity), problems with services (people and equipment), care and parenting strains, and added family strains. Findings from this study indicate that more than one half of the caregiving parents were seriously distressed, and that caregiving had positive effects on some siblings and negative effects on others. This chapter moves toward recognizing diversity in responses to caregiving demands and thus paves the way for future research that can distinguish characteristics of caregivers who suffer ill effects from those who thrive despite their caregiving duties.

In Chapter 6, Brennan and Moore present a study of caregivers of persons living with AIDS, broadening the definition of what is meant by the term *family caregiver.* The nature of AIDS is such that family caregivers are a diverse group, ranging from the traditional (parents providing care to adult children) to nontraditional or emergent family types where nonrelated persons (lovers and/or close friends) provide care. Both caregivers and care receivers discussed in this study cover almost the full spectrum of the life course. The disease examined in this chapter, AIDS, is unique in being life-threatening as well as stigmatizing and having an unpredictable but inevitable trajectory of decline. The chapter highlights the adaptive tasks and problems of caregiver/care receiver dyads who have different relationships, such as elderly parents who must cope with the dual stigma of the lifestyle of their offspring and the devastating effects of the illness. The chapter considers stages in the caregiving process that correspond to illness-adaptive tasks and calls attention to potential caregiving situations in which there is double jeopardy as both caregivers and care receivers may be ill.

All too often, caregiving research with one chronic illness does not build on related research with other illnesses. In Chapter 7, Biegel, Song, and Chakravarthy make use of a theoretical framework adapted from research with caregivers of Alzheimer's disease patients to examine burdens of caregivers of persons with chronic mental illness. After reviewing the literature concerning the extent, and predictors, of caregiver burden, the authors present findings from their cross-sectional study of middle-class caregivers who are support group members. The study examines the simultaneous effect of multiple independent variables upon caregiver burden. Findings indicate that client behavioral problems, poor caregiver health, and inadequate social support were important predictors of caregiver distress. The authors call for a reorientation in the way that mental health professionals involve family members in the treatment of persons with chronic mental illness.

Continuing the discussion of family caregivers of persons with mental illness, this time from an intervention perspective, in Chapter 8 Kane discusses psychoeducational interventions for family caregivers of this population. The chapter presents a systematic review and analysis of these interventions and demonstrates the important roles that they can play in assisting family caregivers. The chapter discusses changes in perceptions of family caregivers with this population over time. Too often in the past, family caregivers of persons with mental illness have been blamed as causal agents of the disease. Such blaming has added to the usual burdens of caregiving and has affected caregivers' relationships with mental health professionals. Kane's historical perspective on this issue represents a continuing effort in the literature to correct past abuses.

Much of the caregiving literature has examined caregiving outcomes such as caregiver burden, physical illness, or depression. There has been much less examination of the process of caregiving itself. Given and

Given's empirical study of caregivers of middle-aged adults with cancer, presented in Chapter 9, sheds much light on the nature of caregiving with this population. The authors discuss the family disruption that takes places when illness strikes during midlife and the unique problems of caregivers and care receivers who face special role demands during this lifespan stage. Further, the authors demonstrate that caregiving tasks and processes are shaped by a number of variables including the site of the cancer, the stage of the disease, and the treatment modalities. In fact, the treatment itself is considered as a source of stress in addition to the illness. In line with the emergent interest in the concerns of care receivers, the chapter provides a focus on patient needs and patient roles. The chapter moves toward providing an integrative model of cancer care across formal and informal systems and patient outcomes.

The final chapter in Part II, by Young and Kahana, discusses caregiving issues with persons who have had a heart attack. This chapter advances dyadic perspectives of caregiving by the presentation of a conceptual model for understanding outcomes in heart disease; the model is tested in an empirical study of older heart attack victims and their families. Four alternative outcomes, both symmetrical and asymmetrical, are provided: both caregiver and care-receiver thrive, both caregiver and care receiver have negative outcomes, the caregiver has a negative outcome but the care receiver thrives, or the care receiver has a negative outcome but the caregiver prospers. Findings indicate that the patterns of dyadic mental health outcomes are diverse, with health of the patient and the amount of caregiving assistance being important predictors of outcome across patient-caregiver dyads.

The third part of the volume, "The Interface Between Formal Care Providers and Caregiving Families," emphasizes that caregiving does not occur in a vacuum and that family caregivers are very much affected by their connection, or lack of connection, with macrolevel systems. In Chapter 11, Fischer and Eustis add to our understanding of the nature of the relationship between informal and formal caregiving through a qualitative empirical examination of an understudied area, the relationship between family caregiving and paid home care. The chapter examines caregiving with adults ranging in age from 27 to 99 years who have a variety of disabilities. The authors indicate that interactions between paid caregivers and family caregivers can be conceptualized into three types: alliance, conflict, and separate worlds. They find that Litwak's substitution theory only partially explains paid caregiving because there is so much informality in the formal role of paid caregivers. Findings demonstrate a number of similarities between paid home-care workers and family caregivers in relation to the scope and nature of the work, with paid caregivers often performing above and beyond the call of duty. In fact, sometimes paid caregivers become quasi-family members. However, there are also differences: Paid home-care workers lack the emotional complexity and legitimacy of family relationships. The authors describe the roles of paid helpers and family caregivers as interlocking, each providing what the other does not. Although services for the clients studied were not fully adequate, the authors indicated that most clients make do.

Studies indicate that families place high levels of trust in their family physician. Yet the relationship of the family physician to family caregiving has been little examined. In Chapter 12, Medalie reviews alternative medical practice models and their implications for assisting family caregivers. He shows how physicians, who are part of the formal service delivery system, can assist caregivers by presenting a comprehensive model of patient-caregiver-physician interactions. The chapter uses an ideographic, case study approach to provide insights into physical health risks to caregivers with their potential of becoming hidden patients. A principal audience of this chapter is physicians, with the author advocating that physicians can play an important gatekeeping role in caregiving. Medalie's work, however, also can help nonphysician caregivers become aware of the important roles physicians can play as caregiving allies.

In Chapter 13, Kazak and Christakis-Zerr present a systems-oriented approach, anchored in social ecology and systems theory, to caregiving with children with diverse chronic medical conditions. The authors' approach to chronic illness suggests that commonalities related to illness exist at all stages of the lifespan. They discuss the distinct nature and commonalities of parenting and caregiving. The authors believe that to understand caregiving outcomes from a family perspective requires an understanding of the interconnectedness of individual, family, and social institutions. The relevant systems that the authors discuss are organized into categories of microsystems, mesosystems, exosystems, and macrosystems.

In the final chapter of the volume, Noelker and Bass propose the need for an integrative model of the relationship between informal and formal caregiving. The strengths and weaknesses of three existing informal-formal relationship models are presented—hierarchical compensatory model, task-specific model, and supplementation model. For each model, the authors present a conceptual overview, followed by a discussion of empirical support for the model. Limitations of existing models include a focus on only particular types of help, static orientation based on a single factor influencing informal-formal care over time, lack of inclusion of contingencies, narrow range of informal and formal helpers, and little systematic attention to use of services by informal caregivers. The authors then discuss their own research, which proposes a test of an integrative model that addresses these limitations.

REFERENCES

Biegel, D. E., Sales, E., & Schulz, R. (1991). *Family caregiving in chronic illness: Alzheimer's disease, cancer, heart disease, mental illness and stroke.* Newbury Park, CA: Sage.

Birkel, R. C. (1991). A lifespan perspective on caregiving. In D. G. Unger & D. R. Powell (Eds.), *Families as nurturing systems* (pp. 99-108). Binghamton, NY: Haworth.

Burton, L. M., & Sorensen, S. (1993). Temporal context and the caregiver role: Perspectives from ethnographic studies of multigenerational African-American families. In S. H. Zarit, L. I. Pearlin, & K. W. Schaie (Eds.), *Caregiving systems: Informal and formal helpers.* Hillsdale, NJ: Lawrence Erlbaum.

Chiriboga, D. A., Weiler, P. G., & Nielson, K. (1988-1989). The stress of caregivers. *The Journal of Applied Social Sciences, 13*(1), 118-141.

George, L. K. (1990). Caregiver stress studies: There really is more to learn. *The Gerontologist, 30,* 580-581.

Horowitz, A. (1985). Sons and daughters as caregivers to older parents: Differences in role performance and consequences. *The Gerontologist, 25,* 612-617.

Kinney, J. M., & Stephens, M. A. P. (1989). Hassles and uplifts of giving care to a family member with dementia. *Psychology and Aging, 4,* 402-408.

Pearlin, L. I., Mullan, J. T., Semple, S. J., & Skaff, T. (1990). Caregiving and the stress process: An overview of concepts and their measures. *The Gerontologist, 30,* 583-591.

Rustad, L. C. (1984). Family adjustment to chronic illness and disability in mid-life. In M.G. Eisenberg L. C. Suthin, M. A. Jansen (Eds.), *Chronic illness and disability through the lifespan: Effects on self and family.* New York, NY: Springer.

Silliman, R. A., Earp, J. L., Fletcher, R. H., & Wagner, E. H. (1988). Stroke: The perspective of family caregivers. *Journal of Applied Gerontology, 6,* 363-371.

Walker, A. J., & Pratt, C. C. (1991). Daughters' help to mothers: Intergenerational aid versus caregiving. *Journal of Marriage and the Family, 53,* 3-12.

Zarit, S. H., Pearlin, L. I., & Schaie, K. W. (Eds.). (1993). *Caregiving systems: Informal and formal helpers.* Hillsdale, NJ: Lawrence Erlbaum.

Zarit, S. H., Reever, K. E., & Bach-Peterson, J. (1980). Relatives of the impaired elderly: Correlates of feelings of burden. *The Gerontologist, 20,* 649-655.

Zarit, S. H., & Toseland, R. W. (1989). Current future direction in family caregiving research. *The Gerontologist, 29,* 481-483.

PART I

Paradigms for Caregiving

1

Developmental Challenges and Family Caregiving

Bridging Concepts and Research

EVA KAHANA
BOAZ KAHANA
J. RANDAL JOHNSON
RONALD J. HAMMOND
KYLE KERCHER

Some of the most promising and interesting advances in the study of caregiving are likely to occur through expansion of the scope of the caregiving paradigm, in particular through focus on caregiving contexts and processes. Such expansion of the paradigm requires consideration of the personal, social, and temporal contexts of caregiving. In this chapter we attempt to identify some of the emerging directions for expansion of the caregiving paradigm using multiple levels of aggregation (individual and social) and specifying processes involved in caregiving (e.g., social support). We also consider implications of a broader view for models of caregiving and caregiving research. Figure 1.1 provides an overview of the proposed expanded caregiving paradigm. The columns represent the proposed dimensions for expansion of the paradigm and the rows represent different levels of aggregation. In this chapter we move toward consideration of salient aspects of the spatial axis (Who is involved in caregiving?), temporal axis (When are caregivers involved in caregiving?), and transactional axis (What processes are involved in

	SPATIAL AXIS: WHO? (key individuals and groups relevant to caregiving)	TEMPORAL AXIS: WHEN? (time frames relevant to caregiving)	TRANSACTIONAL AXIS: WHAT? (processes involved in caregiving)

PERSONAL CAREGIVING CONTEXT (individual level) — Informal	Family caregivers
	  Major family caregiver
	  (e.g., spouse or adult children)
	  Secondary family caregiver
	  (e.g., other family)
	Nonfamily caregivers
	  Friends, neighbors as caregivers
	
	Care receiver
	
	Caregiver-care receiver dyad
		Length/stage of illness
		
		Age/life stage
		
		Length of caregiving
		
		Cohort/historical influences
			Social support:
			  Perceived/received
			  Given/withheld
			  Negative social interactions

PERSONAL CAREGIVING CONTEXT (individual level) — Formal	Paraprofessional caregivers
	  Paid helper (supervised by care receiver or family)
	  Agency worker (supervised by formal organization)
	
	Professional caregivers
	  Physician
	  Nurse
	  Social worker
		Length of employment
		
		Length of service
		
		Cohort/historical influences
			Compliance
			
			Work of caregiving
			
			Exchange

SOCIAL CAREGIVING CONTEXT (system or group level)			Life stage	Cohesion/conflict

Informal	Primary group
	  Nuclear family
	  Extended family			

	Informal group
	  Neighbor network
	  Friend network
			Cohort/historical influences	Social integration

Formal	Formal group/service delivery system
	  Service organizations—medical
	  Service organizations—social
			Length of service	Financing/access provision
				Control

	Societal institutions
	  Local government
	  State government
	  National government
			Cohort/historical influences	Legislation
				Enforcement

Figure 1.1. Spatial, Temporal, and Transactional Dimensions of the Caregiving Paradigm

caregiving?). We then point the way toward consideration of interactions among components of these axes.

Expansion of the caregiving paradigm in space may be conceptualized along two significant axes: a personal- or individual-based axis and a social- or systems-based axis. These are depicted as different levels of caregiving contexts forming the rows of Figure 1.1. A distinguishing feature of the personal context is incremental consideration of key individuals (e.g., family caregivers, nonfamily caregivers, care receivers), whereas the social context is based on a more system-oriented view of a group (e.g., primary groups, informal groups, societal institutions). We begin our discussion with models that consider roles of key individual caregivers, which we term the "Personal Caregiving Context" in Figure 1.1. The traditional focus of family caregiving research has been on a single individual, the caregiver. Studies have generally focused on burdens of caregiving and the impact of the stress of caregiving on the major provider of aid to a chronically ill relative. Interestingly, the second major actor in the caregiving paradigm, the care receiver, has not been extensively considered in this literature (Montgomery, Stull, & Borgatta, 1986). In considering the caregiving paradigm, our first effort at expansion must be in connection with the caregiver/care receiver dyad moving toward an interactive view of caregiving to involve both the provider and the recipient of aid (Kahana & Young, 1990). In the spatial-temporal-transactional paradigm depicted in Figure 1.1, the caregiving dyad is noted as part of the personal caregiving context, reflecting individual-level analysis (Thompson & Walker, 1982). This is consistent with the social psychological tradition wherein dyads have been studied as two individuals engaged in significant interactions (Houston, 1974). At the same time, we recognize that the dyad also may be considered the smallest unit of a group and also is amenable to group-level analysis. An incremental view of the personal context moves from focus on the individual caregiver, to the caregiving dyad, and to other important formal or informal caregivers.

The social context of caregiving considers the groups within which caregiving is embedded in a holistic or system-oriented manner (the social caregiving context in Figure 1.1). The term *family caregiving* reflects an attempt to further the contextual analysis of caregiving in both theory and research. It implies that informal caregiving represents a process embedded in the structure or institution of the family. It thus expands "in space" the consideration of caregiving from focus on individual caregivers to the family system as a whole. A comprehensive caregiving paradigm involves further expansion of the social context beyond the framework of the family. In terms of structure, families represent the primary social context of caregiving. They are complemented or supplemented by the informal social system of friendship networks and the formal service delivery system (Litwak, 1985). On a broader level, the caregiving system also includes societal institutions (governments) that create and implement policies shaping the provision of care to persons with chronic illness.

The second major axis for expansion of the caregiving paradigm that is proposed here relates to expansion of the paradigm "in time" (i.e., the temporal axis in Figure 1.1). Studies of caregiving generally have considered the temporal context by focusing on the length of illness or the duration of caregiving. In a recent article, Burton and Sorensen (1993) provide a description of the temporal dimensions of assistance provided by a variety of informal and formal caregivers referring to these as "kin time," "peer time," and "social service time," respectively. Kin time relates to timing of assistance by various family members, peer time involves the timing of assistance of friends and neighbors, and social service time relates to scheduling of services with social service agencies.

Another important temporal dimension relates to the way caregiving impacts on life-course development of members of the caregiver/care receiver dyad. The introduction of a temporal dimension provides information on developmental and life-cycle issues on the one hand and points to the dynamic nature of the caregiving process on the other. In an effort to illustrate the value of considering temporal contexts of caregiving, we provide a more detailed discussion of the relationship between individual developmental stages of caregivers and care receivers as well as the caregiving experience later in this chapter. Understanding of the spatial and temporal dimensions of caregiving takes us beyond unidimensional and static views of the caregiving paradigm and permits consideration of the rich and changing social fabric within which caregiving is embedded.

In explicating the caregiving paradigm, emphasis generally has been placed on burdens or outcomes of caregiving with relatively little research attention directed at the *process*. To further clarify the essence of caregiving transactions, we also must expand the caregiving paradigm along a third transactional axis. Figure 1.1 includes a transactional axis to depict relevant processes. The traditional focus on outcomes that has generally been framed in terms of distress or burdens of caregivers is not explicitly included in the model. The most prevalent approach to processes of caregiving has concerned transactions involving social support. Accordingly, it is generally understood that caregivers provide support to care receivers (Kahana & Young, 1990). Alternatively, the adverse effects of caregiving may be ameliorated by supports obtained by caregivers (Malone-Beach & Zarit, 1991). We attempt to look at social supports as they impact on, or are shaped by, caregiving transactions and to further place these supports in a temporal context. The attempts to expand the caregiving paradigm outlined above should serve as an impetus for a broader and more contextually based orientation in caregiving research. The elements in Figure 1.1 are proposed as a beginning rather than a completed blueprint of the expanded paradigm.

We now illustrate directions for expanding the paradigm by turning to a more detailed discussion of key components, focusing on (a) the spatial axis (personal and social caregiving context), (b) the temporal axis (with specific focus on members of the caregiving dyad and the caregiving family), and (c) the transactional axis (elements of the caregiving process focusing on the role of social supports).

SPATIAL AXIS:
PERSONAL AND SOCIAL
CAREGIVING CONTEXTS

Personal Context—
An Individual-Level Incremental Approach

Research on caregiving has focused primarily on stresses endured by a designated family member providing care to a chronically ill relative (Pearlin, 1989). An understanding of the impact of caregiving is generally embedded in the stress-coping-support paradigm. Adverse outcomes of caregiving are analyzed along with resources that may buffer these outcomes. In such models the caregiving situation is seen as a stressful stimulus and the caregiver's adverse reactions are seen as responses. The model is thus unidirectional and unidimensional (Kahana & Young, 1990). More recently, focus also has been directed at care receivers and their experiences in receiving assistance, or "counting on kindness" (Lustbader, 1991). There is now at least partial recognition of the fact that help provided by caregivers to their dependent family members may result in adverse as well as positive outcomes for care receivers (Rook, 1990). Recent efforts in caregiving research have expanded the study of caregiving outcomes from focus only on caregivers or care receivers toward a dyadic view of caregiver and care receiver interactions and outcomes (Kahana & Young, 1990; Montgomery, Stull, & Borgatta, 1986). Such analyses have considered symmetrical outcomes in which both caregivers and care receivers prosper or those in which both experience adverse consequences. Alternatively, asymmetrical outcomes occur in which one member of the dyad suffers ill effects while the other prospers (Young & Kahana, this volume). An important challenge to future research on caregiving relates to exploring relationships and mutual interactions of the caregiver/care receiver dyad. Caregivers of persons with chronic illness typically are defined according to their relationship to the recipient. Persons who are not paid for care are considered *informal* support providers. These are typically family members, but they also can include friends and neighbors of the care recipient. *Formal* support providers (also called formal caregivers) are persons who are paid for their help. Such caregivers include both paraprofessionals who supplement efforts of primary family caregivers in providing "hands-on" help with activities of daily living, and professionals who provide important but more episodic care primarily in meeting health and mental health needs. Paraprofessionals may be usefully subdivided into help hired and supervised by the care receiver or family and those supervised by agencies. This latter distinction has not been extensively considered in the caregiving literature, but it has important implications for the degree of personal control experienced by care receivers vis-à-vis providers of care (Kahana, Kahana, & Riley, 1989). A useful direction for future research on formal caregiving relates to consideration of paid helpers on the one hand and of key professionals, such as primary-care physicians, on the other hand (Medalie, this volume).

The term *family caregiving,* considered in a personal context, helps differentiate between formal caregiving, which involves services provided by unrelated persons, and informal caregiving, which typically occurs in a family context and involves two related individuals. Focus is generally on the primary caregiver who is a member of the family and possibly on secondary family caregivers who supplement the aid provided by the primary caregiver. In studying significant caregivers it is useful to move beyond the family caregiver/care receiver dyad to analysis that also involves a formal care provider, such as the primary-care physician or other key health-care providers (Medalie, this volume). Thus we arrive at an incremental model of major caregivers that encompasses both the most significant formal and informal caregivers (Figure 1.1). An incremental model refers to expansion of the caregiver paradigm from focus on only one individual (typically the major family caregiver) to inclusion of other key individuals. A caregiving triad might thus be considered as consisting of the care receiver, the major family caregiver and a key formal caregiver such as the physician (Haug, 1988). Studies using such a model may collect information from several key caregivers but focus on them as separate individuals in an incremental fashion. This approach is distinct from a group-level analysis that uses a systems approach to understanding social groups involved in caregiving.

The relationship of formal to informal caregivers is well portrayed via the case of chronic debilitating illnesses. Often the extent and complexity of care needed by patients are beyond the capabilities of family or friends. Formal caregivers therefore also are involved in providing these services. However, the personal touches that are necessary to maintain the recipient's emotional well-being may be lacking in encounters with formal service providers (Litwak, 1985). This may be due, in part, to the nonfamilial relation to the recipient and in part to the exigencies of a bureaucratic structure. Family members and friends of the care receiver, on the other hand, are presumed to have an emotional stake in the well-being of the care receiver and, therefore, are well placed to provide the affective support functions and personalized individual care that are sometimes missing from the formal caregivers. At the same time, emotional involvement of informal caregivers also may result in greater interpersonal conflict. The task is to create a fit between these seemingly complementary support sources that best meets the needs of the care recipient (Litwak, 1985). This often is not as simple as it may first appear, and alternative models for exploring roles and relationships of informal and formal caregivers have been advanced in the literature (Noelker & Bass, this volume). Curiously, however, these often involve skipping past the families and exchanging focus from the primary informal caregiver to focus on the primary formal caregiver. We believe that a more holistic or system-oriented approach to the caregiving paradigm is needed to move from individual caregiver to family unit to broader social groupings involved in caregiving.

Social Context—A Systems Approach

The units of analysis for the social context of caregiving are significant "primary groups" i.e., family and friendship networks, along with formal organizations, and societal units involved in caregiving (Figure 1.1). Family caregiving in such a social context refers to the entire family unit or system that is involved in the caregiving process (Brubaker, 1990). This orientation considers the family as the major unit of analysis within which caregiving is embedded. Research using the latter approach may aggregate information about members of the group that is of interest; use individual informants to characterize the larger group; or use collective group products, such as legislation, as the basis of making inferences about the social context.

On a conceptual level the systems approach provides a more comprehensive and differentiated understanding of family caregiving than do more molecular approaches. In fact, students of caregiving increasingly espouse this view. However, on the level of empirical research it has been too difficult to measure the impact of caregiving on the entire family unit or the contributions of the entire family unit to the caregiving task (Biegel, Sales, & Schulz, 1991). Consequently, the family unit or system frequently is referred to in conceptual treatises on caregiving or in introductions to empirical studies (Brubaker, 1990). Exhortations about the value of a systems approach to caregiving typically are followed by data on only the designated family caregiver. Not only is the family system not included in operational definitions of caregiving, but also, as noted above, often the care receiver also is excluded from consideration (Kahana & Young, 1990).

In addition to the family as the primary group involved in caregiving to chronically ill members, informal groups comprised of friendship or neighbor networks can also provide important system-level contexts for caregiving. Neighbors and friends are particularly important in agesegregated settings such as retirement communities where elders live dispersed from their families. In our ongoing study of elders living in a Florida retirement community (Kahana, Kahana, Borawski, & Kercher, 1990), we find that neighbors comprise a significant source of organized informal assistance to residents afflicted with chronic illness.

In terms of the formal group or organizational context, services provided by a hospital or home-health-care agency often constitute a critical organizational base for caregiving. This may be a facilitative role, or alternatively one that sets up bureaucratic barriers to home care.

In either case, the system exerts important influences that go beyond support provision by individual representatives of these groups. Increasing recognition of the importance of caregiving systems is reflected in the publication of a recent volume on this subject (Zarit, Pearlin, & Schaie, 1993).

Societal-level analyses are seldom considered by caregiving researchers. Yet society represents a critical context that facilitates or hinders caregiving by families, informal groups, or formal services. Social customs and sanctions result in visitation of the sick in some cultures and shunning of those afflicted in others. Legal historians long have been concerned with laws that protect dependent groups (Grossberg, 1984). Advances in caring for the disabled have, in fact, come in the form of laws, such as the Americans with Disabilities Act of 1990, that protect the physically challenged from discrimination and ensure their access to services and facilities within their communities. Just as social support and caregiving may be facilitated through legislation and social policies, harm can be inflicted on chronically ill persons through societal neglect or inattention. Deinstitutionalization of the mentally ill, for example, represents a major social policy initiative in the United States that has resulted in withholding of care to physically and mentally frail elderly individuals (Kahana, Kahana, & Segall, 1986).

TEMPORAL AXIS:
OVERVIEW OF TEMPORAL CAREGIVING CONTEXTS

The dimension of time is salient to understanding both the personal caregiving context and the social caregiving context (Aldous, this volume; Burton & Sorenson, 1993). We thus take an initial step toward a comprehensive consideration of time dimensions depicted in Figure 1.1.

Temporal factors influence both the composition (or structure) and the functioning of the caregiving family. Researchers who employ a life-course perspective to study the relationship between family caregiving and general well-being recognize that such a temporally based analytical framework enables them to look at both continuity and change across the life span. Consideration of the temporal dimension also can link caregiving to what has been termed "developmental time." Developmental time relates to the impact of the timing of caregiving roles on individual development of caregivers and care receivers. The temporal axis also allows for study of the interactions of historical time and the life of individuals by emphasizing historical change and the timing of transitions that describe and define individual life trajectories. A critical element in understanding family caregiving is to place it among other roles that families are expected to perform in our society. Whether caregiving has positive or negative effects on the family's well-being will depend in large part on the number and importance of role demands shared by the caregiver and care receiver, on the timing of these demands, and on the contexts in which they occur. The life-course perspective is especially attuned to the historical influences on individual roles, such as the changing demography of people's lives. The extension of life over the past two centuries, along with changing patterns of marital and family dissolution, has resulted in the redefinition, and even creation, of new family roles (Watkins, Menken, & Bongaarts, 1987). Changes in the definition and duration of family roles have important implications for family caregiving across the lifespan of the family. We return to this point later in the chapter.

One unique feature of the life-course perspective is that it focuses on the interplay between transitions and trajectories in roles, events, and identities throughout a person's lifetime. The life course is characterized as a set of interconnected trajectories linked by events such as birth, entry into school, marriage, birth of the first and last child, and so on that mark transitions to and from these trajectories (Elder, 1992).

The periods that would require the most intensive caregiving within a family probably are not contiguous but segmented. It is normal, then, for a caregiver to look forward to a period that is relatively free from caregiving responsibilities after such an intensive period. If this is so, whether or not this respite period is realized may have serious implications for the well-being of the caregiver and the family. This possibility indicates that it is not the caregiving role per se that may be detrimental to a person's well-being, but rather its occurrence in relation to one's stage in the adult lifespan, along with its duration, focus of attention (i.e., if it is care of an infant, children, or elderly parents or a husband), and the timing in relation to the caregiver's age and the other roles he or she may occupy. The potential importance of compatibility of developmental life stages between caregivers and care receivers has been alluded to in our research on grandparent-grandchild relationships (Kahana & Kahana, 1971).

The stresses inherent in family caregiving are tied to another concept central to the life course: the normative versus nonnormative timing of events. Some researchers contend that it is not necessarily the number of roles that most strongly affects a caregiver's well-being, but whether the roles are normative in terms of age and gender (Menaghan, 1989). The concept of being "on time" is present when life events follow a culturally prescribed sequence and duration (Hagestad, 1990; Neugarten, 1964). Becoming caregiver to an elderly spouse represents a normative caregiving situation. "Off-time" events are considered nonnormative and may result in stress caused by the anomic or dissonant nature of the events. Examples include early widowhood, non-emancipation of an adult child with mental illness, or unexpected caregiving responsibilities to a younger adult or middle-aged spouse.

In our culture the most prevalent time of caregiving for chronic illness involves older family members. This type of caregiving may be viewed as normative for middle-aged children, particularly daughters, and for older spouses. Because caregiving to frail elders is a prevalent need, societal supports are more likely to be in place for this genre of caregiving. In addition to such normative aspects, there are also important idiosyncratic aspects of caregiving that are likely to impact on both caregivers' and care receivers' experiences (Birkel, 1990). Accordingly, one's life history in terms of caregiving experiences of family members or circumstances that necessitate assuming caregiving roles for an ill family member will shape one's caregiving behaviors and experiences. As we focus on the caregiving encounter or relationship, we also must bear in mind the individual developmental needs of caregivers and care receivers.

In terms of temporal dimensions of caregiving, age and life stage must be differentiated from cohort and historical influences. These latter dimensions influence values of caregivers as well as resources, structure, and function of family units. Furthermore, the illness necessitating caregiving also is likely to have stages that directly impact on demands on caregivers as well as resources of care receivers, caregivers, and families.

If studying caregiving in the holistic family context poses operational and methodological challenges, these are greatly compounded by the call for introducing a temporal dimension through concern with age and stage. Even if we start only with the caregiver/care receiver dyad, we could consider the age of the caregiver, the age of the care receiver, or the difference in age between the two parties. The question arises, whose age or life stage is to become the anchor of such inquiry? If we move beyond this dyad to consideration of the entire family unit, we must introduce stages in the family life cycle that differ from life stages of either caregiver or care receiver, such as ages of children and their age span, the "empty nest" period, widowhood, and remarriage. Empirical research once again tends to lag behind conceptualization, with caregiving studies being generally categorized based on the age of the care receiver. Accordingly, we have studies of caregiving to chronically ill children, young adults, or the elderly. It is useful to note, as we consider caregiving through the life course, that relationships of caregivers to care receivers often are systematically related to age and to life stage. Thus caregivers to children are typically young adults or middle-aged parents, whereas caregivers to the elderly tend to be divided between adult children and elderly spouses. Consideration of family caregiving throughout the life course involves moving beyond "still-life snapshots" of caregivers or care receivers and provides a major step toward placing caregiving in a social/historical context.

We have selected two areas that illustrate time dimensions of the expanded caregiving paradigm for further consideration: the personal developmental stage of the care receiver and the life-cycle developmental stage of the family as a group. Thus the first illustration is related to the individual-level personal caregiving context, whereas the second is related to the group-level social caregiving context (see Figure 1.1).

Personal Caregiving Context: Developmental Perspectives on Caregivers and Care Receivers

We approach consideration of individual developmental issues using a developmental psychological framework that is consistent with our focus on the individuals who make up the personal caregiving context. This discussion is followed by a more sociologically based analysis of developmental issues relevant to consideration of the primary caregiving group: the family. We thus aim to match disciplinary perspectives with the analytical frameworks considered. Nevertheless, we acknowledge the potential for cross-fertilization of ideas as psychological perspectives are applied to family systems, or as sociological ideas are applied to individual development through the life course.

We now consider the ways in which being a caregiver or care receiver may impact on an individual's ability to fulfill adaptive tasks presented by different lifespan developmental stages. Intrinsic to our discussion are developmental concepts such as stage theory and "on-time" versus "off-time" events as previously mentioned (Neugarten, 1964). To illustrate how chronic illness impacts on developmental experiences of caregivers and care receivers, we selectively draw on the works of classical developmental theorists such as Freud (1922/1976), Erikson (1963), Sullivan (1953), Levinson (1978), Benedek (1959), and Butler (1963). In the interest of brevity, we limit our discussion to psychosocial development. In doing so, we hope to document the usefulness of relating caregiving to the temporal context of individual development. For some life stages such as childhood, our focus is primarily on the care receiver, whereas in adulthood, we consider both the effects of being a caregiver and those of being a care receiver. For care receivers, there are problems associated both with being chronically ill and with the dependency involved in receiving care. These problems sometimes are distinct yet often are intertwined and difficult to separate. Being a care receiver or caregiver may distract the individual from dealing with developmental tasks. In some cases it may threaten the very essence of mastering a developmental stage. It is likely to have an impact on the success of "working through" the stage and perhaps on later stages, thus influencing the personality and coping of the developing person. Erikson's (1963) theory of psychosocial development provides a useful framework for considering developmental challenges found by caregivers and care receivers.

Infancy and Childhood: Care Receiving

The infant born with a disability or medical disorder may have less of an opportunity to master developmental tasks of this stage than would a "normal" child. The infant's feeling of "trust" in the world (Erikson, 1963) and in caretakers may be threatened because the all-powerful parent really may be powerless in ameliorating the child's medical problems and in providing security to the infant. Caregiving to an infant with a medical problem would naturally raise the caregiving parent's anxiety, which in turn would be sensed by the infant (Sullivan, 1953).

Toddlers have been characterized as dealing with the issue of "autonomy" (Erikson, 1963). Parental overprotectiveness may be elicited by the child's illness. The child may be deterred from beginning to develop independence from parental caregivers if he or she must receive care for a chronic illness during this period. The next Eriksonian stage of "initiative" contains important elements of the previous stage of autonomy that are difficult to master in the presence of illness or disability. Increasing psychosexual differentiation characterizing this period may be compromised by the general dependency generated through the disability and the subsequent need for care. Middle childhood is normally a period encompassing cognitive maturation and "cognitive shifts" to higher levels of functioning. Chronic illness and disability are likely to threaten developmental tasks during middle childhood primarily in areas of psychomotor development and peer relations. Peer relations and their effect on development constitute an important aspect of major theories of child development (Sullivan, 1953). The disabled child may have a spectrum of difficulties in coping with this period. Difficulties posed by the illness may impact on the child's self-esteem and self-confidence. They also may cause emotional dependency and the failure to learn the cognitive and social skills of that stage of development. Personality development that accrues from working through this stage also is threatened.

Childhood: Caregiving

We also can consider the child as a potential caregiver to younger siblings and as a possible mother's helper (Midlarsky, this volume). Indeed in traditional societies, children age 6, and even younger, may be expected to help their mother in caring for younger children. Furthermore, if the mother becomes ill, the oldest female child often is expected to help the family carry on. Boys also are expected to contribute to household chores in more traditional societies, but less so in middle-class Western societies.

Preadolescence: Care Receiving

The preadolescent stage, or "chum stage" according to Sullivan (1953), is characterized by the need to find a close friend of the same gender to share and discuss experiences and serve as a mirror to reflect ideas, points of view, and outlooks on the world and on oneself. The preadolescent who is chronically ill or disabled will need to find someone who can relate to him or her along these lines. For this to occur, there has to be sufficient similarity or empathy between two preadolescents to share and compare their worlds. This probably can occur most readily among two care-receiving adolescents. It would be interesting to conduct research determining to what extent chronically ill and healthy preteenagers can effectively interact with one another in terms of the chum stage. This would be compared to interactions between two chronically ill preadolescents.

Adolescence: Care Receiving

During adolescence, physical and psychosexual maturation normally take place, along with feelings of increased power and independence. However, the chronically ill adolescent may not have the same opportunities to develop along these lines because the psychosocial situations necessary to bring about psychosexual maturity and independence may not be readily available to the disabled person. Depending on the nature of the disability and the theory of adolescence invoked, a variety of developmental problems may emerge. Thus one may anticipate unresolved Oedipal problems in a teenage boy who, because of his chronic illness or disability, is heavily dependent on his mother for his everyday functioning (Freud, 1922/1976). Issues of "identity" (Erikson, 1963) may not be easily resolved because the adolescent's task is to "psychologically differentiate" and develop an identity that is different from his or her parents, uniquely his or her own, and that evolved based on the individual's previous childhood identity. Increased dependency of disabled children and adolescents may interfere in the establishment of an identity characterized by independence and self-sufficiency (characteristics that are highly valued by Western culture).

Sullivan's concept of early adolescence is characterized by interest in the opposite sex, but an emotional-social bonding with the same gender. To the extent that the disabled teenager is isolated from other male and female teenagers, this stage may not be worked through. Similarly, Sullivan's stage of "later adolescence," characterized by the integration of sexual desires with social-emotional bonding with the opposite sex, may be compromised because of insufficient interaction of the disabled individual with members of the opposite sex.

Young Adulthood: Care Receiving

Being in a state of care receiving places the young adult in a dependency situation within the family. For a newly married young adult this may compromise the mutual sharing, on an equal basis, of oneself with one's spouse. Using an Eriksonian framework, the stage of "intimacy" is partially or completely replaced with a one-way dependency akin to earlier childhood stages. To the extent that illness compromises sexual performance, an important part of the stage of intimacy may be affected, threatening both self-concept and psychosexual identity. The emotional bonding that is supposed to normally develop from intimate sexual relationships also may be weakened unless compensatory factors are introduced. Levinson (1978) presents a useful exposition of developmental tasks of young adulthood that may challenge the young adult care receiver. Levinson's tasks include defining a dream of adult accomplishment, developing a career, finding a mentor, and establishing intimacy. Disabled young adults who depend on receiving care may have to reshape their dreams of adult accomplishments and aspire for careers in which they have a chance to succeed. Even though some individuals in such situations have come forth with very innovative solutions to overcome disabilities, this may mean having to give up, or seriously modify, a very treasured career aspiration. Such individuals should be given as much support as possible and appropriate to their career aspirations.

Young Adulthood: Caregiving

The stage of young adulthood, in contrast to previous stages, presents greater opportunities for considering caregiver as well as care-receiver roles. The adult is mature, in command of self, and capable of negotiating with authority figures, bureaucracies, service organizations, and the like. Physical, cognitive, and social maturity enable the young adult to successfully perform caregiving tasks. Feelings of enhanced self-esteem and competence ensure such successful coping. However, potentially problematic issues include the effects of being a caregiver on mastery of the intimacy stage of young adulthood. Thus the emotional investment as well as the time involved in caregiving on the part of the young adult to a nonspousal family member may adversely affect the successful working through of the Eriksonian stage of intimacy. Often, successful intimacy is promoted by the young adult moving away from home for a period of several years. When a young adult is immersed in caregiving to a parent or sibling, the above process may very well be compromised. The young adult caregiver may feel guilty over physically or psychologically leaving the family of orientation and the care receiver to invest in his or her new mate.

Midlife: Care Receiving

The individual who is in a care-receiving situation may have definite challenges regarding the fulfillment of Erikson's "generativity" stage. The chronically ill parent, unlike most parents, may not be able to take the child to school, to recreational or sports activities or to teach the child a variety of sensorimotor or cognitive skills. Fathers and mothers may face different challenges that also interact with gender and developmental stage of the child. Thus mothers may not be able to physically care for the school age or adolescent child without a surrogate, whereas fathers are less expected to fill this role, even with increasingly egalitarian expectations of child rearing. Fathers, however, generally are expected to play an active role coaching their school-age child in various sports, and a disabled father will find such a task challenging if not impossible. The image of the chronically ill parent is likely to be altered vis à vis the adolescent or young adult child, weakening parental authority. Traditional concepts of competence may have to be modified so that disabled parents can view themselves as good role models despite their disabilities. The challenge for the growing child of a disabled parent is to be able to identify with certain aspects of the parent while at the same time being able to find other parental figures with whom to identify.

The popular concept of midlife crisis has been challenged by a number of research studies (Costa & McCrae, 1978; Kahana, Kahana, & Meznick, 1976). Nevertheless, current societal conditions facilitate changes in career, marital situation, and lifestyle. Thus middle-aged and older adults can significantly alter their previous lifestyle. Individuals who became chronically ill or disabled in midlife, and who previously wished to engage in lifestyle changes during midlife, may be prevented from realizing such dreams. Depending on the nature of the disability, vis-à-vis the ingenuity and persistence of the disabled adult and his or her caregivers, such dreams can be realized, especially with some modifications.

Midlife: Caregiving

Being an adult caregiver to a child with a disability is within the range of adult child-rearing behavior. At the same time, it presents additional challenges to the parents in their stages of psychosocial development. Parental success at this stage is related to having raised children to become mature and functioning adults. Parents of a child with a disability have to work through their own feelings regarding this stage of "generativity," including possible guilt feelings and feelings of being unfulfilled as a parent. This is especially traumatic if the child has a mental rather than a physical disability. The latter may impact on the later Eriksonian stage of "integrity" and jeopardize achieving the feeling that one's life was basically a gratifying one. Overlapping the generativity-stagnation dimension just described is Benedek's (1959) concept of parenthood as a developmental stage. Benedek argues that parenthood involves reexamining the adult's own childhood-developmental issues and conflicts. Thus if a caregiving parent of a disabled child had to deal in his or her own childhood with the "school bully," that parent may reexperience the entire complex of feelings and unresolved emotions when having to defend his or her disabled child against a possible physical confrontation by other children. Similarly, an adult who, as a child, felt ignored or degraded by his or her peer group may be particularly sensitive or overreactive to a disabled child's compromised social situation or peer relationships. Furthermore, because there is an increased probability that disabled children will have to deal with more challenging peer situations and social interactions, there may be a greater sense of reality to the parent who is reexperiencing Benedek's stipulated developmental stage. These problems, however, can be ameliorated, once they are identified by mental health workers who are sensitive to the issues.

Caregiving during midlife also may result in uplifts that are congruent with a generative or nurturant orientation. At the same time, the middle-aged caregiver to a child (or adult child) or spouse also may face a "double jeopardy," as caring for physically frail elderly parents constitutes a normative expectation at this life stage (Brody, 1985).

Old Age: Care Receiving

Care receivers who are reaching old age can be divided into two groups: those who have been care receivers for a very long time (e.g., since childhood, young adulthood, or early middle age) and those who have become disabled in later life. For the latter group, issues of integrity-despair should be less problematic and easier to resolve than for those who have been disabled over a lifetime. The individual who has not been previously hampered by disability was therefore able to successfully cope with previous lifespan stages. Nevertheless the shock of illness and disability during the older years will require a readjustment period. Elderly care receivers who value their autonomy may be confronted with particular developmental challenges, because they must assume a dependent role in which compliance is the only way to reciprocate for help received.

Old Age: Caregiving

Issues of integrity versus a feeling of general despair have to be worked through as one enters old age. Parents who had to raise disabled children may be haunted by feelings of uncompleted or unsuccessful parenthood at this later stage in life. The older person's feelings of generational continuity or perpetuity through one's children, which may be viewed as an important component of integrity, may be compromised or threatened. If so, these feelings need to be worked through. Challenges to ego integrity may occur among elderly (e.g., 70 or older) who are confronted with caregiving for a spouse or an adult offspring who became disabled (e.g., in a disabling automobile accident). Generativity needs once again are evoked in the older person, along with a threat to the feeling of ego integrity during late life. Feelings of futurity and intergenerational continuity also may be threatened.

Social Caregiving Context:
Perspectives on the Caregiving
Family System in a Life-Cycle Context

From consideration of the impact of caregiving or care receiving during different life stages on individual members of the family, we now turn to exploring the roles of family systems in the caregiving process and the impact of caregiving to a chronically ill member on the family unit as a system. In doing so we move from an illustrative discussion of age and life stage in an informal personal caregiving context, to an illustrative consideration of life stage in a social caregiving context (Figure 1.1). Our discussion thus moves from the individual to the group level with particular attention to the temporal axis of caregiving. Corresponding our disciplinary orientation also shifts from a developmental pyschological to a sociological one.

It is generally accepted, from a cross-cultural and historical perspective, that those who enter into family life expect to produce and rear children. It is also a general expectation that, as parents age and become infirm, the primary caregiving responsibilities fall to their children

(Goode, 1982). From this we can conclude that caregiving, in some form or another, is a fundamental aspect of family life for the vast majority of people. The degree to which a family can be viewed as a resource for its chronically ill family members, and the degree to which caregiving is disruptive to the family unit, depends to a great extent upon the particular circumstances surrounding the caregiving experience. These include the present stage of the family in the family life course and the particular functions of that family during that stage, the severity of the illness/disability of the care receiver, and the types of resource demands placed on the family. As the family approaches each stage, parents and friends offer advice about what to expect and how best to handle the difficulties presented at each stage. Thus, the stressors indigenous to each stage are normative as they are somewhat anticipated and prepared for. However, as is often the case, nonnormative stressors, including unanticipated chronic illness of a family member, also may be present.

McGoldrick and Carter (1982) identified six stages of the family life cycle and the emotional and family status transitions that accompany them. They include unattached young adults, newly married couples, family with young children, family with adolescents, family with young adults, and family in later life. Each stage has characteristic processes and relationships that distinguish it from prior or successive stages. Each stage also presents unique challenges, as well as corresponding needs for various types and sources of resources used by the family to face these challenges. Caregiving responsibilities to a chronically ill family member further complicate the interplay between the normative exigencies of the family life stage, the stresses associated with caregiving, and the adequacy of coping resources available to the family.

The likelihood of becoming a caregiver is greatly influenced by stages of the family life cycle. Unattached young adults typically experience a preparatory phase in which they achieve a differentiation of self in relation to the family of origin, a development of intimate peer relationships, and an establishment of self in work that leads to economic independence. In this stage mate selection generally will occur based primarily on love between a man and a woman (Bowen, 1978; Meyer, 1980). Interestingly, the average age at marriage has been steadily increasing since 1950, with 80% of Americans marrying by age 34 and 95% marrying before they were 45 years old (Henslin, 1990). The fact that singles are marrying later in life suggests that they may have a greater chance of becoming caregivers simply by their availability, especially for the nonspouse females who represented about half of all caregivers. Stone, Cafferata, and Sangl (1987) provide extensive information about demographic characteristics of major family caregivers based on a national survey. Their research indicates that approximately 22% of caregivers were between ages 14 and 44 years and 13% were never married. Nonspouse males represented only 16% of caregivers.

The members of the newly married couple adjust and commit to their new family system by pooling their resources, negotiating roles and responsibilities, and realigning their relationships with extended family and friends to include their spouse's network. The demands of caregiving at this stage are most likely tied to aging parents of one or both new spouses and could strongly affect the couple as they begin to adjust to each other and to their new relationship. Stone and colleagues (1987) also indicate that most caregivers were married (69.5%) and lived with the recipient, and about one third were related in some other way to the care recipient. Most caregivers also were found to be at or below middle income, with one third near poverty. It is easy to see the existing potential of economic disruption that a young couple living in a lower income bracket might face. During this stage the challenges posed by caregiving are related primarily to the possible dissolution of the couple. Both members of the new marital dyad maintain strong ties to their families of origin and their social networks, whose members are not usually common friends to both individuals (i.e., not all of the husband's friends are also friends of the wife).

The arrival of children introduces the couple to the next stage. They accept the new generation of members into their family system by adopting the parenting roles and by realigning their relationships with extended family to include grandparents and, often, great-grandparents (Watkins et al., 1987). In the beginning of the child-rearing stage, caregiving responsibilities can be centered on either the young children, older parents, or both. Families with chronically ill children struggle to reconcile normative expectations for children of a given age in the face of restrictions posed by the child's illness (Patterson, 1988). The compromises that must be made in this process can interfere with normal family activities and place stresses on siblings as well as on parents and on the ill child. Because family activities tend to include all family members, particularly when young children are present, the illness has an impact not only on the child and a designated caregiver such as the mother, but also on the entire family unit. Restrictions imposed on the sick child are likely to become restrictions on the entire family as well.

Caregiving needs of older parents also are likely to impact on marital satisfaction and other characteristics of family roles of the child-rearing family. When children begin to arrive, the couple will go through many adjustments, and some couples adjust better than others (Bahr, 1989). The most important factor affecting the adjustment to children is marital satisfaction prior to the arrival of the child (Worthington & Buston, 1986). Another major influence is support from the father, as most of the care a new baby receives comes from the mother. This is especially important if, due to her participation in the workforce, the mother expects help from the father with household tasks (Belsky, 1985). Fathers and mothers directly involved in both caregiving and income generation may not be able to contribute as much to the care of their children as they would prefer. Caregiving burdens also could lead to lower levels of marital satisfaction.

Adolescence often is viewed as a difficult time of adjustment in our society for all family members involved. Parent-youth conflict is common and may provide an added dimension of stress for parents (Bahr, 1989). Couples with adolescent children begin to refocus on midlife marital and career issues and to shift concern to issues of the older generation. Children begin to establish their independence but still rely heavily on their parents (Goldscheider & Devanzo, 1986; Sebald, 1986; Willits, 1986). Caregiving mothers of adolescents or young adults with chronic illness are at risk of becoming the "woman in the middle," juggling numerous role demands such as wife, mother, homemaker, employee, and possibly grandmother, as well as caregiver to an aging parent (Brody, 1981, p. 479). Caregiver burden is most severe when a single individual is responsible for care to both generations (Montgomery et al., 1985).

The couple then moves to the stage of the family with young adults. In this stage the family accepts multiple exits and entries into the family system and encourages economic independence among the children. There is a renegotiation of the marital dyad, a development of adult-to-adult relationships between parents and children, a realignment of relationships to include in-laws and grandchildren, and the acceptance of the functional decline and eventual death of the parents (Ciernia, 1985; Clemens & Axelson, 1985; Duvall & Miller, 1985; Glick, 1977). In families with young adults much of the role strains and conflicts that result from the combination of caregiving and parenting demands would be reduced. The children become more independent and enter the first stage of their own family-of-procreation life course. This means they are likely to have multiple entries to and exits from their parents' home as they establish their own economic independence. The parental couple, meanwhile, renegotiates the marital dyad in a similar fashion to newlywed couples, with the exception that they both can contribute more years of experience and maturity to the negotiation process than do newlyweds. These older couples are also at increased risk of developing personal health problems (Atchley, 1991). Caregiving at this stage, however, would conflict less with parenting than it does in earlier stages. With no children present in the home, the couple has more time to spend with each other. This stage presents a need for some readjustment in activities, roles, and priorities. Caregiving responsibilities may interfere with the couple's renegotiation of roles and responsibilities, particularly because wives during this period may be caught between caregiving responsibilities for their parents as well as their spouses. As the couple launches their children from the nest, challenges to the marital dyad once again center around issues related to the dissolution of the marriage. If, for example, one or both partners have remained in the marriage only for the sake of the children, divorce may now take place (Hammond & Muller, 1992). However, because past behavior is an excellent predictor of future behavior, and because personality traits remain rather constant throughout the lifespan (Costa & McCrae, 1989), these renegotiations of existing family roles will be consistent with previous patterns during the lifespan.

The family in later life is characterized by an acceptance of shifting generational roles. Socialization processes vary and become more consultative in nature as the couple reaches this later life stage. As older couples increasingly face illness of at least one spouse, they must maintain their personal and/or couple functioning and interests in the face of physiological decline. When older husbands and wives both develop chronic illness, they may alternate roles between caregiver and care receiver. Members of the older generation must align their personal roles toward concerns more central to the role of the middle generation and make room in the family system for their wisdom and experience. They also must deal with the losses of spouse, siblings, and peers as well as prepare for their own eventual decline and death (Brubaker, 1985; Treas & Bengtson, 1987). Challenges of caregiving or care receiving may thus represent cumulative stresses for older members of the family.

Research by Stone and colleagues (1987) documents that about 35% of all caregivers are 65 years of age or older. The significant risks of caregiving in this stage are those that threaten the limited resources that the couple uses to maintain its physical, social, emotional, intellectual, and spiritual way of life. Grandparenting and great-grandparenting roles take on a less central, still important focus within the family structure. Older couples assume a more or less supportive role and maintain frequent contacts and visits with their family (Atchley, 1991). Previous research suggests that the quality of contact between older parents and their adult children contributes more to both parties' life satisfaction than do other factors (Houser & Berkman, 1984). Excessive caregiving burdens may tax the limited resources available to older couples and adversely affect their caregiving and family role performance. In late life, as both spouses become increasingly frail, the responsibility of caring for ill or aging parents typically reverts back to the adult children. Support usually is sought from sources external to the marital dyad, particularly because elderly spouses and friends are likely to pass away during this period. Types of support are both affective and instrumental, and there is evidence that caregiving relationships during this stage are not strictly unilateral, going from the younger to the older generation, but that a great deal of reciprocity occurs (Kahana, Midlarsky, & Kahana, 1987).

Understanding the family life cycle as a significant caregiving context has great heuristic value. However, few empirical studies of caregiving have utilized such a framework. Consideration of processes involved in family caregiving is required as a useful first step in initiating research on caregiving families within a developmental context. We now turn to an illustrative discussion of one major example of interpersonal processes involved in family caregiving: that of social support. In doing so we move to the transactional axis of caregiving (Figure 1.1).

TRANSACTIONAL AXIS: PERSPECTIVES ON THE PROCESS OF CAREGIVING

Theoretical understandings regarding caregiving generally are embedded in a stress-coping-support model. The variables of major interest in such models have been on outcomes such as burden or psychological distress of the caregivers and the nature of the care receiver's illness defining caregiver demand and constituting the major stressor in the paradigm (Pearlin, 1989).

With attention directed at consequences of caregiving, the processes or transactions involved in providing aid to the chronically ill generally are given little attention. In the simplest terms the caregiving transactions may be reduced to caregiving hours, with little attention paid to the currencies of caregiving or the transactions that take place during these hours. In Figure 1.1 we attempt to designate what actually might be exchanged between caregivers and care receivers during the process of caregiving. We call this the transactional axis.

Exchange theory (Dowd, 1980) suggests that patterned interactions or exchanges of valued social supplies occur in all dyadic social interactions. In the case of caregiver/care receiver exchanges, social supports may be given and compliance may be the exchange currency exacted from the care receiver (Lustbader, 1991).

Social support generally has been advanced as the most promising and well researched concept for understanding caregiving transactions (Pearlin, 1989). It generally is viewed as a buffer in the stress paradigm that may moderate the adverse effects of caregiving on those providing care. Alternatively, it also may be viewed as the buffer that enhances well-being of care receivers in the face of stresses posed by their illness. We will return to a closer examination of the value, as well as the limitations, of the social support construct for understanding caregiving transactions throughout the life course.

First, however, we want to acknowledge the potential value of alternative transactions relevant to caregiving, both on the individual and the system level. On an individual level (the personal caregiving context in Figure 1.1), Corbin and Strauss's (1988) analysis of the "work of caregiving" presents a promising avenue for understanding caregiving transactions in a qualitative framework. Aspects of symbolic meaning attached to caregiving relationships also have been analyzed by clinicians such as Silverstone and Hyman (1982) and Lustbader (1991).

On a system level (the social caregiving context in Figure 1.1), a very different set of processes may pertain to caregiving. Family cohesion or family conflict may reflect important aspects of family functioning in response to challenges of caregiving. Social integration of both the caregiver and the care receiver in the family system may have important implications for the family's effectiveness in providing care and may influence the outcomes of caregiving for both the individual and the group (Zarit & Pearlin, 1993).

On a system level, pertinent societal processes relate to the enactment and enforcement of legislation that creates services or programs for the chronically ill. The service delivery system brings such services to the consumer (caregiving dyad or family) by financing programs and creating or controlling access to the program by setting eligibility criteria and ultimately delivering services. At present the caregiving literature is just beginning to address such system-level processes (Harrington, 1993; Noelker & Bass, this volume).

In our efforts to illustrate the value of considering the transactional caregiving axis, we now return to a more detailed consideration of social support as a fundamental caregiving transaction. Social support has been designated as the major process variable to explain the beneficial effects of caregiving on care receivers. Conversely, social support also is seen as buffering the adverse effects and burdens on caregivers (Kahana & Young, 1990). An important area of interest to social support researchers is how social support may alleviate some of the stresses inherent in the caregiving relationship. This research centers on the role of social supports in the classical stress paradigm and has attempted to develop a prototype of how such supports operate. Some research in this area over the past two decades has drawn criticism for its lack of conceptual and methodological clarity; researchers have disagreed on which dimensions of support are the most important (O'Reilly, 1988; Pearlin, Menaghan, Lieberman, & Mullan, 1981; Thoits, 1982). The absence of consensus about the dimensions of support, as well as a lack of formal standardized operational definitions for these dimensions, have, in part, contributed to a lack of consistent results being reported in the literature on caregivers' social supports.

Although there is no single accepted definition of social support, it is useful to think of support in terms of the relationship between the difficulties of life experienced by an individual and the resources mobilized to cope with those difficulties. Generally, social support is the provision of resources (i.e., affect, information, or tangibles) by others (the social network) to an individual who is experiencing some level of difficulty. This definition suggests a conceptual distinction between (a) types of support (i.e., functional dimensions) (Cobb, 1976, 1979; Ensel & Lin, 1991; Gottlieb, 1981; House, 1981) and (b) sources of support (i.e., structural dimensions) (Mitchell, 1969; Wellman, 1981). The National Academy of Sciences panel concluded that research on types of social support usually includes one or more of the following: affective (emotional) support (i.e., behavior of a member of the support network, such as empathy, love, caring, or trust directed toward the central individual in the network), instrumental support (i.e., help that is directly rendered to the individual to help him or her to deal pragmatically with a situation, including material and economic aid), informational support (i.e., help given to others to help themselves by providing them with information that they may use to resolve a problem situation), and social integration (the extent to which a person is embedded in a social network) (Cohen, Horowitz, Lazarus, et al., 1982). These dimensions of support are characteristics of the *functions* of the interaction between an individual and the network.

With regard to sources of support, a distinction is made between the behavioral elements of social support and the structural elements (O'Reilly, 1988; Wellman, 1981). This distinction is variously referred to as the content versus context of support, types versus source (as we have mentioned), or structure versus functions of support. However it is characterized, the *social network* should be considered the baseline determinant of social support, because social support cannot exist without the presence of others. Sociologists generally define social networks as a set of linkages among a defined group of people, whose characteristics can explain the social behavior of the people within the group (Mitchell, 1969). Social networks are important because they form the context in which the needs of the care-receiving individual are met. It is through these social contacts and relationships that the reciprocal influences of individuals on their environment, and environmental influences on the individual, are played out (Sarason, Sarason, & Pierce, 1990).

Figure 1.1 gives us the opportunity to discuss the transactional axis in relation to the temporal and spatial axes. One example that is relevant to the current discussion is the issue of life stages and social support, which represents the interplay between the temporal axis and the transactional axis. It is useful to think of the couple as the basic unit of a social relationship in the framework of the family. In this way, a family may be understood as the collectivity of individuals who are emotionally, economically, and legally attached, through kinship or emotional bonds, to a wedded couple. As we discussed above, families evolve through several stages of development during their journey through the life span. Each stage presents the family with challenges and difficulties that must be overcome if it is to survive. The type, source, and amount of support provided vary across life stages, and in relation to the type, source, and amount of stress encountered due to challenges at each stage (Antonucci, 1985; Antonucci & Akiyama, 1987; Schulz & Rau, 1985).

One of the most prevalent needs of caregivers is the need for some sort of respite from the intense demands of caregiving. Young, single caregivers need some form of respite from caregiving responsibilities to have time to pursue intimate peer relations. Support may come from parents or adult siblings who give babysitting services, or from formal care providers such as day-care or adult day-health-care or home-health-care agencies that augment the care provided by the primary caregiver with skilled nursing or child care. With respect to social supports available to child-rearing couples faced with care of a chronically ill child, family ties are typically still strong, but the friendship network shrinks in size and includes friends common to both partners. These friends are usually couples in the same life stage who are experiencing similar challenges. At this point the primary source of support shifts away from external sources and centers on the spouse. The types of support sought are more instrumental (e.g., help with child care, laundry, and housework) than in the previous stage, but affective and informational support also are sought. For the young wife providing care to a chronically ill child, esteem support from her spouse may be overwhelmingly important; for a middle-aged mother providing care to her elderly parents, information support may be particularly useful.

During the middle years in which members of the "sandwich generation" may be faced with multiple caregiving roles, the interaction between type and source of support is most apparent. In cases where the woman cannot help with housework or health care for both households, these instrumental supports are likely to be sought first from the woman's siblings, and then from sources outside the family that are geographically convenient. Formal service providers often are contacted to fill in the gaps left by families who have competing demands and cannot fulfill both. Affective and informational support for the caregiving woman, on the other hand, are likely to be sought primarily from the spouse along with the woman's siblings. Older adults who need care for chronic illness generally receive support from a spouse and from adult children. When informal sources of aid prove insufficient, these elderly increasingly turn to formal service providers and to paid helpers in addition to relying on family members.

Caregiving poses multiple stresses and challenges to those providing care. It is clear that those providing care to persons with chronic illness may require and benefit from instrumental assistance (e.g., an alternative caregiver takes over caregiving duties to provide respite to the primary caregiver); esteem or affirmation support, which helps reinforce caregiver self-esteem and continued motivation for providing care; and informational support to enable caregivers to be more effective and better informed about resources available to both the recipient and the provider. Temporal expansion of the caregiving paradigm allows examination of the process of caregiving, as it is exemplified by the activation of a social support network, particularly in view of nonnormative life events. If caregiving responsibilities are needed at a time when they are not normally expected (e.g., a stroke or heart attack in a young person) these challenges are even more stressful (Gurin & Brim, 1984). Not only are these events statistically infrequent (and so most people are unprepared for them), but also the support network that a caregiver would usually approach for aid may not be able to give timely or appropriate support if the events are temporally nonnormative (Schulz & Rau, 1985). In cases such as this the questions of adaptation of the family caregiver to a perceived or real lack of support, as well as the support network's positive or negative reaction to nonnormative demands for aid, are very important.

Expansion of the caregiving paradigm in space (i.e., emphasizing the caregiving dyad) reminds us that social support is equally important for the caregiver and recipient. Recent research on caregiving has begun to focus on the dyadic nature of the caregiving relationship by (a) studying care receivers' outcomes in conjunction with caregiver variables (Rook, 1984), (b) including measures of burden experienced by the care recipient (Noelker & Kercher, 1991), and (c) concentrating on the care receivers' perceptions of conflict within the relationship (Johnson, 1993).

Not all effects of social support or social interaction, however, are positive. Unavoidable stresses and strains on individuals result from the responsibilities and obligations inherent in social relationships. Being upset by the network tempers the network's ability to promote a respondent's mental and physical health (Rook, 1984). For the chronically ill care receiver, needing help with formerly simple tasks often is upsetting, especially if the recipient feels that the help is given perfunctorily or begrudgingly. Those who are dependent on others for life or living are very attuned to the emotional messages presented to them (Drew, 1986). Caregivers may be openly resentful or argue with each other, or with the recipient, about caregiving issues. Conversely, formal caregivers have been criticized for performing caregiving tasks without any emotional interaction at all (Drew, 1986). Frail elderly people may have needs that are not being met by their caregivers even though the caregivers are doing all in their power (Kahana & Young, 1990). Such receivers may perceive that the caregiver is withholding care as a means of punishment, or out of neglect. Caregivers also may provide so much support that they induce dependencies, that is, they "overcare" (Coyne, Wortman, & Lehman, 1988).

A growing body of research finds that social support networks may have adverse effects on both care receivers and caregivers, and that these effects often are more powerful and enduring than positive effects. Negative effects of a support network include increased psychological distress symptoms (Johnson, 1991), reduced satisfaction with the support network (Melichar, Okun, & Hill, 1990), and increased depression in the central figure of the network (Pagel, Erdly, & Becker, 1987; Rook, 1984, 1989). Negative aspects of the social network also have resulted in greater dependence in ADL and inhibited personal adjustment after stroke (Norris, Stephens, & Kinney, 1990). Being upset with the social support network, in contrast to being satisfied with the network or finding network members helpful, is more strongly associated with caregiver burden and depression (Pagel et al., 1987; Strawbridge, 1991).

Another potentially negative aspect of social support is that persons (particularly a primary caregiver) who are closely involved with someone in distress may become emotionally overinvolved, develop resentful or hostile feelings toward him or her, or develop symptoms of psychological distress. These effects are especially likely in cases of protracted, intensive care (Eggert, Granger, Morris, & Pendleton, 1977; Noelker & Townsend, 1987). Evidence from the family therapy literature suggests at least four possible ways that family involvement may adversely affect caregivers' and care receivers' psychological and adaptational well-being. First, emotional overinvolvement may interfere with a caregiver's ability to perform instrumental tasks, such as feeding, toileting, or more serious tasks such as cardiopulmonary resuscitation (CPR). Second, family members unwittingly may emphasize the care recipient's dependence and thereby decrease the care recipient's ability to perform self-care activities even though he or she may be perfectly capable. Third, over a period of time, issues about the relationship itself may become more important to the participants than the care activities that initially brought them together. For example, a care recipient who loves to snack between meals and a caregiver who constantly forbids this may be involved in a power struggle that has little to do with the requirements of the recipient's diet. Finally, as caregivers experience problems that may be unrelated to the caregiving role, if they are overinvolved with the care recipient, the stress caused by these problems may project onto the caregiver and increase his or her distress (Coyne et al., 1988).

As indicated in the above discussion, the concept of social support is one useful approach to understanding the "what" of caregiving transactions. Nevertheless, it should be noted that this concept still stops short of answering the question of how caregiving is accomplished, nor does it necessarily address the relational quality of the transaction.

Specification of processes involved in the stress paradigm in general and caregiving in particular represents an unmet challenge in the field. Ecological models (Lawton & Nahemow, 1973; and Kahana, 1975, 1981) represent one useful approach to understanding the interactions involved in the caregiving process. The applicability of congruence models to family caregiving has been noted in our earlier work (Kahana & Young, 1990). Focusing on the caregiver/care receiver dyad, it is suggested that to the degree that needs of the care receiver are met by actions of the caregiver, care receiver well-being would be maximized. Conversely, to the extent that care receiver needs or demands exceed resources of the caregiver, caregiver burden and poor caregiver well-being would follow.

The use of congruence models can better inform consideration of the role of social supports as processes of caregiving. Thus, for example, it may be argued that negative social supports (Rook, 1990) are, for the most part, not inherently negative. Instead they reflect an incongruence between behaviors of the caregivers and preferences and needs of the care receivers. Accordingly, what caregivers may define as protective behaviors aimed to assist persons with chronic illness may be viewed by care receivers as unwelcome actions that make them dependent (Coyne et al., 1988). Such incongruent caregiving behaviors may be particularly problematic at certain points in the care receiver's development, such as adolescence.

CONCLUSIONS: TOWARD NEW FRONTIERS IN CAREGIVING RESEARCH USING THE EXPANDED PARADIGM

In our exposition of the expanded caregiving paradigm we selectively focused on issues and orientations that have been touched upon in prior conceptual and empirical work on caregiving. In our conclusions we look toward fresh frontiers for expansion that are much broader. We thus suggest that there is much open territory for future exploration.

In our discussion of the spatial axis of the expanded caregiving paradigm, we focused exclusively on the social world of individuals and groups. A useful alternative formulation in this area relates to consideration of the physical environment. There has been little emphasis on the role of the physical environment in facilitating or limiting functioning of care receivers or well-being of caregivers (Calkins, 1982). Physical barriers in the home environment have been identified in Noelker's (1987) work as contributing to poorer functioning among care receivers along with increased burden for caregivers. The potential role of environmental modifications in assisting physically and/or cognitively impaired elders has been acknowledged (Pynoos & Ohta, 1991). However, only very limited empirical research explores the effectiveness of such modifications as a buffer in reducing caregiver or care receiver stress (Namazi, Rosner, & Calkins, 1989). Research on caregivers to patients with dementia living in the community by Namazi and colleagues (1989) suggests that caregivers find such modifications effective and beneficial to both themselves and the patients they care for. This brief foray into consideration of an alternative approach to understanding the caregiving paradigm underscores the potential for alternative formulations that may be possible in each area of context and process upon which we have commented. The advantage of a comprehensive paradigm, with broad spatial and temporal parameters, is that it may provide a general road map with opportunities for developing more exact specifications of diverse locations. It is also noteworthy that alternative formulations suggest alternative methodologies. Thus, for example, the social support formulations of process generally have been explored in quantitative research. Alternatively, the biographical approach focusing on the work of caregiving arises from a qualitative tradition (Gerhardt & Brieskour-Zinke, 1986).

In our discussion of the temporal axis of the expanded caregiving paradigm we considered individual developmental issues relevant to the personal caregiving context for understanding the caregiver/care receiver dyad. Here we relied heavily on conceptual orientations of lifespan developmental psychologists. In contrast, our exposition of temporal issues relevant to the social caregiving context (the caregiving family) was anchored in a sociological orientation. We thus demonstrated the contributions of multiple disciplines for understanding the expanded caregiving paradigm. Future research directions in this area might apply the dimension of time, for example, to understanding social policies relevant to health-care delivery, or housing policies that might impact on the chronically ill and their caregivers.

In our discussion of the transactional axis of the expanded caregiving paradigm we focused on social supports as potentially useful ways of approaching the caregiving process. It is important to note, however, that other useful conceptualizations of the caregiving process are also possible and observable. Such an alternative view to understanding the process of caregiving is presented in the work of Corbin and Strauss (1988), who focus on the nature of work involved in caregiving. These qualitative researchers subdivide caregiving tasks into those related to managing the illness, including controlling symptoms and carrying out regimes. Second, caregiving tasks also are related to general lifestyles of the care receivers, in particular dealing with activity limitations and social isolation. Finally, one may consider "biographical work" related to one's identity. These relate to coming to terms with the illness, dealing with the possibility of death, and arriving at a self-conception in light of the illness. It is noteworthy that all of these types of tasks involve varying degrees of active work by caregivers as well as care receivers. In Corbin and Strauss's conception, development or biography thus represents a central construct for understanding the caregiving process.

It is our hope that by pointing to some of the directions for expansion of the caregiving paradigm, we may be opening up new and creative avenues for research in this area. Our overview of directions for expanding the caregiving paradigm to include contextual factors reveals that each contextual factor considered introduces greater complexity. We believe progress toward comprehensive caregiving models requires the development of taxonomies that provide systematic understanding of important contextual and process variables. Once we succeed in delineating parameters of key contextual and process factors we will be in a position to design studies that explicate elements of the paradigm and cumulatively offer a more comprehensive understanding of caregiving than that available in current research in this field.

REFERENCES

Antonucci, T. (1985). Personal characteristics, social support and social behavior. In R. Binstock & E. Shanas (Eds.), *Handbook of aging and the social sciences*, (2nd ed., pp. 94-128). New York: Plenum.

Antonucci, T. C., & Akiyama, H. (1987). Social networks in adult life and a preliminary examination of the convoy model. *Journal of Gerontology, 45*, 519-527.

Atchley, R. C. (1991). *Social forces and aging*, 6th ed. Belmont, CA: Wadsworth.

Bahr, S. J. (1989). *Family interaction*. New York: Macmillan.

Belsky, J. (1985). Exploring individual differences in marital change across the transition to parenthood: The role of violated expectations. *Journal of Marriage and the Family, 47*, 1037-1044.

Benedek, T. (1959). Parenthood as a developmental stage. *Journal of the American Psychoanalytic Association, 7*, 389-417.

Biegel, D. E., Sales, E., & Schulz, R. (1991). *Family caregiving in chronic illness*. Newbury Park, CA: Sage.

Birkel, R. C. (1990). A lifespan perspective on care-giving. *Prevention in Human Services, 9*, 99-108.

Bowen, M. (1978). *Family therapy in clinical practice*. New York: Aronson.

Brody, E. M. (1981). Women in the middle and family help to older people. *The Gerontologist, 21*(5), 471-480.

Brody, E. M. (1985). Parent care as normative family stress. *The Gerontologist, 25*(1), 19-29.

Brubaker, T. H. (1985). *Later life families*. Beverly Hills, CA: Sage.

Brubaker, T. H. (1990). A contextual approach to the development of stress associated with caregiving in later-life families. In M. A. P. Stephens, J. H. Crowther, S. E. Hobfoll, & D. L. Tennenbaum (Eds.), *Stress and coping in later-life families* (pp. 29-47). New York: Hemisphere.

Burton, L. M., & Sorenson, S. (1993). Temporal context and the caregiver role: Perspectives from ethnographic studies of multigeneration African American families. In S. H. Zant, L. I. Pearlin, & K. W. Schaie (Eds.), *Caregiving systems: Formal and informal helpers* (pp. 56-61). Hillsdale, NJ: Lawrence Erlbaum.

Butler, R. N. (1963). The life review: An interpretation of reminiscence in the aged. *Psychiatry, 26*, 65-76.

Calkins, M. (1988). *Design for dementia: Planning environments for the elderly and the confused*. National Health Publisher.

Ciernia, J. R. (1985). Death concern and businessmen's midlife crisis. *Psychological Reports, 56*, 83-87.

Clemens, A. W., & Axelson, L. J. (1985). The not so empty-nest: The return of the fledgling adult. *Family Relations, 34*, 259-264.

Cobb, S. (1976). Social support as a moderator of life stress. *Psychosomatic Medicine, 38*(5), 300-314.

38 PARADIGMS FOR CAREGIVING

Cobb, S. (1979). Social support and health through the life course. In M. W. Riley (Ed.), *Aging from birth to death* (pp. 93-106). Boulder, CO: Westview.

Cohen, F., Horowitz, M., Lazarus, R., et al. (1982). Panel report on psycho-social stress. In G. Elliott & C. Eisdorfer (Eds.), *Stress and human health: Analysis and implications for research.* New York: Springer.

Corbin, J. M., & Strauss, A. (1988). *Unending work and care: Managing chronic illness at home.* San Francisco: Jossey-Bass.

Costa, P., & McCrae, R. (1978). Objective personality assessment. In M. Storandt, I. Siegler, & M. Elias (Eds.), *The clinical psychology of aging.* New York: Plenum.

Coyne, J. C., Wortman, C. B., & Lehman, D. R. (1988). The other side of support: Emotional overinvolvement and miscarried helping. In B. H. Gottlieb (Ed.), *Marshalling social support: Formats, processes, and effects* (pp. 305-330). Newbury Park, CA: Sage.

Dowd, J. (1980). *Stratification among the aged: An analysis of power and dependence.* Monterey, CA: Brooks/Cole.

Drew, N. (1986). Exclusion and confirmation: A phenomenology of patients' experiences with caregivers. *IMAGE: Journal of Nursing Scholarship, 18*(2), 39-43.

Duvall, E. M., & Miller, B. C. (1985). *Marriage and family development,* 6th ed. New York: Harper & Row.

Eggert, C., Granger, V., Morris, R., & Pendleton, J. (1977). Caring for the patient with a long-term disability. *Geriatrics, 22,* 102-114.

Elder, G. L., Jr. (1992). Life course. In E. F. Borgatta & M. L. Borgatta (Eds.), *Encyclopedia of sociology,* (Vol. 3, pp. 1120-1130). New York: Macmillan.

Ensel, W. M., & Lin, N. (1991). The life stress paradigm and psychological distress. *Journal of Health and Social Behavior, 32,* 321-341.

Erikson, E. H. (1963). *Childhood and society,* 2nd ed. New York: Norton.

Freud, S. (1976). Group psychology and the analysis of the ego. In J. Strachey (Ed. and Trans.), *The complete psychological works of Sigmund Freud* (Vol. 18). New York: Norton. (Original work published 1922)

Gerhardt, U., & Brieskour-Zinke, M. (1986). The normalization of hemodialysis at home. *Research in the Sociology of Health Care, 4,* 271-317.

Glick, P. C. (1977). Updating the life cycle of the family. *Journal of Marriage and the Family, 39,* 5-13.

Goldscheider, F. K., & Davenzo, J. (1986). Semiautonomy and leaving home in early adulthood. *Social Forces, 65,* 187-201.

Goode, W. J. (1982). *The family,* 2nd ed. Englewood Cliffs, NJ: Prentice Hall.

Gottlieb, B. H. (1981). Preventive interventions involving social networks and social support. In B. H. Gottlieb (Ed.), *Social networks and social support.* Beverly Hills, CA: Sage.

Grossberg, M. (1984). *Governing the hearth.* Chapel Hill: University of North Carolina Press.

Gurin, P., & Brim, O. G., Jr. (1984). Change in self in adulthood: The example of the sense of control. In P. B. Baltes & O. G. Brim, Jr. (Eds.), *Life-span development and behavior,* (Vol 6, pp. 291-334). New York: Academic Press.

Hagestad, G. O. (1990). Social perspectives on the life course. In R. Binstock & L. George (Eds.), *Handbook of aging and the social sciences* (3rd ed., pp. 151-168). San Diego, CA: Academic Press.

Hammond, R. J., & Muller, G. O. (1992). The late-life divorced: Another look. *Journal of Divorce and Remarriage, 17*(3/4), 135-150.

Harrington, C. (1993). Social health maintenance organizations: An innovative financing and service delivery model. In S. H. Zarit, L. I. Pearlin, & K. W. Schaie (Eds.), *Caregiving systems: Formal and informal helpers* (pp. 173-193). Hillsdale, NJ: Lawrence Erlbaum.

Haug, M. R. (1988). Power, authority, and health behavior. In D. S. Gochman (Ed.), *Health behavior: Emerging research perspectives* (pp. 325-336). New York: Plenum.

Henslin, J. M. (1990). *Social problems,* 2nd ed. Englewood Cliffs, NJ: Prentice Hall.

House, J. S. (1981). *Work, stress, and social support.* Reading, MA: Addison-Wesley.

Houser, B. B., & Berkman, S. L. (1984). Aging parent/mature child relationships. *Journal of Marriage and the Family, 46,* 295-299.

Johnson, J. R. (1991). *The effects of social support and social interaction on psychological distress in an aging veteran population.* Unpublished doctoral dissertation, Department of Sociology, University of Washington.

Johnson, J. R. (1993, November). *Factors associated with negative interactions between family caregivers and elderly care receivers.* Paper presented at the Annual Meeting of the Gerontogical Society of America, New Orleans, LA.

Kahana, B., & Kahana, E. (1971). Theoretical and research perspectives on grandparenthood: A theoretical statement. *Aging and Human Development, 2,* 261-268.

Kahana, B., Kahana, E., & Meznick, J. (1976). *Midlife crisis: Fact or myth?* Paper presented at the Annual Meeting of the Gerontological Society of America.

Kahana, E., Kahana, B., Borawski, E., & Kercher, K. (1990). Adaptation to frailty among dispensed elders. *University Center on Aging and Health Newsletter, 10*(1), 9-14.

Kahana, E., Kahana, B., & Riley, K. (1989). Person-environment transactions relevant to control and helplessness in institutionalized settings. In P. S. Fry (Ed.), *Psychological perspectives of helplessness and control in the elderly* (pp. 121-146). New York: Elsevier North-Holland.

Kahana, E., Kahana, B., & Segall, M. (1986). Stepping stones: Long distance moves among the aged. *Newsletter: The University Center on Aging and Health, 8*(3), 9-13.

Kahana, E., Midlarsky, E., & Kahana, B. (1987). Beyond dependency, autonomy and exchange: Prosocial behavior in late-life adaptation. *Social Justice Research, 1*(4), 439-459.

Kahana, E., & Young, R. (1990). Clarifying the caregiving paradigm: Challenges for the future. In D. E. Biegel & A. Blum (Eds.), *Aging and caregiving: Theory, research and policy* (pp. 76-97). Newbury Park, CA: Sage.

Lawton, M. P., & Nahemow, L. (1973). Ecology and the aging process. In C. Eisdorfer & M. P. Lawton (Eds.), *Psychology of adult development and aging* (pp. 619-674). Washington, DC: American Psychological Association.

Levinson, D. J. (1978). *The seasons of a man's life.* New York: Knopf.

Litwak, E. (1985). *Helping the elderly: The complementary roles of informal networks and formal systems.* New York: Guilford.

Lustbader, W. (1991). *Counting on kindness.* New York: Free Press.

Malone-Beach, E. E., & Zarit, S. H. (1991). Current research issues in caregiving to the elderly. *International Journal of Aging and Human Development, 32,* 103-114.

McGoldrick, M., & Carter, E. A. (1982). The family life cycle—Its stages and dislocations. In F. Walsh (Ed.), *Normal family processes* (pp. 167-195). New York: Guilford.

Melichar, J., Okun, M., & Hill, M. (1990). Negative daily events, positive and negative ties, and psychological distress among older adults. *The Gerontologist, 30,* 193-199.

Menaghan, E. C. (1989). Role changes and psychological well-being: Variations in effects by gender and role repertoire. *Social Forces, 67,* 693-714.

Meyer, D. (1980). Between families: The unattached young adult. In E. A. Carter & M. McGoldrick (Eds.), *The family life cycle: A framework for family therapy* (pp. 71-91). New York: Gardner.

Midlarsky, E., & Kahana, E. (1988). Altruistic lifestyles among the old: A contributory model of late life adaptation. *Gerontology Review, 1,* 51-58.

Mitchell, J. C. (1969). The concept and use of social networks. In J. C. Mitchell (Ed.), *Social networks in urban situations: Analyses of personal relationships in central African towns* (pp. 1-50). Manchester, England: Manchester University Press.

Montgomery, R. J. V., Gonyea, J. C., & Hooyman, N. R. (1985). Caregiving and the experience of subjective/objective burden. *Family Relations, 34,* 19-26.

Montgomery, R. J. V., Stull, D. E., & Borgatta, E. F. (1986). Measurement and analysis of burden. *Research on Aging, 7,* 137-152.

Namazi, K. H., Rosner, T. T., & Calkins, M. P. (1989). Visual barriers to prevent ambulatory Alzheimer's patients from exiting through an emergency door. *The Gerontologist, 29,* 699-702.

Neugarten, B. (1964). *Personality in middle and later life.* New York: Atherton.

Noelker, L. (1987). Incontinence in elderly cared for by family. *The Gerontologist, 27,* 194-200.

Noelker, L., & Kercher, K. (1991, November). *Perceived burden on well-being of elderly receiving family care.* Paper presented at the Annual Meeting of the Gerontological Society of America, San Francisco.

Noelker, L., & Townsend, A. L. (1987). Perceived caregiving effectiveness: The impact of parental impairment, community resources, and caregiver characteristics. In T. H. Brubaker (Ed.), *Aging, health, and family* (pp. 58-79). Newbury Park, CA: Sage.

Norris, V. K., Stephens, M. A. P., & Kinney, J. M. (1990). The impact of family interactions on recovery from stroke: Help or hindrance? *The Gerontologist, 30,* 535-542.

O'Reilly, P. (1988). Methodological issues in social support and social network research. *Social Science Medicine, 26*(8), 863-873.

Pagel, M. D., Erdly, W. W., & Becker, J. (1987). We get by with (and in spite of) a little help from our friends. *Journal of Personality and Social Psychology, 53,* 793-804.

Patterson, J. (1988). Families experiencing stress: The family adjustment and adaptation model. *Family Systems Medicine, 6*(2), 202-239.

Pearlin, L. I. (1989). The sociological study of stress. *Journal of Health and Social Behavior, 30,* 241-256.

Pearlin, L. I., Menaghan, E. G., Lieberman, M. A., & Mullan, J. T. (1981). The stress process. *Journal of Health and Social Behavior, 22,* 337-356.

Pynoos, J., & Ohta, R. J. (1991). In-home interventions for persons with Alzheimer's disease and their caregivers: Special issue: The mentally impaired elderly: Strategies and interventions to maintain function. *Physical and Occupational Therapy in Geriatrics, 9,* 83-92.

Rook, K. S. (1984). The negative side of social interaction: Impact on psychological well-being. *Journal of Personality and Social Psychology, 46,* 1097-1108.

Rook, K. S. (1989). Strains in older adults' friendships. In R. G. Adams & R. Bleizner (Eds.), *Older adult friendship.* Newbury Park, CA: Sage.

Rook, K. S. (1990). Stressful aspects of older adults' social relationships: Current theory and research. In M. A. Stephens, J. Crowther, S. Hobfoll, & D. Tennenbaum (Eds.), *Stress and coping in later-life families* (pp. 173-192). Washington, DC: Hemisphere.

Sarason, B. R., Sarason, I. G., & Pierce, G. R. (1990). *Social support: An interactional view.* New York: John Wiley.

Schulz, R., & Rau, M. T. (1985). Social support through the life course. In S. Cohen & S. L. Syme (Eds.), *Social support and health* (pp. 129-150). New York: Academic Press.

Sebald, H. (1986). Adolescence shifting orientation toward parents and peers: A curriculum trend over recent decades. *Journal of Marriage and the Family, 48,* 5-13.

Silverstone, B., & Hyman, H. K. (1982). *You and your aging parents.* New York: Pantheon.

Smyer, M. A., & Birkel, R. C. (1991). Research focused on intervention with families of the chronically mentally ill elderly. In E. Light & D. B. Lebowitz (Eds.), *The elderly with chronic mental illness* (pp. 111-130). New York: Springer.

Stone, R., Cafferata, G. L., & Sangl, J. (1987). Caregivers of the frail elderly: A national profile. *The Gerontologist, 27,* 616-626.

Strawbridge, W. (1991). *The effects of social factors on adult children caring for older parents.* Unpublished doctoral dissertation, Department of Sociology, University of Washington, Seattle.

Sullivan, H. S. (1953). *The interpersonal theory of psychiatry.* New York: Norton.

Thoits, P. (1982). Conceptual, methodological, and theoretical problems in studying social support as a buffer against life stress. *Journal of Health and Social Behavior, 23,* 145-159.

Thompson, L., & Walker, A. J. (1982, November). The dyad as a unit of analysis: Conceptual and methodological issues. *Journal of Marriage and the Family,* 889-925.

Treas, J., & Bengtson, V. L. (1987). The family in later years. In M. B. Sussman & S. K. Steinmetz (Eds.), *Handbook of marriage and family* (pp. 625-628). New York: Plenum.

Watkins, S. C., Menken, J. A., & Bongaarts, J. (1987). Demographic foundations of family change. *American Sociological Review, 52,* 346-358.

Wellman, B. (1981). Applying network analysis to the study of support. In B. H. Gottlieb (Ed.), *Social networks and social support* (pp. 171-200). Beverly Hills, CA: Sage.

Willits, W. L. (1986). Pluralistic ignorance in the perception of parent-youth conflict. *Youth and Society, 18,* 150-161.

Worthington, E. L., & Buston, B. G. (1986). The marriage relationship during the transition to parenthood: A review and a model. *Journal of Family Issues, 7,* 443-473.

Zarit, S. H., Pearlin, L. I., & Schaie, K. W. (Eds.). (1993). Social interpretation of both caregiver and care receiver in family systems. *Caregiving systems: Informal and formal helpers.* Hillsdale, NJ: Lawrence Erlbaum.

2

Someone to Watch Over Me

Family Responsibilities and
Their Realization Across Family Lives

JOAN ALDOUS

It has been more than six decades since Ira Gershwin penned the lyrics for "Someone to Watch Over Me," to music by his brother, George. Nothing in the interim has changed the sentiment for most people. "There's a somebody," they fervently hope, who "turns out to be someone to watch over me." Events occur when even the stoutest heart quivers and longs for care and comfort from a concerned other. And it is to their families that most people turn when they are in difficulties. The particular focus of this chapter, therefore, is on families and their caregiving activities throughout the lives of family members.

This is an examination of how families as groups vary in their capacity over time to meet the unexpected insults to physical and mental well-being that their members suffer. It is not concerned with the particular disabilities that flesh is heir to; this is the province of the health-care professionals. The concern here is with the fairly typical problems that families face at particular stages in their existence. These specific times on the family clock may present difficulties for all

AUTHOR'S NOTE: This chapter is a revision of the plenary address given at the Conference on Family Caregiving Across the Life Span, Case Western Reserve University, October 22, 1990. It could not have been completed without the research and bibliographic help of Jane Maguire, Cindy Sutton, Marek Szopski, and Robert Woodberry. My thanks also go to Linda Williams, who saw it through previous drafts.

families but especially for those also having the responsibility of watching over ailing members. The chapter begins with relevant definitions. This section is followed by a summary of the demographic changes that affect caregiving and the persons looked after at particular periods in family histories. A closer examination of these periods and their characteristics with reference to caretaking across family careers is next. In the discussion, the ambivalent and often negative emotions family caregivers feel toward the ailing are not ignored. The chapter's conclusion traces the implications of the family development analysis for the caregiving endeavor in intimate groups and for research on these activities.

DEFINITIONS

It is family members whom people expect to watch over them and whom they turn to for help when they are "under the weather." It should be noted that nowadays the term *family* encompasses a wide variety of groups. Most of these groups are captured by defining **family** to include cohabiting groups of some duration composed of persons in intimate relations based on biology, law, custom, or choice and usually economically interdependent.

The common term used for the activities of these family groups on behalf of needy members is *caregiving*. **Caregiving** refers to the physical work or financial assistance involved but also includes the accompanying comfort that family members provide. This emotional support incorporates the idea of caring about someone, the "concern for" and "taking charge of" the welfare of others when they are troubled or unwell, that lies behind the search for someone to watch over us. That family person or persons is a caretaker in being a caregiver. In other words, the provider's services are accompanied with the sentiment and sensitivity to the recipient's needs and feelings that indicate a strong desire to benefit the sufferer.

Persons count on caring and the care work to which it gives rise to be found in intimate family relations, especially those involving women. In fact, caring and caregiving often are seen as the defining characteristics of women. Watching over others involves the warm feelings and quiet domesticity persons have come to expect women to display in their customary home settings. In contrast to this traditional depiction of women's roles, men's identity has been seen as wrapped up in doing things for themselves and by themselves, often in public places (Graham, 1983, pp. 13, 15, 18). Yet men, too, expect someone to watch over them, and that someone in most cases is a woman: a wife, a daughter, or a mother. And what about women? They also look to other women— mothers, sisters, or daughters—to care for them. Thus an interest in family caregiving over time more often has less to do with families than it does with women in families.

It is well to note that just as the neutral term *caregiving* hides its ties to one gender, so, too, our knowledge of when families provide such services obscures reality. In one recent review of the research on care providers, the authors concluded that "most" of the work on the caregiving burden "primarily" concerned those helping the frail elderly or dementia patients (Raveis, Siegel, & Sudet, 1988-1989, p. 43). A survey of the entries in a recent *Family Caregiver Bibliography* bears out this judgment (Biegel, Farkas, & Fant, 1989). Where it was possible from the title of the reference to determine what age group was studied, more than half (58.3%) dealt with persons at the end of the life span. Less than one fifth (17.6%) dealt with children, and a bare fourth (24.1%) centered on the ages between youth and old age.

There are good reasons that special attention is devoted to the elderly, as they are more likely to be infirm, but the disproportionate numbers of articles and books devoted to their condition limits the discussion of the caregiving picture throughout family lives. Consequently, in this chapter, although the primary focus is on caregiving as it affects older families, I also cover the challenges families face during the length of their particular histories. To make the task manageable, there is a demarcation of periods within family lives. I use family development analysis to determine the internal problems families are apt to face, along with the external circumstances that are more likely to affect them at certain periods on the family calendar (Aldous, 1990). These circumstances that families must face at certain times are usually quite apart from the conditions requiring them to undertake the responsibilities we think of as family caregiving. However, a reckoning of years in terms of family time will give an idea of the groups' changing caregiving capacities for members of all ages. This schema of family stages making up the **family career** will be useful in determining periods when members are likely to need someone to watch over them. These family time markers will not necessarily fit all families, and a discussion of class and ethnic time variations appears where appropriate.

The terms *generation* and *cohort,* with their references to time, also often appear in the analysis. They refer to the consequences of family lives. **Generations** measure time in terms of forebears and descendants—one's parents and grandparents, one's children and grandchildren. **Cohort,** in contrast, refers to persons born around the same period in the various families.

DEMOGRAPHIC CHANGES

To place the predictable problems families face in the chapters of their family sagas in historical context, it is necessary to look at recent demographic changes that have affected families and their ability to give care.There has been a rise in cohabitation rates—half of the recently marrieds have cohabited, but most persons eventually marry (Bumpass & Sweet, 1989). Ninety-five percent of all women who are 40 years of age and older are married. Even among the slower-to-marry younger cohorts, estimates are that 90% will marry some time. However, among black women, the number marrying is lower. It is likely to be 80% (Norton & Moorman, 1987, pp. 4-5). Another change is today's high divorce and remarriage rates. Young couples married in the 1980s experience odds that suggest that only one of three will stay together until separated by death (Castro Martin & Bumpass, 1989). Figure 2.1 indicates just how the life course of families has gone beyond the one track of yesteryear. Compared with the past, family units are more subject to couple divisions and subsequent switches to single-parent lines, often followed by remarriages with different couple and child arrangements. While these couple transfers are occurring and while members are settling into the new patterns, young families are less able to assist their elders and are more in need of assistance themselves.

We also should not overlook the considerable number of unmarried women who start their families by bearing children. For white women 24 to 34 years of age, the birth rate to unmarried women doubled between 1974 and 1986, accounting for 16% of all births to whites in 1986. The proportion was 61% among blacks (Bumpass & McClanahan, 1989). Poverty more often characterizes single-mother families, and this is especially true among unmarried mothers. They are less likely to be awarded child support from fathers (Robins & Dickinson, 1984).

However, there is somewhat more childlessness. It is 14.7% among women 40 to 44 years old in 1988 instead of the 10.2% in 1976 in the

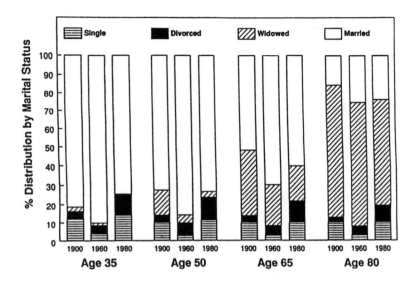

Figure 2.1. Percent Distribution of Cohort by Marital Status

SOURCE: Watkins, Menken and Bongaarts: 1987. "Demographic Foundations of Family Change." *American Sociological Review, 52,* p. 353.

same age cohort (U.S. Bureau of the Census, 1989a, p. 10, Table G). As a consequence, there will be more elderly in the future without children to take over family caregiving responsibilities.

For those with children, fertility is down. Although the 3.7 children per woman that was the average during the 1900s was almost reached during the 1950s, the average number of children per woman in the 1980s had slipped to 1.8 (National Center for Health Statistics, 1987, p. 7, Table 1). Thus cohorts with children who follow the parents of the baby boom generation will still have fewer children to turn to for caregiving than in the past. However, racial differences affect fertility rates. These are higher among African Americans and Hispanics, the families most subject to poverty and so less capable of supplying financial assistance to others.

Childbearing also is being postponed. First births to women 30 to 34 years old were up by 140% during the years 1970 to 1986. One of seven first births in 1986 were to women 30 years of age or older (Ventura, 1989). In turn, these older women are more likely to have elderly parents when their children are adolescents. Also subject to divorce, older mothers, in addition to their own needs, face competing demands for attention from preceding and following generations. Caring for adult children has become a responsibility for a number of families in the middle years. By the mid-1980s, 45% of 20- to 24-year-olds and 14% of 25- to 29-year-olds were at home compared with 37% and 9% for the same age cohorts 15 years earlier (Glick & Lin, 1986).

Parents of the 1950s baby boom generation, who are now approaching or are in their post-65 years, will have several children among whom to choose to help out. This is not true of younger cohorts, who, as shown above, are having smaller families. They will have smaller numbers of siblings in their own generation, and in the next generation, they will have fewer children.

If fertility is down, the demographic factor of increased longevity has added more vertical linkages up and down family lines (Bengtson, Rosenthal, & Burton, 1990). As members of "beanpole families," fewer persons will be related within the generations, but the representatives in each generation will be longer lived, making for longer family lineages of living members. The irony is that although more families are disrupted due to divorce, remarriage, and divorce again, there are longer existing intergenerational linkages among families.

However, it is well to note that there is little evidence of unusually long lineages, say five generations or more. Findings from a recent Boston study (Rossi & Rossi, 1990) showed the model lineage depth at all ages to be three generations. More respondents had no ascendants or descendants than were members of five-generation lineages. In the first case, it was 2% of those in their 20s, and in the second, 1.7% for the same age group. For the overall sample, 6% were in an isolated generation, and less than 1% were in a five-generation linkage (Rossi & Rossi, 1990, p. 146).

Figure 2.2 shows the startling demographics of fertility decreases and longevity increases. By 1960, adults were spending more time with parents over age 65 than with children under 18 (Bengtson et al., 1990, p. 265). In 1980, women could expect to spend 18 years with one or more parents over 65, more than 2.5 times the 7 years women in 1800 spent with one or both elderly parents (Watkins, Menken, & Bongaarts, 1987, p. 349, Table 2). These long-lived parents are more likely to be the so-called "oldest-old," that is, persons 85 years of age and older. Their numbers increased by 281% during the 30 years between 1950 and 1980, while the general population during the same period grew by

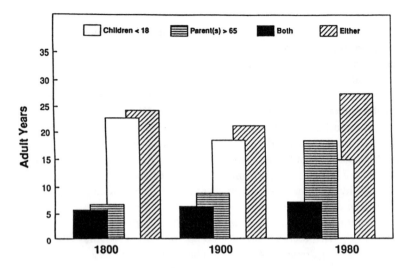

Figure 2.2. Adult Years Lived With Children Under 18, Parents Over 65, Either, or Both

SOURCE: Watkins, Menken and Bongaarts: 1987. "Demographic Foundations of Family Change." *American Sociological Review,* 52, p. 353.

62% (Gilford, 1988, pp. 52, 53). This group of the very old are those most likely to need care from others in order to cope with daily routines.

In any discussion of longevity trends, we should not overlook the increased survival of infants at the beginning of life as well as of seniors at the end of life. At both extremes of the life course, medical technology has cut mortality rates. One third more infants born after five months' gestation were surviving in 1987 than in 1950 (National Center for Health Statistics, 1990, p. 107, Table 15). Such less-than-full-term infants, however, are more likely to be of low birth weight and to have higher rates of congenital malformations than full-term infants (Taffel, 1989, p. 7, Table C). They are more likely to be in need of family care.

The increasing number of AIDS (acquired immunodeficiency syndrome) sufferers also will put heavy demands on families as well as on public services. There were some 33,000 (33,512) newly reported AIDS cases during the year from July 1989 through June 1990, up from 8,249 reported cases five years earlier. The total number of reported persons with AIDS in 1990 was 139,765 (Leighton, 1991, Table 1, Table 7; U.S. Bureau of the Census, 1989b). These individuals presently are more likely to be in the productive years beyond childhood and before 50 years of age (87.7% of the total reported cases). Again, middle-aged parents and young people just starting out in jobs or beginning their own families will be the ones most likely to be called upon for help.

Another trend affecting family caregiving is the increased proportion of women in the paid labor force. Today, there are fewer nonelderly women of any age who are devoting their time primarily to domesticity and are available for family caregiving. In 1988 at least two thirds of women from the age of 20 to the age of 54 and more than two fifths (42.3%) of women 55 to 64 were employed (U.S. Department of Labor, 1989, p. 72, Table 16). These working women include married women with children, the women who traditionally were homemakers while their husbands were breadwinners. More than three fifths (62.9%) of families with children under 18 have both mothers and fathers working for wages. Among single-mother families, the proportion of women employed is two thirds (67.2%) (Hayghe, 1990, p. 18, figures calculated from Table 4). This wholesale entrance of wives and single mothers into the labor force is generally due to economic necessity. Whether at the childbearing and child-rearing stages, the youth-launching period, or the years after, women are earning money to pay for family necessities and children's education.

An overall perspective on these trends is that women, the main sources of caregiving, most often are involved in the changes. They are having fewer children at older ages, and more often there is not a father present in these families. Women also are likely to have added wage-earning roles outside the home to their family responsibilities whether or not they are presently married and whether or not they have children. At the end of family lives, there are more parents who are living longer, and they are more often women. These changes in fertility, mortality, and labor-force participation rates affect the family personnel needed and available for watching over disabled members.

FAMILY TIME PERIODS AND THEIR CHALLENGES

For the purpose of giving an overview of the divisions in family time and their expected challenges, it is appropriate to begin with a formation period when families get started, followed by childbearing and child-rearing divisions (see Table 2.1). Children then become mature and start leaving home, eventually leaving a parent or parents alone in their middle years to sustain the family. With their aging and death, this family's life comes to an end.

TABLE 2.1 Family Challenges According to Family Stages

Stage	Challenges
I. Formation	Staying together
	Divorce
	Remarriage
II. Child Rearing	Unwed parenthood
	Child care and child-support payments
	Unemployment/meager wages
III. Children Leaving Home	Providing resources for higher education
	Supplying housing and child care for divorced and unwed parents
	Supplying housing and support for adult children who are not self-supporting
IV. The Middle Years	Financial support and services to adult children
	Caregiving to aged parents
	Divorce
V. Final Years	Emotional and daily care necessities
	Maintaining financial necessities

Stages I and II, The Formation and Child-Rearing Periods

Internal Problems

Although most people continue to marry, the overriding problem newlyweds must cope with, which affects their ability to focus on other families' concerns, is simply staying together. Well over half (56%) of all persons born in the early part of the 1950s, the vanguard of the baby boomers, will divorce (Norton & Moorman, 1987, p. 12, Figure 5). Marital breakups occur fairly early in marriage with 40% of the separations taking place fewer than five years after the wedding day (Bumpass, Sweet, & Castro Martin, 1990, p. 750).

The difficulty these divorces create for the former partners and their relatives can be considerable. As one woman said when announcing tearfully that her daughter's marriage after 2 years was on the rocks, "Julie can't sleep at nights, and I can't either. I worry about the neighborhood where she had to move now that she has only her own paycheck to live on." The emotional and economic stress that couples and their kin experience when partners split up is accentuated if children are present. And in the first half of the 1980s, almost three fourths (69%) of marital separations involved children (Bumpass et al., 1990, p. 750). Rather than being caregivers, single parents, themselves, are turning to their parents for solace and help with children.

Women's economic status after divorce tends to fall by about one third (30%), because child-support payments are not large and often are unmet (Hoffman & Duncan, 1988, p. 641). A 1987 survey indicated that about half (51.3%) of the mothers received the full amount of the award; but a fourth (24.7%) received only partial payments, and a fourth (23.9%) received nothing at all from the awarded payment (U.S. Bureau of the Census, 1990a). This situation of unmet payments should improve as provisions of the 1988 Family Support Act calling for the automatic wage withholding of all child-support orders take effect, beginning in 1994.

Remarrying is one means for divorced women to repair their families' financial situation. Somewhat more than 70% of separated women will remarry after divorce. However, women over 30 and women with children are less likely to remarry (Bumpass et al., 1990, pp. 751, 753). These remarriages, in turn, are more likely to dissolve than are first marriages. Among white women married between 1980 and 1985, for example, remarried women are 25% more likely to divorce than women in their first marriages (Castro Martin & Bumpass, 1989, p. 47).

External Circumstances

Unemployment, as well as divorce and unmarried parenthood, contributes to the hardships that accentuate the tumult and turmoil of the family formation years. In times of economic downturn, young families, including those with preschoolers, are most likely to be affected by layoffs and poverty. Wage-earners who have recently started their own families are also newcomers in the workplace. They lack the seniority that keeps workers employed during economic downturns and the savings to tide them over hard times. Black families and single-mother families are even more likely than white families and families with fathers to face unemployment and poverty. Their joblessness and financial hardships also last for longer periods (Moen, 1983).

It is also true, as Figure 2.3 shows, that workers 25 to 34 years old, who are likely to be in the first stages of family life, have taken a pay cut in the past 10 years. This is especially true of those with less education (Levy & Michel, 1991, pp. 19-20, Table 3.1). In constant dollars, the median income of white males of this age group in 1991 was about $22,389. In 1979 it was greater than $5,000 more ($28,131). Among young black males, the fall in median income was from $19,064 in 1979 to $15,790 in 1991, a loss of a little more than $3,000. Black female workers ages 25 to 34 in 1991 were earning $12,249. In 1979 the median income for this group was approximately $1,500 more ($10,666). Only young, white females earned more in 1987 ($11,332), still a skimpy amount, than did the 25- to 34-year-olds in 1979 ($9,810) ("Who Earned What," 1989). Thus, even during good times, young families possess thin wallets from which to find money for financial caregiving.

To summarize their conditions, families in the first years are subject to the transitions of marriage; childbirth, sometimes outside of marriage; child rearing; separation; divorce; and, in many cases, remarriages in the context of limited incomes. All of these signposts in family lives represent breaks with the past and require new learning in getting along with and without intimate others and establishing different sentimental ties. These turning points make it harder for young families to undertake caregiving responsibilities for others because they are in need of emotional and financial support themselves.

Caregiving Among Young Families

The touchy area of finances provides one good example of just how important family aid is. Researchers using data from a 1985 national survey found that almost 99% of the money going from one household to another went to relatives (U.S. Bureau of the Census, 1988, p. 6, Table E). Although persons giving regular money payments to individuals living in other households constitute less than 4% (3.7%) of adults in the population 18 years of age and over, one of the ironies of caregiving is that young families are disproportionately involved in the transfer of money. It is young adults (25-44) who are most apt to be giving money to this 5.8% of the population (U.S. Bureau of the Census, 1988). They made up 63% of the givers.

The contributors are more likely to be men, and their contributions take the form of child-support payments to the living reminders of failed intimacy. These payments make sense, as men on average earn more than women and are less likely to have custody of children. However,

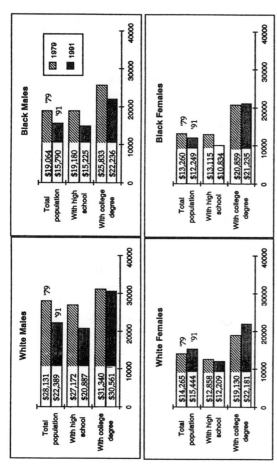

Figure 2.3. Median Income, Workers Ages 25 to 34, in Constant 1987 Dollars

1979 figures from U.S. Bureau of the Census of Population, Vol. 1, Characteristics of the Population, PC 80-1 September 1981: 447-474, Table 296. In the data "4 years of college" and "4 years of high school" are taken as equivalent to "college degree" and "high school degree," respectively.

1991 figures from U.S. Bureau of the Census, Current Population Reports, Series P-60, No. 180, Money Income of Households, Families, and Persons in the United States: 1991, U.S. Government Printing Office, Washington, DC, 1992: 116-143, Table 29.

NOTE: All data constant in 1991 dollars. Constant 1991 dollars calculated with the Consumer Price Index in U.S. Bureau of the Census, Statistical Abstracts of the United States: 1992 (112th edition). Washington, DC, 1992: 466, No. 738.

almost half (45.6%) of those men providing child support were married (U.S. Bureau of the Census, 1988, pp. 2, 6, last figures based on Table G). Child support, therefore, often flows from one young family to another.

Thus we see that past marital histories account for the preponderance of younger, usually less well off, families being involved in monetary aid. Because these payments take the form of child support, the particularly hard-pressed, single-parent families with children are more apt to be recipients (U.S. Bureau of the Census, 1988, pp. 1, 2, 6). Financial help, therefore, tends to be concentrated on the younger generation, who have children, or is given by parents in the preceding generations to adult children.

Aid across family boundaries involves care as well as the money gifts that enable families to buy care. Information from a recent (1987-1988) national representative sample provides a useful supplement to what we know about monetary transfers. Interestingly, other forms of aid, such as household services, child care, and emotional support between parents and adult children living in different homes, showed much the same patterns as financial support. Daughters, however, are more involved in exchanges with parents than sons, due primarily to their greater receipt of child care and advice. The often struggling young parents received child care and money help at this family formation stage of family histories. The "haves" in monetary terms, however, were more apt to give and to receive various forms of help than the "have-nots" (Eggebeen & Hogan, 1990, pp. 221-222).

The most struggling among young families with children are single mothers, especially African Americans, with one or more children under 5. More of these young (18-29) African-American mothers (34%) live with parents than do their white counterparts (21%). But in general, these young single mothers are not receiving financial or service support from their parents, and contrary to the findings from small-scale studies, this is especially true of African-American mothers. Almost a third of them (31%) and somewhat more than one fifth (23%) of white single mothers receive no parental assistance at all (Eggebeen & Hogan, 1990, pp. 228-229; see also Hogan & Eggebeen, 1991).

Data on financial aid, as well as services given by one family to another, suggest that much of it is concentrated among the needy beginning families. Monetary payments represent continuing obligations usually of men to children they have fathered but with whom they are no longer living. The prevalence of remarriage indicates that many of these men have established new family ties and so are splitting their paychecks to fulfill responsibilities in several households. Support from parents to adult children in young families lacking legal suasion to obtain child support is more casual and of a less sustained nature. Consequently, the limited assistance available to needy young families comes most often from others in the same leaky financial boat.

Stage III, The Leaving Home Period

When we look at families whose children are old enough to be getting ready to leave home, we can see how previous hard times carry over to affect the events in this family chapter. Traditionally, low- and middle-income families have worked to ensure a better life for their children. Lacking the property to provide a lifetime of security for children, parents have tried to see that children received a decent education. And access to higher education is increasingly important for the future financial status of young people. In 1986, men 25 to 34 years old with 4 years of college earned half again as much as did 25- to 34-year-old men with 4 years of high school (Levy & Michel, 1991).

One of the current problems families with adolescents face is making it possible for their children to get a higher education in a time of rising tuition costs. Yet from the previous information on income difficulties in the earlier child-rearing period, we can understand why investment in the future of young adults will be less in single-mother families, families in which parents are themselves young, and African-American families. Research also indicates that stepparents, now more common due to divorce, contribute less than birth parents in two-parent families to young people for education. Children's expectations of how much post-high school training they will receive are affected by parental incomes. These influence contributions to children's educational expenses after high school graduation (Goldscheider & Goldscheider, 1988).

This internal, expectable need of youths for financial help from families to obtain an education limits a family's ability to meet unexpected caregiving demands. Mothers and fathers are both in the labor force to provide for their families. But if families still lack resources, the children in the younger generation are ill prepared to take on the responsibilities of getting a job and forming their own families. Under these circumstances, emergency caregiving to family members can fall by the wayside.

In addition, quite contrary to the plans of many parents who thought they had prepared their children for independence, young adults are returning home or never leaving it. They are at home because they cannot afford to set up their own households. A less prosperous economy leads to lower pay and higher unemployment rates. Youths are postponing marriages, and housing costs are high. The numbers of unwed mothers are up, and divorces are common among those who have married.

Staying at home or returning there makes monetary sense. One of the financial and caring contributions parents can give to lower paid youths, to children attending local colleges and universities, to offspring whose marriages have failed, and especially to single adults with children is to provide temporary housing, and in the case of young mothers or fathers to care for grandchildren. Yet middle-aged women are apt to be in the labor force and less available for child care and caregiving of all types.

Having young adults at home also can throw into disarray cherished plans and expected changed routines of middle-aged parents. As one husband remarked during an interview in a study of midlife couples, "having young adults lingering in the household is not easy" (Aldous, 1985, p. 131). He stated emphatically when asked about youths returning home, "Gosh, I wouldn't want it at all. I think if they moved back it would be difficult. Somehow I would feel I had to tell them what to do, and you can't tell them what to do when they are 30." And a wife exclaimed, apropos of the female caregiving role, "Oh, God, I wouldn't like it. It would be awful. I'm tired of waiting on people."

Stage IV, Families in the Middle Years

Some of the mixed feelings those in the middle period of family life feel toward having their grown-up children still at home comes from their responsibility for meeting the needs of aged parents. Watching over parents has become an expectable task for the middle-aged (Robinson & Thurnher, 1979). This responsibility transfer forces children to develop a new filial maturity (Blenkner, 1965). The former hierarchical relation between parents and children reverses (Williamson, 1981). To the middle-aged, it means the loss of parental authorities to whom they can turn and depend upon in times of hardship. To the elderly, it means a loss of the power and independence acquired during their adult years.

This seismic upheaval in the power balance between aging parents and their middle-aged children is wrenching for both generations, as the following incident suggests. One woman on a recent visit to her 85-year-old mother, who lived some distance away, noticed how dirty the kitchen floor was. She offered to wash it. The mother replied that she didn't need to. When the daughter insisted, the mother then asked how she planned to wash the floor. The daughter replied that her husband would buy her a mop at the nearby mall. The mother then retorted indignantly, "You mean after 65 years that floor is not going to be scrubbed?" This is a good example of how the younger generation, in attempting to maintain some order in their elders' lives, can be rebuffed. The elders resent having decisions made for them, especially because they often recognize the need for the actions to be taken but can no longer themselves carry them out.

The disruption in long-term, intimate relations the middle-aged experience when taking on responsibility for their elders while continuing to shelter their adult children can be capped by a failed marriage. Divorce per 1,000 married women from 35 to 54 years of age doubled in the years from 1970 to 1987. In the earlier year, the rate for 35- to 44-year-old women was 11 per 1,000. It was 22 per 1,000 in 1987. Among women 45 to 54 years of age, the rate increased during the same years from 5 to 10 per 1,000 (Glick, 1992, Table 1). Divorce at this period forces former wives and husbands to turn away from taking care of other generations to seek solace for themselves.

So what do we know about intergenerational exchanges with the elderly, such as widows, and the infirm? The exchange balance in terms of services and money does shift toward the benefit of older people. Middle-aged persons 45 to 64 years of age are somewhat more likely to give financial aid to their parents (50%) than to their children (40%) (U.S. Bureau of the Census, 1988, p. 2). Adult children do help out more with money and advice when parents are ill, but very old parents and widows who appear to be getting along all right do not receive much additional financial or other help from children. Moreover, all this and other support from the middle-aged tends to be episodic and concentrated during the period of need. Its limited nature is due to potential caregivers' lack of finances and to competing demands. Parents who have a number of children to prepare for adulthood, or to succor if adult independence proves elusive, are less apt to help out their own parents (Eggebeen & Hogan, 1990, p. 229).

But looking more specifically at these caregivers of the substantial proportion of the infirm or disabled who are elderly, one can see the importance of intergenerational ties. National survey data show that more than one third (37.4%) of older people who need help to carry out at least one important daily activity depend upon a child. A roughly comparable number of the caregivers (35.6%) are spouses of the dependent person. The children giving help also tend to have their own families, as more than half are married (daughters, 55.7%; sons, 52.8%). They are usually in their middle years, 45 to 64 (daughters, 62.6%; sons, 55.6%), the years when their own children are leaving home. However, not an inconsiderable number of these offspring are themselves elderly. Twelve and one half percent of daughters and 8.4% of sons who provide care are 65 years of age or older. Whether spouses, offspring, other relatives, or outsiders, those who are caring for the frail elderly are overwhelmingly women (77.5%) (Stone, Cafferata, & Sangl, 1987, pp. 16-17, Table 1).

Even though this is the expected pattern, some of the demographic trends noted above are complicating the lives of these caregivers. First of all, a substantial number of women have competing family responsibilities. One fourth of them still had children under 18 at home, and from the previous discussion, we could predict that some would be helping adult children. Others had experienced the breakup of their own marriages. This was true of almost a third of the daughters (14.2% widowed and 16.2% separated or divorced) and one fifth of the sons (19.5% divorced) (Stone et al., 1987, pp. 16-17, Table 1). These problems the middle-aged face diminish their ability to give assistance. We know from other studies that children of the elderly in disrupted marriages tend to perceive less need and to provide less help to elderly parents, due in major part to job responsibilities (Cicirelli, 1983).

The world of work affected a sizeable number of daughters in the national study of the caregivers of the frail elderly. Two fifths (43.5%) of the daughters and more than half (55.1%) of the sons faced conflicts between jobs and families (Stone et al., 1987, pp. 16-17, Table 1). The offspring handled these conflicts in different ways. More daughters (12%) quit their jobs than did sons (5%). Daughters also were more likely than sons to have rearranged their job schedules (34.9% vs. 27.7%) or to work fewer hours (22.8% vs. 15%) (Stone et al., 1987, p. 20, Table 3).

The greater disruption of women's lives due to caregiving is consistent with conventional gender role expectations. Women traditionally were family caregivers because, if middle class, they were not usually job holders. It was assumed that they had more flexible schedules than men did and more free time. This was coupled with their greater involvement in nurturing roles. Although these expectations of women nowadays make for very real conflicts, we can see why sons who have some responsibility to watch over infirm parents usually face fewer competing responsibilities.

Sons are the caregivers of last resort, playing the role only when no daughters are available. With the smaller families of today, sons are more likely to have to take on this responsibility. However, sons more often turn to their own spouses to fill in for them than daughters do to their spouses, so that again women are involved. Daughters also give more overall services, especially those that require personal care, than do sons. Understandably, as compared with daughters, sons report less stress from caring for an elderly person or from guilt at neglecting competing demands from the families they are part of (Horowitz, 1985; Young & Kahana, 1989).

Stage V, Families in the Final Years

In the finale of family life, it is true that the elderly can expect lower incomes, poorer health, and the death of a long-time partner. And as shown above, they are more likely to need care from other family members. However, today's aging families enjoy a number of advantages over those of previous eras (Aldous, 1987). Table 2.2 shows that more of the current cohorts of the elderly, who are less affected by today's high divorce rates, are apt to be married than in the past. This is due to increasing health and longevity (Busse & Maddox, 1985, p. 127). Their general poverty level (11.4% in 1989), thanks to Social Security and other government transfer payments, is not too different from that of the working-age population, 18 to 64 (10.2% in 1989). About 1 in 10 of persons in poverty were elderly, although they constituted some 1 in 5 of "near poor" persons whose incomes were between 100% and 125% of their respective poverty thresholds (U.S. Bureau of the Census, 1990b, p. 2, Table 2).

These healthy, hale, and well-fixed older people would seem to be able to provide financial and physical aid to disrupted families of children and grandchildren. However, the evidence is that they are unlikely to give financial aid. Just 7% of such contributors are 65 or older and their money goes overwhelmingly to their middle-aged children (U.S. Bureau of the

TABLE 2.2 The Marital Status of Older Americans by Age and Sex in Percentage, 1950-1989

Marital Status	Male 55-64	Male 65-74	Male 75+	Female 55-64	Female 65-74	Female 75+
			1950^a			
Never married	9.2		8.1	7.2		8.0
Married						
(Spouse present)	78.6		62.8	62.9		34.3
(Spouse absent)	2.8		2.9	2.2		1.7
Widowed	7.3		23.9	25.2		55.3
Divorced	2.2		2.2	2.2		0.7
N^b	6,686		5,755	6,659		6,480
			1960			
Never married	6.7	6.1	5.6	6.8	7.3	7.7
Married						
(Spouse present)	82.4	77.0	55.3	63.1	44.5	20.3
(Spouse absent)	3.6	2.6	2.4	3.2	2.2	1.2
Widowed	4.5	12.9	35.2	23.9	44.3	69.3
Divorced	2.8	1.3	1.4	2.9	1.8	1.5
N	7,582	4,755	2,390	8,224	5,580	3,231
			1989			
Never married	5.6	4.9	4.4	4.4	4.5	5.8
Married						
(Spouse present)	80.5	78.4	66.7	65.3	51.4	24.3
(Spouse absent)	2.6	2.7	2.7	2.9	1.8	1.4
Widowed	3.3	8.9	23.4	18.0	36.6	65.6
Divorced	8.0	5.1	2.8	9.4	5.7	2.9
N	10,088	7,880	4,199	11,311	9,867	7,077

SOURCES: The 1950 and 1961 data are from the U.S. Bureau of the Census, 1962, Marital Status and Family Status: March 1961, *Current Population Reports*, Series P-20, No. 114 (31 January), pp. 7-8, Table 1. The 1989 data are from the U.S. Bureau of the Census, 1989, Marital Status and Living Arrangements: March 1989, *Current Population Reports*, Series P-20, No. 445 (August), p. 9, Table 1.
[a]The 1950 data were not divided into the 65-74 and 75+ age groups.
[b]Numbers are in thousands.

Census, 1988, p. 2). Moreover, data from the 1987-1988 National Survey of Families and Households with respondents 55 and older, including some preretirement persons, showed more than one third not to be involved in any giving to adult children not living at home. Parents were particularly unlikely to be givers to stepchildren (Eggebeen, 1991), a family composition type likely to become more common in the future.

True, aged women and members of minority groups continued to be financially troubled due to spotty employment and lower wages during their working lives. But future cohorts of women, with their higher employment rates, should be better off. They will be eligible themselves for Social Security and private pension payments.

Summary

The challenges families face over the course of their existence vary according to the period involved. In the formation and child-rearing stages, families are the most hard pressed with respect to caregiving resources. Trying to maintain marriages, starting parenthood, divorcing, remarrying, and preparing youths to leave home in the economic context of stagnant or falling wages and troublesome unemployment rates make these family life stages careseeking rather than caregiving periods. The middle years find married couple families in better shape financially to help the needy, younger families. However, the longer periods children remain home, or return home as adults to stay, cut down the time employed mothers and fathers have to devote to elderly parents. And if their own marriages are in danger, families in the middle years may be seeking solace from kin in other generations. Finally, elderly couples are increasingly in sound financial and health circumstances to enjoy their declining years. They are able to remain independent and to assist their descendants longer prior to reaching the final period when frail health may make them turn to other family members for care.

SOME DIFFICULTIES

There is a contradiction here, however. Although the previous discussion centers on how family members, particularly daughters, care for dependent relatives, families watch over disabled members who do not live with them only episodically. The needy, whether the sick or the poor, cannot always count on family ties to ensure caring, and the members who do provide aid may do so unwillingly. Thus we read about daughters who complain, as one did, that she had "had a bellyful" of her elderly mother, because the mother was demanding and forgetful (Robinson & Thurnher, 1979, p. 590). We can also find examples of dislike bordering on hatred among caregivers of the disabled at the beginning instead of the end of life. A mother of one handicapped child stormed, "Not only did I not get the baby I wanted, but now I've got one that rocks all day, and who acts like he hates me" (Trout, 1983, p. 341).

Nurturing others quite clearly occurs, although affection as its basis may be lost. Instead, feelings of family obligation provide a substitute motivation when nursing the disabled becomes a long-term duty (Jarrett, 1985). Under these pressures the caregivers are likely to be in the same house as the person they are watching over. Not only is this true of spouses, but also three fifths of daughters and sons taking care of elderly parents are sharing a home with the care receiver (Stone et al., 1987, p. 16, Table 1). However, this constant presence of the dependent person, though simplifying the logistics of providing assistance, adds to the burden of the care for families in the child-present stages. In some cases the stress, financial costs, and weariness resulting from care of the frail and the handicapped can, at some point, lead to marital splits. As one father of a disabled child shouted as he left his family, "My father didn't make any Mongoloid, and neither did I!" (Trout, 1983, p. 343). But by and large, despite the physical fatigue and emotional distress long-term care of disabled members within the family entails, it is from their families that members receive help.

FINAL THOUGHTS

To summarize the discussion, there are times on the family clock when calls for caregiving assistance are particularly inopportune. Families just starting out must focus on the two internal concerns: first, the couple's staying together and, second, making a living. These two tasks, to say nothing of parenthood, require the active cooperation of both partners. Few extra hours or dollars are left to care for disabled relatives. This is doubly the case for remarried couples, who have added responsibilities for a second (or third) family or for child-support payments or child custody for the offspring of previous unions. Not surprisingly, these families, along with those of single mothers, look to previous generations for aid.

Families with older children, those who are approaching high school graduation or are of college age or older, also must negotiate common obstacles to caregiving. Financially, they are trying to pay for increasingly expensive—but increasingly necessary—higher educations to prepare youths to be self-supporting adults. Women are in the labor force along with men to make this goal a reality. And parents in the launching stage can find this a prolonged period as adult children facing job difficulties, failed marriages, or childbirths out of marriage are slow to leave or have to return home.

Families whose children are relatively set in adult roles can enjoy a breathing space from caregiving demands. Even then, however, requests from young families for child care or financial loans keep them aware of relatives' continuing needs to be watched over. In their middle years, families find their increasing freedom from parenting the now-established younger generation being narrowed by the needs of their elders.

Today, older individuals are better off and more likely to be married than in the past. If they choose, they can help out children and grandchildren with money and services. But they are living longer and, as a consequence, are more likely to suffer the disabilities of very old age. Presently, their needs for care when old threaten the work lives and competing family responsibilities of their daughters and, to a lesser degree, their sons. When these cohorts of baby-boomer parents are replaced by parents from the baby-bust generation, there will be fewer daughters to share the caregiving burden. In addition, fewer children will be unaffected by troubled marital histories and the attendant emotional, financial, and child-care hardships that make concern for others difficult. The aged also will have seen their own partnership trajectories disrupted by divorce and shifted through remarriage. Elderly men touched by divorce may be especially isolated from supportive networks due to their loss of contact with offspring (Furstenberg, Peterson, Nord, & Zill, 1983).

What is lacking in this analysis of family caregiving, according to the fairly typical stages in family development, is knowledge of how young families are coping with contemporary problems and why the caretaking balance between the elderly and other generations is lopsided. As far as the first knowledge gap is concerned, the material on caregiving continues to be sketchy with respect to the young. It was pointed out above that limited research is available on how families are coping with handicapped youngsters whom medical science is now able to keep alive (Holroyd & Guthrie, 1986; Kazak, 1987). There have been a few studies comparing parents of premature babies and those whose infants were full term (Crnic, Greenberg, Ragozin, Robinson, & Basham, 1983; Zarling, Hirsch, & Landry, 1988). How families deal with children having chronic disabilities also has not been widely studied (Marcenko & Meyers, 1991). The so-called crack babies and other human debris resulting from drug abuse continue to make newspaper headlines, but studies of them do not often appear in research publications. The comparative newness of the problem, its nature, and its incidence among the poor and minority populations as well as other disadvantaged groups help to account for the dearth.

AIDS is another growing health problem whose incidence among adults also is seen by large segments of society as due to immoral behavior. But its deadly outcome and appearance among heterosexual and non-drug-using persons make it difficult to ignore. As discussed earlier, its victims up to now have been primarily young adults who, because of disadvantaged backgrounds or lifestyles affecting the onset of the disease, have families with few resources or are estranged from relatives. Who, aside from functionaries in public health facilities, is watching out for these afflicted remains a question worthy of more research attention (Shelp, DuBose, & Sunderland, 1990).

Both AIDS and drug-abuse sufferers provide an apropos test case for the caregiving function of families. With respect to the latter problem, some would argue that the failure of families to provide benign child-raising settings is implicated in drug use. But even if one argues that many families are unable to protect their members from dangerous elements, the issue remains of just how active families can be on behalf of members afflicted by AIDS or drug abuse. Particularly for long-term and deep-seated conditions, young families or those with older children present are often at a disadvantage as caretakers for all the reasons analyzed above.

A second research gap concerns the caregiving activities of older families. There does not appear to be much giving to younger generations among preretirement or aging families. There are exceptions. We read of grandmother caretakers of children abandoned by their parents although somewhat less than 4% of children live with their grandparents (Norris, 1991). However, the evidence given earlier suggests that the older generation, despite its better financial situation, is doing disproportionately less for relatives than are younger families. Is it because they limit their "watching over" to the more needy of their offspring, retaining their freedom from responsibility, as some research (Aldous & Klein, 1991) would suggest? Or are they saving their finances and energies for the lengthened years they see ahead of them? As was discussed above, many spouses are taking care of the frail elderly. What is not clear is whether the able-bodied near-elderly and the "young old" see the intergenerational balance sheet of caregiving as balanced by this possible future devotion to ailing spouses, thereby leaving children carefree, or by their earlier activities on behalf of children and their own parents, or whether caregiving in families is distinguished by the absence of reciprocity considerations. This is the ideal picture of family dealings, but, as we have seen, families are often episodic and sometimes unwilling when caregiving is concerned.

All persons, female or male, old or young, poor or rich, continue to seek out someone to watch over them. If they are lucky they find this someone in their family circle. Here, intimacy adds to the bonds of affection although these bonds can become chains when the care in caregiving is lost. As we have seen, however, the ability of families to be caregivers waxes and wanes with changes in family time.

In this decade before the second millennium, a fair judgment of families as caregivers for infirm members is probably that the public and policy makers expect too much. As sociologists, Eggebeen and Hogan concluded that on the basis of their analysis of intergenerational caregiving, though families clearly can help, "family exchanges alone are inadequate to deal with problems of teen pregnancy, single parenthood, aging parents or poor health" (Eggebeen & Hogan, 1990, p. 230). Without attention being devoted to the strengths and weaknesses of family caregiving over time, the number of persons looking in vain for someone to watch over them will continue to grow. Caregiving within the family circle can be an affection-filled repayment of prior tender attentions. However, the reasons families do not always respond to caregiving requests or, having responded, at times feel overwhelmed by onerous demands may have less to do with irresponsibility than with competing loyalties. Rather than leaving families to compensate for inadequate public services, attempts to make it easier for relatives to care for dependents, whether children or elders, at home or on the job, should be further explored and encouraged.

REFERENCES

Aldous, J. (1985). Parent-adult child relations as affected by the grandparent status. In V. L. Bengtson & J. F. Robertson (Eds.), *Grandparenthood: Research and policy perspectives* (pp. 117-132). Beverly Hills, CA: Sage.

Aldous, J. (1987). New views on the family life of the elderly and near elderly. *Journal of Marriage and the Family, 49*, 227-234.

Aldous, J. (1990). Family development and the life course: Two perspectives on family change. *Journal of Marriage and the Family, 52*, 571-583.

Aldous, J., & Klein, D. M. (1991). Sentiment and services: Models of intergenerational relationships in mid-life. *Journal of Marriage and the Family, 53*, 595-608.

Bengtson, V., Rosenthal, C., & Burton, L. (1990). Families and aging: Diversity and heterogeneity. In R. H. Binstock & L. K. George (Eds.), *Handbook of aging and the social sciences* (3rd ed., pp. 263-287). San Diego, CA: Academic Press.

Biegel, D. E., Farkas, K., & Fant, K. (1989). *Family caregiver bibliography.* Cleveland, OH: Case Western Reserve University, School of Applied Social Sciences.

Blenkner, M. (1965). Social work and family relationships in later life with some thoughts on filial maturity. In E. Shanas & G. F. Streib (Eds.), *Social structure and the family: Generation relations* (pp. 46-59). Englewood Cliffs, NJ: Prentice Hall.

Bumpass, L., & McClanahan, S. (1989). Unmarried motherhood: Recent trends, composition, and black-white differences. *Demography, 26*, 279-286.

Bumpass, L., & Sweet, J. A. (1989). National estimates of co-habitation. *Demography, 26*, 615-625.

Bumpass, L., Sweet, J. A., & Castro Martin, T. (1990). Changing patterns of remarriage. *Journal of Marriage and the Family, 52*, 747-757.

Busse, E. W., & Maddox, G. L. (1985). *The Duke longitudinal studies of normal aging, 1955-1980: Overview of history, design, and findings.* New York: Springer.

Castro Martin, T., & Bumpass, L. (1989). Recent trends and differentials in marital disruption. *Demography, 26*, 37-51.

Cicirelli, V. G. (1983). A comparison of helping behavior to elderly parents of adult children with intact and disrupted marriages. *Gerontologist, 23*, 619-625.

Crnic, K. A., Greenberg, M. T., Ragozin, A. S., Robinson, N. M., & Basham, R. B. (1983). Effects of stress and social support on mothers of premature and full-term infants. *Child Development, 54*, 209-217.

Eggebeen, D. J. (1991, March). *Family structure and intergenerational exchange.* Paper presented at the Population Association of America Annual Meeting, Washington, DC.

Eggebeen, D. J., & Hogan, D. P. (1990). Giving between generations in American families. *Human Nature, 1*, 211-232.

Furstenberg, F. F., Jr., Peterson, J. L., Nord, C. W., & Zill, N. (1983). The life course of children of divorce: Marital disruption and parental contact. *American Sociological Review, 48*, 656-688.

Gilford, D. M. (Ed.). (1988). *The aging population in the 21st century: Statistics for health policy.* Washington, DC: National Academy Press.

Glick, P. C. (1992). Marriage and divorce rates. In E. F. Borgatta & M. L. Borgatta (Eds.), *Encyclopedia of sociology* (pp. 1188-1199). New York: Macmillan.

Glick, P. C., & Lin, S. (1986). More young adults are living with their parents: Who are they? *Journal of Marriage and the Family, 48*, 107-113.

Goldscheider, F. K., & Goldscheider, C. (1988, April). *The intergenerational flow of income: Family structure and the status of black Americans.* Paper presented at the Population Association of America Annual Meeting, New Orleans, LA.

Graham, H. (1983). Caring: A labour of love. In J. Finch & D. Groves (Eds.), *A labour of love: Women, work and caring* (pp. 13-31). London: Routledge & Kegan Paul.

Hayghe, H. (1990). Family members in the labor force. *Monthly Labor Review, 113*(3), 14-19.

Hoffman, S. D., & Duncan, G. J. (1988). What are the economic consequences of divorce? *Demography, 25,* 641-646.

Hogan, D. P., & Eggebeen, D. J. (1991). *The structure of intergenerational exchange in American families.* Unpublished manuscript.

Holroyd, J., & Guthrie, D. (1986). Family stress with chronic childhood illness: Cystic fibrosis, neuromuscular disease, and renal disease. *Journal of Clinical Psychology, 42,* 552-561.

Horowitz, A. (1985). Sons and daughters as caregivers to older parents: Differences in role performance and consequences. *Gerontologist, 25,* 612-617.

Jarrett, W. H. (1985). Caregiving within kinship systems: Is affection really necessary? *Gerontologist, 25,* 5-10.

Kazak, A. E. (1987). Families with disabled children: Stress and social networks in three samples. *Journal of Abnormal Child Psychology, 15,* 137-146.

Leighton, S. (1991). *AIDS in the workplace: Municipal policies affecting public safety personnel.* Washington, DC: National League of Cities.

Levy, F., & Michel, R. C. (1991). *The economic future of American families.* Washington, DC: Urban Institute Press.

Marcenko, M. O., & Meyers, J. C. (1991). Mothers of children with developmental disabilities: Who shares the burden? *Family Relations, 40,* 186-190.

Moen, P. (1983). Unemployment, public policy, and families: Forecasts for the 1980s. *Journal of Marriage and the Family, 45,* 751-761.

National Center for Health Statistics. (1990). *Prevention Profile. Health, United States, 1989.* Hyattsville, MD: Public Health Service.

National Center for Health Statistics, Public Health Service. (1987). *Vital Statistics of the U.S., 1987: Vol. 1. Natality* (DHHS Publication No. PHS 89-1100). Washington, DC: Government Printing Office.

Norris, M. L. (1991, September 9-15). Grandmothers reach across one generation to save another. *Washington Post National Weekly Edition,* pp. 33-34.

Norton, A. J., & Moorman, J. E. (1987). Current trends in marriage and divorce among American women. *Journal of Marriage and the Family, 49,* 3-14.

Raveis, V. H., Siegel, K., & Sudet, M. (1988-1989). Psychological impact of caregiving on the careprovider: A critical review of extant research. *Journal of Applied Social Sciences, 13,* 40-80.

Robins, P. K., & Dickinson, K. P. (1984). Receipt of child support by single parent families. *Social Service Review, 58,* 622-641.

Robinson, B., & Thurnher, M. (1979). Taking care of aged parents: A family cycle transition. *Gerontologist, 19,* 586-593.

Rossi, A. S., & Rossi, P. H. (1990). *Of human bonding.* New York: Aldine de Gruyter.

Shelp, E. E., DuBose, E. R., & Sunderland, R. H. (1990). The religious structure of religious communities: A neglected resource for care of people with AIDS. *American Journal of Public Health, 80,* 970-972.

Stone, R., Cafferata, G. L., & Sangl, J. (1987). *Caregivers of the frail elderly: A national profile*. Washington, DC: Department of Health and Human Services, Public Health Service, National Center for Health Services Research and Health Care Technology Assessment.

Taffel, S. M. (1989). Trends in low birth weight: United States, 1975-85 [Special issue]. *Vital Health Statistics, 21*(48).

Trout, M. D. (1983). Birth of a sick or handicapped infant: Impact on the family. *Child Welfare, 62,* 337-349.

U.S. Bureau of the Census. (1988). Who's helping out? Support networks among American families. *Current Population Reports,* Series P-70, No. 13. Washington, DC: Government Printing Office.

U.S. Bureau of the Census. (1989a). Fertility of American women: June 1988. *Current Population Reports,* Series P-20, No. 436. Washington, DC: Government Printing Office.

U.S. Bureau of the Census. (1989b). Marital status and living arrangements: March 1989. *Current Population Reports,* Series P-20, No. 445. Washington, DC: Government Printing Office.

U.S. Bureau of the Census. (1990a). Child support and alimony: 1987. *Current Population Reports,* Series P-23, No. 167. Washington, DC: Government Printing Office.

U.S. Bureau of the Census. (1990b). Poverty in the United States: 1988 and 1989. *Current Population Reports,* Series P-60, No. 171. Washington, DC: Government Printing Office.

U.S. Department of Labor, Bureau of Labor Statistics. (1989). *Bulletin 2340: Handbook of labor statistics*. Washington, DC: Government Printing Office.

Ventura, S. J. (1989). Trends and variations in first births to older women, 1970-86. *Vital and Health Statistics,* Series 21, No. 47.

Watkins, S. C., Menken, J. A., & Bongaarts, J. (1987). Demographic foundations of family change. *American Sociological Review, 52,* 346-358.

Who earned what. (1989, December 18-24). *Washington Post National Weekly Edition,* p. 7.

Williamson, D. S. (1981). Personal authority via termination of the intergenerational hierarchical boundary: A "new" stage in the family life cycle. *Journal of Marital and Family Therapy, 7,* 441-452.

Young, R. F., & Kahana, E. (1989). Specifying caregiver outcomes: Gender and relationship aspects of caregiving strain. *Gerontologist, 29,* 660-666.

Zarling, C. L., Hirsch, B. J., & Landry, S. (1988). Maternal social networks and mother-infant interactions in full-term and very low birthweight, preterm infants. *Child Development, 59,* 178-185.

3

Altruism Through the Life Course

ELIZABETH MIDLARSKY

A baby wails. Barely a moment later, a toddler appears from another part of the supermarket, bearing a teddy bear, a cookie, and his blanket—offering all to assuage the infant's distress.

Even after the untimely death of her husband, Donna continues to care for her father-in-law, who is paralyzed and aphasic following a series of strokes. She has three young children and is barely making ends meet, but continues to give tender care to all of her charges.

Sandra and Donald are 70-year-old retired professionals who could have "followed the sun" to a retirement haven, as suggested in many magazines for the "mature." Instead, they commute each day to Harlem, to care for children afflicted with AIDS.

What do these people have in common? At least during the process of helping, all appear to be focusing on the needs of someone other than themselves. Their intentions are to relieve suffering and bring happiness to others. At the moment of helping they are relatively unconcerned with extrinsic rewards for themselves. Although positive expressions of this kind often have posed a "problem" for philosophers and social theorists (Oliner et al., 1992; Wallach & Wallach, 1983), they abound in the society around us.

Indeed helping—in all of its diverse manifestations, including caregiving—is a critical facet of human interaction. As in the case of other interpersonal behaviors, however, apparently identical acts of caregiving and other forms of helping may be prompted by different motives and may have widely diverse consequences. Motivation may be egoistic, stemming from the anticipation of extrinsic positive consequences, such as money or praise, or because extrinsic negative consequences are expected if one fails to comply with implicit or explicit norms or demands. It may come from the egoistic desire to manipulate the other, to outdo the other to enhance one's own status, or to do the "right thing" so as not to lose face in the community. On the other hand, the caregiver may be motivated—as in the instances cited above—by genuine empathic concern, wherein the comfort or safety of another is the foremost consideration. In the latter instance, the caregiving may be said to be altruistically motivated. When the empathic concern also encompasses a comprehension of the other's need, then the need is more likely to be met. When, however, helping is motivated less by concern for the other than by a desire to underscore the incompetence or dependency of the other, or the need to manipulate the other (Jung, 1987), then in many instances the benefits are undermined.

During the past few years, the literature on caregiving has burgeoned. A parallel, virtually nonintersecting literature on altruism has burgeoned, as well, in roughly the same period of time. Whereas caregiving refers to the context or domain of certain help-giving behaviors, the term *altruism* refers to the interpersonal orientation or motivation underlying helping behavior in general and caregiving in particular. Thus each literature has a great deal to offer the other. An understanding of the nature, antecedents, and consequences of caregiving is critical for those who wish to fully comprehend altruism—a domain of inquiry in which theory often emerges from studies of short-term or one-shot helping of strangers. Conversely, the meaning and consequences of caregiving, both to the helper and to the recipient, may depend at least in part on the motivation (altruistic or other) for the behavior. Our understanding of caregiving that is altruistically motivated thus may be enriched and expanded by the literature on altruism and helping.

The aim of this chapter is first to explore the development of altruism through the life course, and then to examine the implications of altruism for caregiving and for its outcomes. I begin with a discussion of the ways in which both "altruism" and "life course" will be employed in this chapter and then review research and theory on the development of altruism from infancy through late life. In a final section, implications for caregiving are discussed.

DEFINITIONS

Altruism

Altruism, described as "generosity without hope of reciprocation" (Wilson, 1978, p. 149), is a form of behavior in which the actor is oriented to the needs of the other rather than to selfish needs. In the extreme, altruism can take the form of action that ultimately will lead to self-destruction, as in the case of heroism during wartime. The many acts of daily self-sacrifice that occur when, for example, people tend to the needs of the acutely or chronically ill are less dramatic than "altruistic suicide" but are no less critical for the maintenance of society. Furthermore, because chronically ill or disabled people require vast expenditures of time and effort, the human costs may be comparable to the costs inherent in dramatic rescue efforts.

Altruism often is equated with helping but is not, in actuality, always coterminous with helping. It even may be argued that there are instances in which the most altruistic course of action is to desist from helping despite one's own urges to "do something" in response to neediness (Brickman et al., 1982; Midlarsky & Hannah, 1985). According to A. Comte, who has been credited with coining the term, altruism is "consideration, concern, and affection for other people as opposed to self-love or egoism." Altruistic acts, in turn, are characterized by "constructive consideration and interest in others" (Wolman, 1973). When helping results from altruistic—or other—motives, it can take various forms. The two studied most frequently by altruism researchers are sharing of resources, also termed generosity or charitableness, and rescue. A third, nurturance, is more directly concerned with caregiving in the family context.

In addition to the focus on the other, the term *altruism* is reserved for helping that, although costly for the helper, is *not* performed because the actor expects extrinsic rewards or reciprocation, because it is mandated by one's social roles, or because of coercion by others. The benefactor *chooses* to act because of the desire to benefit another, whatever the cost to oneself. Indeed, an important determinant of helping—particularly unreciprocated helping—is the perceived dependency of others for reasons of illness or disability.

This is not to say that helping ultimately must be entirely unrewarding in order to be considered altruistic. People who generally care for and about others may reap diverse benefits, albeit benefits that are subtle and not directly sought. Helping others may take the altruist's mind off his or her own troubles, may enhance the sense of competence and mastery, and may increase social integration—because kind people are nice to know (Midlarsky, 1984, 1991)! In the definition employed here, to be considered altruistic, the behavior must entail at least some degree of self-sacrifice and must be voluntarily and unintentionally undertaken to benefit others despite the fact that no extrinsic gain is expected. What is important is the focus on the other, and that the individual's primary (if not sole) reason for undertaking the act is that the actor wishes, and intends, to alleviate the suffering and/or enhance the well-being of the other.[1]

The distinction between altruism and other forms of motivation is important for caregiving, for pragmatic as well as theoretical reasons. The spirit in which care is tendered may be an important determinant of the way in which it is applied, and therefore of its effects, on both the caregiver and the care recipient.

Life Course

Having defined altruism, let us now consider what is meant by life course. This term is used to refer to the temporal progression of life from beginning to end—the sequence and timing of life stages (O'Rand & Kriecker, 1990). To fully explore the development of altruism, or any other human characteristic, it would be desirable to chart its evolution, and all of its vicissitudes, along the path of life. Unfortunately, however, current approaches to the study of human development impede efforts to develop a coherent picture of altruism through the life course. As Levinson (1986) has noted:

> Every discipline has split the life course into disparate segments, such as childhood or old age. Research has been done from such diverse theoretical perspectives as biological aging, moral development, career development, adult socialization, enculturation, and adaptation to loss or stress, with minimal recognition of their interconnectedness. The resulting fragmentation is so great that no discipline or viewpoint conveys the sense of an individual life and its temporal course. (p. 3)

This problem has been exacerbated by the fact that the preponderance of altruism researchers appear to have implicitly assumed that the roots of adult character formation are found in childhood and adolescence (Eisenberg & Mussen, 1989) and perhaps in the biological substratum as well (Wilson, 1978). Even so, few studies have been done on the very early years of life or on adolescence. Even the studies of altruism in school-age children are primarily cross-sectional rather than longitudinal. The fields of human development and gerontology have in common their relative inattention to early and middle adulthood. Few investigators of the phenomena of adulthood employ a developmental perspective, despite the seminal theoretical work by Erikson (1950, 1969) on the organic connection between the individual from birth to death with the world around him or her. Notwithstanding the paucity of systematic research, in this chapter the existing work is woven into a picture of the development of altruism through the life course and is discussed in the sections that follow.

DEVELOPMENTAL PERSPECTIVES

To behave altruistically, one undoubtedly must possess certain competencies, both perceived and actual (Midlarsky, 1984). The competencies associated with mature caregiving—which include the ability to correctly perceive a need from the perspective of the other, to feel genuine concern, to develop an intention, and to act effectively—are products of normal socialization. Normal socialization, in turn, assumes that the helpless infant is nurtured and protected until adulthood, and that the caregiver attends to emotional as well as physical needs. In Freud's (1954) words, "the original helplessness of human beings is the primal source of all moral motives" (p. 379). Under conditions of normal caregiving, the individual's fundamental nature and experiences interact in a positive way with the stages of cognition and personality, as these last two evolve.

A precondition for altruistic motivation is, first of all, the concern for others. A first question, then, is when does the concern for others emerge? The answer can be found, in point of fact, in human interactions all around us. It has long been obscured, though, by a *zeitgeist* reflective of the convergence of several theoretical orientations. These have included classical psychoanalysis, Watsonian behaviorism, and certain interpretations of Darwin's theory.

According to Freudian theory, the innate predisposition of humankind—personified at birth by the id—is aggressive, hedonistic, irrational, and utterly self-centered. Although altruism is necessary for the individual's survival within the community, at the core of all seemingly altruistic acts is guilt (and self-interest) (Freud, 1954). John B. Watson adopted Locke's idea that all human beings begin life as tabulae rasae. In contrast to Freud's view of the newborn as a "nasty beast," for the behaviorists "the infant does not start life with preformed ideas, such as that of original sin" (Bell, 1979, p. 823). Helpful acts, like other behavior, could readily be learned by the malleable organism, but Watson's rejection of consciousness rendered any consideration of ethics—and hence of altruism—meaningless. According to Watson's heir, B. F. Skinner, all feelings, perceived "motives" and feelings come from the same roots: "control exerted by the social environment" (Skinner, 1971, p. 105) through the manipulation of extrinsic reinforcements. The classical interpretation of Darwin's (1859) principles, "natural selection" and "survival of the fittest," is that only competitiveness and selfishness can be biologically based. Emerging from these and other theories was the conception that human beings had either no basic nature at all or a nature that was derived from the lower animals and therefore assumed to be negative and self-centered.

Altruism in Animals

Challenges to the skepticism about altruism have come from observations of actual behavior. The predominant emphasis in the literature on altruism within subhuman species has been on such normative activities as help by parents toward their children (Rushton, 1980; Wilson, 1975; Wright, 1971). As a case in point, the eusocial (or "truly social") insects such as bees, wasps, and ants cooperate in caring for the young; also, the young assist parents (Wilson, 1971). Furthermore, animals do engage in behaviors that far transcend such "normative" acts. There is considerable evidence that many species of animals engage in cooperative defense, food sharing, rescue behavior, and care of the wounded, helpless, ill, and disabled.

Thus, for example, as early as 1871, Darwin (1871) provided numerous examples of apparent altruism in the animal world. These included the defense of cows and calves by bull bisons; warnings about animal predators by rabbits, sheep, and monkeys; and caretaking and grooming by chimps—all of which appeared to be intentional acts that were costly in terms of time spent or danger incurred. Porpoises have been observed helping a species mate (Hebb & Thompson, 1954), a weasel was seen lifting and carrying a wounded companion, and even the large (and clumsy) Molucca crabs have spent several hours working to rescue a comrade who had fallen on his back, by lifting him to an upright position. Several monkey species show great care and concern for their companions, going to great lengths to protect one another from enemies and harsh weather and tending their wounded in battle until there is no question that they are beyond help (Kropotkin, 1914). Wolves, instead of ravaging and destructive, tend to be generally loyal and cooperative (Fiennes, 1976). In the laboratory setting, Nissen and Crawford (1936) found equitable food-sharing among young chimpanzees, even when self-sacrifice was involved.

In addition to rescue or protection under conditions of extreme stress, or in cases of injury or acute illness, animals extend compassionate care to their chronically ill or disabled comrades. In Kropotkin's (1914) notable review of the accounts by many naturalists, we learn of species in which the old routinely are the first to dine on a fish kill, guarded by the young. We also read of

> a blind pelican which was fed, and well fed, by other pelicans upon fishes which had to be brought from a distance of thirty miles. . . . rats . . . feeding a blind couple. . . . two crows feeding in a hollow tree a third crow which was wounded; its wound was several weeks old. . . . Indian crows feeding two or three blind comrades. (p. 59)

Why is the animal evidence important? It is certainly not sufficient proof that altruism is a powerful instinct at the human level. Rather, we can argue that the common observation of the compassion in many subhuman species counteracts the notion that only aggression, competitiveness, and egoism are natural, with apparent acts of self-sacrifice representing a thin veneer of civilization upon a genetically "bestial" nature. According to Midgley (1978), an important problem with theories about the biological substratum of human nature is that they have been founded on an incorrect view of animal nature as irrational and antisocial. This is a view "which was formed by seeing animals not as they were, but as projections of our own fears and desires" (p. 25). Indeed, to the extent that we have an animal nature, this nature may include elements of compassion and empathic concern—including caregiving for the ill and disabled among us.

Infancy and Early Childhood

In addition to evidence of positive behavior in certain animal species, human infants have been observed to be more social than several theories would have us believe. At an age at which Freud postulated that the id—an intrinsic "nasty beast"—was the sole facet of personality, and behaviorists postulated a "blank slate," human beings already exhibit a rudimentary form of empathy: arousal based on another's distress.

Newborn infants only 18 hours old were found by Martin and Clark (1982) to cry when they heard a tape of another newborn crying. To determine whether the babies had just confused another's crying with their own, the researchers also played a tape of the babies' own cries. Results indicated that the newborns were less likely to cry at the sound of their own distress than at the distress of another. Indeed, those already crying continued when they heard another cry, but stopped when they heard a tape of their own crying.

In studies conducted with 2- to 3-day-old infants, Simner (1971) found that newborns are more apt to cry spontaneously and to cry for a longer time when they hear another newborn crying than when they hear white noise or a synthetic cry with similar acoustic properties. These results were replicated by Sagi and Hoffman (1976). A total of more than 250 infants were the subjects in these studies. Because empathy is a predispositional variable often found to motivate genuine altruistic behavior, the finding that infants may be disturbed by the distress of another attests to the intrinsic nature of altruism.

As the child grows and develops, the response to others becomes more differentiated and complex. The young infant, however upset by the distress of another, cannot respond in any other way than by crying—and certainly cannot provide help, altruistic or not. By age 6-12 months, the child has an increased behavioral repertoire and responds to emotional distress in other infants either by not responding or by crying, frowning, or looking to its parent for help. In a more positive vein, the child can show affection to its caretaker and can share with others.

According to cognitive, object relations, and other developmental theorists, interpersonal arousal and even helping cannot be viewed as "other oriented" (i.e., altruistic) until the sense of self and other are developed and differentiated. This development also is generally conceived as a multistage process. Concomitantly, at around 1 year of age, children become increasingly aware of themselves as differentiated from others. As the distinction between self and other becomes apparent, the child is more competent to move beyond expressions of generalized distress that provide no help to others, to positive actions that do have the potential to help. From about 13 or 14 months to about 20 months, children show even less distress and attempt to comfort others by touching, patting, kissing, or hugging. In the period from about 18 to 24 months, helping attempts become even more frequent. Examples include verbal expressions of sympathy, shielding the distressed individual from harm, and offering and bringing of objects that the child associates with comfort. The child often will give help that is inappropriate or ineffective, as when it brings its bottle or blanket to a distressed older sibling, but the compassion behind the act is quite apparent, nevertheless. This general sequence of events, from undifferentiated distress at the suffering of others to comforting and helping by the age of 2, has been observed in several studies (Dunn & Kendrick, 1979; Rheingold & Emery, 1986; Zahn-Waxler & Radke-Yarrow, 1982).

What happens in cases wherein there is serious illness in the family, particularly on the part of the caretaker of the young child so that the normal course of events is disrupted? As noted above, whatever the innate predisposition to help, it is the attachment to and identification with a nurturant caregiver throughout childhood that may serve as the spur and paradigm for genuine altruism throughout the life course. Although an impaired caregiver may provide numerous opportunities for empathic arousal, failure to achieve a secure attachment to a caring adult may have adverse effects on the development of altruism. A study by Zahn-Waxler, Cummings, McKnew, and Radke-Yarrow (1984) indicates that this may indeed be the case. A two-year longitudinal study of 2-year-old children of a manic-depressive parent found that these children manifest heightened emotional distress when observing distress reactions by others, but manifested lesser amounts of altruistic interaction with their peers.

Research on helping during the preschool years indicates that help-giving occurs with considerable frequency. Behavior of the type generally observed in the home between the child and its family is extended to peers and teachers when the child enters nursery school. In Murphy's (1937) early study in a nursery school, in which naturalistic observations were conducted for more than 3 months, children were seen to become very upset at signs of distress, to comfort and sympathize with other children, and to aggress against the cause of any harm. More recently, Sawin (1980) studied reactions of 3- to 7-year-old children to a crying child, in a study conducted on the playgrounds of child-care centers. Sawin found a wide range of empathic and sympathetic reactions, with only 7% showing no reaction, and only 2% making directly unsympathetic responses.

Although preschool-age children have been observed to comfort others, why is this comfort given? The behavior can be considered altruistic only if it is primarily intended to help the others, rather than become the source of one's own extrinsic rewards. Are the motives of this early behavior hedonistic—designed to alleviate the child's own distress—as predicted by the cognitive-developmental theorists? Does the behavior represent compliance with explicit or implicit demands? On another level, does helping others have one meaning to all of these young children, or is more than one kind of motive possible (Bryant & Crockenberg, 1980)? A study of behavior in nursery school pupils by Eisenberg-Berg and Neal (1979) was designed to address the question of motivation. During observations made over a 3-month period, whenever a child helped, shared, or comforted another he or she was asked the reason for the behavior. Explanations referred to the recipient's needs or the child's own desire to help. In some cases, the child mentioned the benefits to both from the exchange, or cited friendship or the desire for social approval.

These preschool-age children, then, do engage in prosocial behavior. This is *not* to say, though, that altruism predominates as a motivator of that behavior. A variety of naturalistic studies in which observations were made of both antisocial and prosocial responses noted that altruism increases with age. Depending on the stringency of the definition of altruism, the relative frequencies of altruistic and aggressive acts favor aggression, or the relative frequencies of altruism and aggression are quite similar to one another (Murphy, 1937; Yarrow & Waxler, 1976).

What is noteworthy about these results is that they depict even the youngest children as both egoistic and altruistic. Furthermore, the altruism that is exhibited is based on emotional arousal by, empathic concern for, and increased understanding of the needs of others as differentiated from the self. Although many helping acts are effective in alleviating distress, other such acts by these youngsters are ineffective and even inappropriate. The ineffectiveness may come from the fact that the empathic concern of young children is relatively primitive, lacking the refinements concomitant with further development.[2] That is, one may *wish* to be helpful, but may entirely misjudge the nature of what is needed. Even so, there has been an accumulation of data that disputes the portrait of young children as unsocialized and therefore "bestial." Whatever the outcome of the sociobiology debate, naturalistic observations indicate that the concern for others appears even at the dawn of life, thus disputing the notion that egoism and aggression are more "natural" than empathy and altruism.

It is probably the case, as indicated by developmental theorists, that empathic concern is enhanced and refined as the child matures. It also may be the case that the child whose experience with being the recipient of parental nurturance is disrupted by the parent's illness may develop lesser degrees of altruistic motivation. Nevertheless, the data on what appears to be an intrinsic basis for empathic concern provide a fascinating challenge to theories in which altruism is not a serious possibility before 5 to 7 years of age.

Childhood and Adolescence

If altruism represents an imposition of societal needs or norms on a basically egoistic, aggressive (or "blank") human being, then altruism must ipso facto develop through the early years. Childhood is prime time for such development because it is a period of growth, expansion, and learning. The child's growth in size, strength, and knowledge may lead adults to attribute more responsibility to it for the care of others, especially if the family includes younger siblings or persons with disabilities (Hannah & Midlarsky, 1985). According to the literatures of developmental and social psychology, many of the factors associated with altruism, including perceived competence, empathy, and moral judgment, show increases throughout childhood (Eisenberg, 1982; Hoffman, 1981; Midlarsky, 1984); the general prediction is that with increases in personal predictors associated with altruism, altruism must increase as well (Midlarsky & Hannah, 1985).

Altruism has been observed in children and adolescents by numerous investigators, both in and outside the family context. In the literature on altruism and helping there has been little emphasis on the systematic investigation of helping within the family. An important ethic within U.S. society, in fact, is that the "normal" family is one in which the school-age child is encouraged to grow in competence not only through school achievement and peer relationships but also through play. Indeed, play is viewed as a central function of childhood that prepares the child for later life (Clarke-Stewart & Koch, 1983). The importance of caretaking and helping roles as preparation for adulthood has received far less attention in our society.

Nevertheless, studies indicate that children do help throughout the younger years of life. To begin with, observations of family life frequently have suggested that children (especially girls) help their parents during childhood. The fact that little is written on this topic probably is attributable to the assumption that except in unusual situations, children do not provide altruistically motivated help to their parents. When they do help, it is further assumed that the helping may represent compliance to a parental demand, reciprocation of love received, ingratiation to ensure future care, or expiation of some "bad" behavior. In situations wherein the child's help-giving is a voluntary response to a parental need—as in the case of parents with physical or mental disabilities—it is at least theoretically possible that such helping is prompted by empathic concern, and by altruism. The virtual absence of systematic data mitigates against evaluation of these possibilities, however.

Altruistic helping among child siblings has only recently been receiving attention (Hannah & Midlarsky, 1985). The long neglect of the positive facets of sibling interactions may be derived from theoretical orientations and popularized accounts of sibling interactions that emphasize the "naturalness" and primacy of sibling rivalry (Levy, 1937; White, 1975). Nevertheless, though sibling rivalry is certainly a facet of sibling relationships, it is far from the sole facet. Cicirelli (1976) found a high level of empathy among siblings, and Bryant and Crockenberg (1980) observed that helpfulness occurs among elementary-school-age siblings, with the older more often helping the younger child. In a study on the development of specialized roles within the family, Bossard and Boll (1955) discovered eight types of roles adopted by children from families with six or more siblings. These roles included the responsible role (parental substitute), popular and well-liked (charm is emphasized), socially ambitious, studious, self-centered, isolate, irresponsible, unwell, and unliked. Pepler, Corter, and Abramovitch (1982), observing siblings in naturalistic settings, found that although aggressive interchanges did occur, altruistic interchanges predominated.

During childhood, altruistic activity is observed in extrafamilial relationships as well. But does altruism *increase* during this period of life? On the basis of the existing literature, the best response is that it depends on the kind of altruism that is being studied: helping (or rescuing), sharing (or generosity), or nurturing (caregiving).

A "yes" can be given in the case of *generosity*. In laboratory studies in which children were given nuts or coins and then told to share them, Ugurel-Semin (1952) found that between the ages of 4 and 16, children became less selfish. Handlon and Gross (1959) used the same experimental method and found that school-age children shared unselfishly to a significantly greater extent than did preschoolers. In an experiment controlling for the possibility that the children's preference for the reinforcer may decrease with age, Midlarsky and Bryan (1967) found that elementary school pupils were increasingly more likely to share M&Ms with age. Green and Schneider (1974) performed a cross-sectional study in which the subjects were 25 boys in each of four age groups: 5 to 6, 7 to 8, 9 to 10, and 13 to 14. The amount of candy shared was found to increase with age. Several other laboratory studies also have indicated that the amounts donated to hypothetical others increase with age, at least from about 4 to 16 (e.g., Dremen, 1976; Emler & Rushton, 1974; Hull & Reuter, 1977).

How is the literature on generosity or sharing relevant to our understanding of caregiving for people with illnesses or disabilities? The helping that generally is referred to as "generosity" concerns the giving of help to unknown others, and these "others" often are described as children who are suffering from some illness or disability. That is, investigators of altruistic phenomena often appear to assume that giving (often anonymously) to a stranger is more altruistic (because strangers often cannot reciprocate) and that neediness based on illness or disability will promote higher rates of giving (Midlarsky & Suda, 1978). Unfortunately, however, because no study that I found has systematically investigated the role of these factors, no conclusion can be reached about whether the relationship to the recipient (stranger vs. nonstranger) or the nature of the need (acute vs. chronic illness or disability vs. other source of need) has main or interactive effects on generosity across the years of childhood and adolescence.

In contrast to sharing, which generally increases with age, the relationship between age and *helping* (and rescue) is quite complex, when one combines evidence from the existing studies. Overall, however, although there are ebbs and flows, and in the end the differences are not very large, helping in adolescents is higher than in children. Looking at the research data, in the Green and Schneider (1974) study, which investigated altruism in the four age groups from 5 to 14, helping was observed as well as the sharing of candy mentioned above. Among boys faced with a situation in which pencils were "accidentally" dropped, helping increased until the age of 9 or 10, at which point almost all of the boys helped. Investigations of rescue behavior by Staub yielded a curvilinear relationship between age and helping of a child (an injured stranger) in distress. Helping increased from kindergarten to the middle of the elementary school period and then declined to its lowest point among seventh-graders (Staub, 1970, 1971).

A study by Midlarsky and Hannah (1985) investigated emergency intervention by children and adolescents, on behalf of a stranger who suffered an injury. Results replicated Staub's finding of a curvilinear relationship between helping and age. First-graders and seventh-graders were least likely to help, and helping peaked in the fourth grade. After reaching its lowest point in the seventh grade, helping increased again in high school.

Whatever the *number* of people helping, though, the *reasons* are what indicate the nature of the motives, whether altruistic or not. Interview data from this study indicated that among the first-graders, the primary reasons for reticence were fears of possible incompetence. Seventh-graders were most often fearful of social disapproval. In contrast to the primarily narcissistic concerns expressed by the two groups in whom helping was at the lowest ebb, motives for reticence among the tenth-graders, who also manifested a shift in the direction of helpful behavior, involved concern for others. That is, tenth-graders reticent about helping their peers primarily emphasized the potential embarrassment or social disadvantage that may result from being helped. These results suggest that just as reasons for helping others are more altruistic as children mature (Bar-Tal, Raviv, & Shavit, 1981; Eisenberg, 1982), the motives for inhibiting helping behavior may become more altruistic as well.

The third type of prosocial behavior is *nurturance* (or caregiving), often within the family context. Like sharing or generosity, which seems to increase with age, the few studies of the relationship between age and nurturance within the family indicate an increase in this form of behavior with age as well (Whiting & Whiting, 1973).

In addition to varying with age, the amount and type of nurturance vary with other factors—including the degree and nature of the need-based dependency of the recipient. Thus, for example, Zahn-Waxler and Radke-Yarrow (1982) found that when children are exposed to serious illness in their parents, they experience anxiety and stress, but they also exhibit caregiving behavior.

Voluntary, intrafamilial caregiving by children and adolescents is most likely to occur when the dependency of the recipient is obvious, as in the case of older children with their younger siblings (Berman, Sloan, & Goodman, 1979; Feldman & Nash, 1979). The greatest amount of both voluntary and involuntary caregiving by children in this society, however, probably occurs among children with disabilities and with chronic illnesses (Hannah & Midlarsky, 1985). To cite one example, McAndrew (1976) reported that 75% of children over the age of 7 who had a sibling with cerebral palsy or spina bifida were expected to provide help.

In most of the research conducted on siblings of children with chronic diseases or disabilities, comparison groups of children with nonhandicapped siblings were not included, so that we cannot determine whether or not responsibilities exceeded those that are more typically given to siblings. However, several studies indicate that such may be the case. Swirean (1976) compared siblings of hearing-impaired or normal 4-year-olds on indices of helping within the family context. Results indicated that siblings of hearing impaired preschoolers had significantly greater child-care and general home responsibilities than did siblings of the normal preschoolers. McHale and Gamble (1989) found that all siblings spent about 2 hours per day engaged in activities with their brothers or sisters. However, siblings with retarded brothers or sisters spent more time in caretaking activities and engaged in more different caretaking behaviors than did siblings with nonhandicapped brothers or sisters. In a similar study, McHale, Sloan, and Simeonsson (1986) found that siblings with retarded or autistic brothers or sisters were more likely to engage in teaching, protection, and helping than were siblings of nonhandicapped brothers or sisters.

Also investigating caregiving behavior, but using observational techniques, Stoneman, Brody, Davis, and Crapps (1988) found that older female siblings with a mentally retarded brother or sister had more child-care responsibilities and engaged in a teacher/helper role more than older brothers with a mentally retarded brother or sister, and more than both male and female siblings with a nonhandicapped brother or sister.

Are all of the caregiving siblings of ill and disabled children altruistic? Probably not, at least not at the outset. Although a subset of the normal siblings may have voluntarily offered help on the basis of their altruistic dispositions, most probably began to help in compliance with parental requests, or demands. As the sibling helping typically consisted of imposed caregiving rather than of a voluntary response to empathic concern, it probably is not surprising that many older sibling caregivers have been described as managerial and dominant, behaviors that may impede growth and encourage passivity in the handicapped sibling (Hannah & Midlarsky, 1985; Summers, Summers, Ascione, & Braeger,

1989). Indeed, a hallmark of nonaltruistic helping—that is, involuntary compliance, with little empathic concern—is its relative inefficacy in meeting the needs of the recipient (Midlarsky, 1990).

What if, however, even the initially most reluctant caregiver were taught to give help that is effective in meeting the needs of the recipient? If the caregiver has a modicum of desire to promote the welfare of the recipient, then knowing that one has successfully enhanced the recipient's well-being may be quite satisfying. Indeed, there is both theoretical and empirical support for the notion that whatever the initial motivation, when helping behavior results in a successful outcome, the probability of subsequent helping increases (Midlarsky, 1984, 1991).

To test the notion that increases in perceived competence as a helper lead to increased helping among siblings of handicapped children, I performed an experiment in which siblings of children with disabling orthopedic conditions were randomly assigned to one of three county-sponsored camps (and a waiting list control). The camps were described as opportunities for siblings who are typically cast in a helping role to have a vacation. One camp was purely recreational. In the second camp, in addition to the recreational activities, children were given information about the nature of the siblings' condition, the importance of the medical treatment and their own helping role, and information about how to obtain respite for themselves. Children in the third camp were given the recreational activities and information, as well as extensive training on how to provide help for their siblings in a growth-promoting way. In interviews held on the last day of camp, all of the children manifested significant increases in positive affect. In addition, the participants in the helping skills camp (Camp 3) showed increases in helping and perceived helping effectiveness, self-esteem, and satisfaction with helping activities, and decreases in agonistic and dominant behavior over a 1-year follow-up period. None of the other groups manifested these changes over the 1-year period following the camps.

In sum, then, the literature on altruism and helping shows increases through the years of childhood and adolescence. Most of the studies that indicate such a trend, however, have been experimental investigations of the predictors of one-shot helping, usually of strangers. The preponderance of the literature on nurturance, or caregiving within families, tends to use observational or self-report methods and rarely investigates age trends. In general, though, the results of those studies suggest that children whose parents or siblings are ill or disabled tend to help, with older siblings often among the most actively helpful children observed within families, at least within U.S. society. Are these children altruistically motivated? Recent evidence suggests that siblings of children with orthopedic handicaps may be motivated to help their siblings, and that their helping increases concomitantly with an increase in their helping skills. In accordance with my model of the benign cycle wherein competence → helping → competence (Midlarsky, 1984), effective helping by these normal siblings may provide the basis for a lifetime of altruistic endeavor.

Adulthood

Even a cursory reading of the altruism literature reveals the implicit assumption that the development of altruism is complete by the end of childhood. Thus, whereas developmental psychologists study altruism during the years of childhood and adolescence, with some exceptions adult altruism generally is considered to be the province of social psychologists. The latter group investigates factors that elicit helping behavior, and not its development.

The general assumption that appears to be made by researchers may, however, be unwarranted, as altruism actually may develop throughout the course of life. Personality and motivation are far from immutable in a lifespan replete with kaleidoscopes of experience that have the potential to facilitate the developmental process. Experiences such as parenting and participation in diverse helping roles in adulthood may increase empathy, altruistic motivation, and subsequent altruistic behavior (e.g., Wundheiler, 1985-1986). Education, occupation, and caretaking experience in adult life affect moral judgment—and possibly altruistic action as well. According to Kohlberg (1973), stages 5 and 6, the highest stages of moral judgment, emerge only during adulthood following experiences that encourage the individual to face moral choices and resolve the dilemmas in ways designed to ensure the welfare of another—if they are to emerge at all.

Theories of adult development primarily developed by ego psychologists allow for the possibility of increases in altruism throughout adulthood. The concept of maturity for these authors includes the nature of *ego* development. To the extent that a strong ego permits one to become free of the constraints imposed by social roles, and to feel empowered to make genuinely voluntary choices, then there is a potential for continued increases in *genuine* altruism as defined in this chapter.[3]

According to the ego psychologist Erik Erikson (1950), for example, in early adulthood the individual moves through stages in which concern steadily can expand beyond the self with successful resolution of life crises. Thus, it is only after the achievement of identity in adolescence that the individual can sustain loyalties. In early adulthood, resolving the struggle between intimacy and isolation in favor of intimacy means the individual is now able to commit him- or herself to work and to love others freely. At middle age, successful resolution of the midlife crisis results in a broadening of concern about other people, including posterity, and societal institutions. In recent years, Erikson has added a ninth stage, expected to occur in later life, in which caring and contribution are extended to all of humankind (Erikson, Erikson, & Kivnick, 1986).

In Loevinger's (1976) theory of ego development, the adult is assumed to move through stages in which the focus is first on personal relationships, then on conformity to social roles, and later in life, on conscientiousness and the establishment of personal values. According to both of these theories of adult development, then, as the individual increasingly resolves personal issues and becomes relatively free from personal and social constraints, both values and behavior may shift in the direction of concern for others—or altruism. Even the increase in life expectancy in humans has been viewed as tied, by evolutionary mechanisms, to the benefits provided by older persons to younger adults engaged in reproductive activities, because of the altruism and wisdom embodied by older adults (Rockstein, Cheskyi, & Sussman, 1977).

The studies that have been conducted on altruistic development in adulthood provide evidence in support of lifelong increases in altruism. As predicted by Loevinger (1976), ego functioning increases with age, and there are concomitant decreases in impulsiveness and in the use of "immature defense mechanisms." From adolescence through later life, there are increases in the use of "mature defenses," including altruism (Haan & Day, 1974; Vaillant, 1977). There also appear to be age-related increases throughout adulthood in social interest, an Adlerian construct that bears marked resemblance to altruism. According to Crandall (1981), "among people in the age range of around 20 to 65, the data indicated small but significant correlations for both sexes, with men showing a somewhat higher relationship" (p. 85).

Riley and Foner (1968) found that in comparison with younger adults, self-reports by older adults indicate that they have higher moral values; in a longitudinal study, Schaie and Parham (1976) found that "humanitarian concern" increased over the lifespan. Additional evidence of the shift of concern from self to others through the adult years comes from the finding by Veroff, Douvan, and Kulka (1981) that older adults were more likely than were younger adults to show concern for moral values.

There is also evidence that the increase in altruistic *values* and *concerns* is reflected in *behavior.* In a study using well-standardized self-report measures of altruism and aggression in people 19 to 60 years of age, altruistic behavior was found to increase, and aggressiveness decreased (Rushton, Fuller, Neale, Nias, & Eysenck, 1986). Convergent evidence of increases in altruism through the lifespan comes from naturalistic experiments on two types of altruistic activity: rescue, or helping behavior, and generosity.

In an effort to explore donation behavior across the lifespan, two experiments were conducted in randomly selected shopping malls and parks, known to be frequented by individuals of diverse ages (Midlarsky & Hannah, 1989). In each experiment people had an opportunity to donate to a fund for infants with birth defects. Results indicated that when the costs of giving were controlled so that they were comparable for people of different ages, then generosity increased from age 5 through extreme old age.

The research on rescue behavior began with announcements of first-aid classes, including thorough training in emergency intervention techniques such as cardiopulmonary resuscitation (CPR). In response to the announcements, middle-aged (34-64) and older (65+) adults were more likely to sign up for first-aid classes than were young adults (18-34). Older adults also were more likely to express altruistic reasons for enrolling ("I may learn to save a life!") than were younger adults ("I've always wanted to learn CPR," or "I was curious"). In a second study, in which people were individually exposed to an emergency situation, first-aid training increased rescue attempts only among the elderly. Furthermore, older adults who were trained in first aid were the most competent helpers of all and were most highly motivated to help others (Midlarsky, 1992). In-depth interviews with a subsample indicated that those with the highest expressed motivation attributed their concerns to caregiving roles in their own families—roles that were described as most engrossing by the oldest adults. The preponderance of respondents in the study who were 65 years of age and older had a close family member, friend, and/or neighbor to whom they were frequently or continually giving help for health-related reasons.

CONCLUSIONS REGARDING
THE DEVELOPMENT OF ALTRUISM

The results of this brief review seem counterintuitive at first blush. Altruistic infants and older adults seem to belie the fact that in many cases both groups are dependent on caregiving by others. Resolution of this apparent paradox resides in the distinction between *altruism* (a motive, trait, or predisposition) and *caregiving* (a behavior with many possible motives). It is not only *possible* for members of "recipient" classes to be altruistic; altruism and helping among individuals characterized as "dependent" may be both natural and an antidote to the stigma and self-abnegation that can result from that status. Thus the infant who appears helpless has the power to elicit loving and caregiving responses from others and to respond to the distress of the caregiver. In the case of young children, the very fact that the child, already equipped with at least rudimentary empathic arousal (Sagi & Hoffman, 1976), receives nurturance from others may encourage the child to emulate and even initiate altruistic behavioral sequences. To the extent that the child enjoys the growing sense of competence likely to result from helping others, there is an increased probability that altruistic behavior will recur (Midlarsky, 1984). By the same token, competent older adults may be more altruistic than younger people both because of increased altruistic predispositions with age, and higher levels of ego development and moral judgment, and because helping others increases the sense of competence and well-being (e.g., Kahana, Midlarsky, & Kahana, 1987). What all of this implies is that sometimes the greatest kindness that one can do for an individual in need of help—such as an ill or disabled family member—is to provide opportunities for that individual to be of help.

Whatever the age of the individual, there also is evidence that helpful behavior—particularly when it is altruistic in nature—may be beneficial to the caregiver as well as to the recipient! As I have argued elsewhere (e.g., Midlarsky, 1991), the absorption in efforts to alleviate the distress of another has several benefits. Helping others (a) provides distraction from the helper's own concerns, (b) provides a sense of value congruence and meaning, (c) increases the helper's sense of personal control and competence, (d) leads to increased satisfaction and happiness, and (e) is a wonderful antidote to loneliness because helpers—*particularly* helpers who are genuinely concerned about other people—often are appreciated and become integrated into the social world around them.

IMPLICATIONS OF ALTRUISM
FOR CAREGIVING IN FAMILIES

Why are theory and research on altruism important for our understanding of caregiving? First, consider that the literature on caregiving seems to emphasize, above all, the burdens of the caregiver. A typical statement is that "distress is characteristic in all caregiving situations" (Schulz, Williamson, Morycz, & Biegel, 1992, p. 157). However, to the *altruistic* caregiver, whose nurturance is based on a focus on others' needs and gratification, this sense of burden actually may be reduced. Thus, for example, the most altruistic older adults in my own studies also were among the most satisfied (cf. Kahana et al., 1987). Indeed, it is when the caregiver is not altruistic that problems of inequity and imbalance in the relationship should be most keenly experienced, as in cases of chronic illness or disability, wherein continual and one-sided helping may be required.

In addition to the problems faced by the caregiver, however, a number of authors have noted problems experienced by the help recipient. The "dilemma of caregiving" (Thompson & Pitts, 1992) is that by being a recipient, one is enacting a dependent, needy role (Midlarsky, 1991; Spacapan & Oskamp, 1992). The nonaltruistic caregiver is most prone to evoking adverse reactions by the recipient. Prompted, perhaps, by a sense of duty, the nonempathic, and nonaltruistic, caregiver may become angry and resentful at what seem to be unremitting demands. With reluctance may come a tendency to dominate, criticize, overprotect, patronize, and infantilize the recipient—all of which serve to emphasize the power imbalance in the relationship. Feelings of discouragement may be hidden under an appearance of relentless optimism, in the face of which the recipient cannot comfortably express his or her true fears. When comfort and caring are lacking from the equation, such "help" and "protection" can lead to excessive disability (Hyman, 1971). Indeed, expressions of hostility and criticism by the family predict poorer outcomes in schizophrenics (Karno et al., 1987) and in women with rheumatoid arthritis (Manne & Zautra, 1989). The adverse consequences for the recipient, in turn, are likely to increase the burden on the caregiver.

When the caregiver is motivated by the genuinely selfless, other-oriented, empathic phenomenon we call altruism, both the benefactor and the recipient are likely to benefit. The recipient will benefit because genuine and (usually) appropriate help should promote a sense of psychological well-being and, where possible, also may promote improvements in physical well-being. The altruistic helper certainly may experience at least some degree of stress in the course of prolonged and arduous caregiving. Nevertheless, the altruistic helper also may experience value congruence and may achieve a sense of mastery when helping has the hoped-for effects.

SUMMARY AND CONCLUSIONS

In considering altruism through the life course, this chapter has reviewed evidence that a rudimentary form of altruism appears to exist in animals and in young children. Nevertheless, altruism continues to evolve and develop from birth to death.

The bifurcation of altruism research into (a) work by developmental psychologists studying childhood and adolescence and (b) the study of factors eliciting altruism (presumably fully developed) in adults by social psychologists makes discussion of lifespan development a challenging task. Far more research is needed, especially as we face the prospect of a shrinking population of children and a concomitant increase in older adults.

I hope, though, that this chapter at least has piqued the reader's curiosity about the development of altruism and the rich insights that further investigation may yield about antecedents and outcomes of *altruistic* caretaking—for the caregiver as well as for the recipient.

NOTES

1. What is the source of altruistic motivation? The two major theoretical responses are that in order to be altruistic, an act must be based on either (a) moral reasoning or cognitions (e.g., Power, Higgins, & Kohlberg, 1989) or (b) empathic concern for others (Blum, 1980; Gilligan, 1982). Still another perspective is that a comprehensive theory of altruism must consider both empathy and moral cognitions (Hoffman, 1981). Recent empirical studies on personality predispositions associated with altruistic actions indicate that altruists may be characterized by high levels of moral judgment, or empathy, and in some instances by high levels of both (but in virtually no cases by low levels of both variables) (Midlarsky, 1990). In this chapter I take the position that for caregiving in families, altruism motivated by empathic concern is most salutary, because in empathy-based altruism the needs of the dependent person, rather than abstract moral principles, are of foremost concern.

2. According to Hoffman (1981), the empathy that is the precursor to caregiving comprises two discriminable mechanisms. One is a form of primitive arousal, or *personal distress* about the plight of the other, and is essentially reflexive in nature. The second is the more flexible, less reflexive mechanism exhibited in what is termed *empathic concern*. It is empathic concern, the more flexible form of empathy—and which includes cognitive elements—that is subject to development and refinement.

3. A great deal of helping is done by people who are in a position to help by virtue of their social roles. Yet the quality, motivation, and meaning of helping by people occupying those roles vary widely. Some helping (for example, by parents, nurses, teachers, and firefighters) may be altruistic, whereas in other instances it is not. Hence, a teacher may prepare homework for a sick child because her role—not to mention her job description—demands that she do so. However, a warm and cheerful note attached to the homework each day, or telephone calls to tell the child that he or she is missed—motivated by an understanding of nonacademic needs—go beyond the usual role requirements. Such actions, when motivated by empathic concern and *not* by the "teacher role," may be altruistic. Similarly, one hospital nurse may check on her patients at the scheduled times and another, equally harried, may check in even at unscheduled times, demonstrating a greater concern for individual needs than for the exigencies of her role.

REFERENCES

Bar-Tal, D., Raviv, A., & Shavit, N. (1981). Motives for helping behavior. *Developmental Psychology, 17,* 767-772.

Bell, R. (1979). Parent, child, and reciprocal influences. *American Psychologist, 34,* 821-826.

Berman, P. W., Sloan, V., & Goodman, V. (1979, March). *Development of sex differences in response to an infant and to the caretaker role.* Paper presented at the Society for Research in Child Development meetings, San Francisco.

Blum, L. (1980). *Friendship, altruism, and morality.* London: Routledge.

Bossard, J., & Boll, E. (1955). Personality roles in the large family. *Child Development, 26,* 71-78.

Brickman, P., Rabinowitz, V., Karuza, J., Jr., Coates, D., Cohn, E., & Kidder, L. (1982). Models of helping and coping. *American Psychologist, 37,* 368-384.

Bryant, B., & Crockenberg, S. (1980). Correlates and dimensions of prosocial behavior. *Child Development, 51,* 529-544.

Cicirelli, V. (1976). Siblings teaching siblings. In V. L. Allen (Ed.), *Children as teachers* (pp. 99-111). New York: Academic Press.

Clarke-Stewart, A., & Koch, J. (1983). *Children.* New York: John Wiley.

Crandall, J. (1981). *Theory and measurement of social interest.* New York: Columbia University Press.

Darwin, C. (1859). *On the origin of species by means of natural selection.* London: Murray.

Darwin, C. (1871). *The descent of man.* London: Murray.

Dremen, S. (1976). Sharing behavior in Israeli school children. *Child Development, 47,* 186-194.

Dunn, J., & Kendrick, C. (1979). Interaction between young siblings in the context of family relationships. In M. Lewis & L. Rosenblum (Eds.), *The child and its family.* New York: Plenum.

Eisenberg, N. (1982). The development of reasoning regarding prosocial behavior. In N. Eisenberg (Ed.), *The development of prosocial behavior* (pp. 219-250). New York: Academic Press.

Eisenberg, N., & Mussen, P. (1989). *The roots of prosocial behavior in children.* New York: Cambridge University Press.

Eisenberg-Berg, N., & Neal, C. (1979). Children's moral reasoning about their own spontaneous prosocial behavior. *Developmental Psychology, 15,* 228-229.

Emler, N., & Rushton, J. P. (1974). Cognitive-developmental factors in children's generosity. *Journal of Social and Clinical Psychology, 13,* 277-281.

Erikson, E. H. (1950). *Childhood and society.* New York: Norton.

Erikson, E. H. (1969). *Ghandi's truth.* New York: Norton.

Erikson, E. H., Erikson, J., & Kivnick, H. (1986). *Vital involvement in old age.* New York: Norton.

Feldman, S., & Nash, S. (1979). Changes in responsiveness to babies during adolescence. *Child Development, 50,* 929-949.

Fiennes, R. (1976). *The order of wolves.* London: Constable.

Freud, S. (1954). *The origins of psychoanalysis.* New York: Basic Books.

Gilligan, C. (1982). *In a different voice.* Cambridge, MA: Harvard University Press.

Green, F., & Schneider, F. (1974). Age differences in the behavior of boys on three measures of altruism. *Child Development, 45,* 248-251.

Haan, N., & Day, D. (1974). A longitudinal study of change and sameness in personality development. *Aging and Human Development, 5,* 11-39.

Handlon, J., & Gross, P. (1959). The development of sharing behavior. *Journal of Abnormal and Social Psychology, 59,* 425-428.

Hannah, M., & Midlarsky, E. (1985). Siblings of the handicapped. *School Psychology Review, 14,* 510-520.

Hebb, D., & Thompson, G. (1954). *A textbook of psychology.* Philadelphia: W. B. Saunders.

Hoffman, M. L. (1981). Is altruism part of human nature? *Journal of Personality and Social Psychology, 40,* 121-137.

Hull, D., & Reuter, J. (1977). The development of charitable behavior in elementary school children. *Journal of Genetic Psychology, 131,* 147-153.

Hyman, M. (1971). Social isolation and performance in rehabilitation. *Journal of Chronic Disease, 25,* 85-97.

Jung, J. (1987). Toward a social psychology of social support. *Basic and Applied Social Psychology, 8,* 57-83.

Kahana, E., Midlarsky, E., & Kahana, B. (1987). Beyond dependency, autonomy, and exchange. *Social Justice Research, 1,* 439-459.

Karno, M., Jenkins, J., de la Selva, A., Santana, F., Telles, C., Lopez, S., & Mintz, J. (1987). Expressed emotion and schizophrenic outcome among Mexican-American families. *Journal of Nervous and Mental Disease, 175,* 143-151.

Kohlberg, L. (1973). Continuities in childhood and adult moral development revisited. In P. Baltes & K. Schaie (Eds.), *Lifespan developmental psychology* (pp. 179-204). New York: Academic Press.

Kropotkin, B. (1914). *Mutual aid: A factor of evolution.* Boston: Extending Horizons Books.

Levy, D. (1937). Sibling rivalry. *American Orthopsychiatric Research Monograph,* No. 2.

Levinson, D. (1986). A conception of adult development. *American Psychologist, 41,* 3-13.

Loevinger, J. (1976). *Ego development.* San Francisco: Jossey-Bass.

Manne, S., & Zautra, A. (1989). Spouse criticism and support. *Journal of Personality and Social Psychology, 56,* 608-617.

Martin, G., & Clark, R., III. (1982). Distress crying in neonates. *Developmental Psychology, 18,* 3-9.

McAndrew, I. (1976). Children with a handicap and their families. *Child, 2,* 213-237.

McHale, S., & Gamble, W. (1989). Sibling relationships of children with disabled and nondisabled brothers and sisters. *Developmental Psychology, 25,* 1-9.

McHale, S., Sloan, J., & Simeonsson, R. (1986). Sibling relationships of children with mentally retarded, autistic, and nonhandicapped brothers and sisters. *Journal of Autism and Developmental Disorders, 16,* 399-414.

Midgley, M. (1978). *Beast and man.* Ithaca, NY: Cornell University Press.

Midlarsky, E. (1984). Competence and helping. In E. Staub, D. Bar-Tal, J. Karylowski, & J. Reykowski (Eds.), *Development and maintenance of prosocial behavior* (pp. 291-308). New York: Plenum.

Midlarsky, E. (1990). *Heroes of the Holocaust* (Final report, NIA grant #R15 AG06535). New York: Columbia University, Teachers College, Center for Lifespan and Aging Studies.

Midlarsky, E. (1991). Helping as coping. In M. Clark (Ed.), *Review of personality and social psychology* (pp. 238-264). Newbury Park, CA: Sage.

Midlarsky, E. (1992, November). *Older adults as helpers in health emergencies.* Paper presented at the Gerontological Society of America meetings, Washington, DC.

Midlarsky, E., & Bryan, J. H. (1967). Training charity in children. *Journal of Personality and Social Psychology, 5,* 408-415.

Midlarsky, E., & Hannah, M. (1985). Competence, reticence, and helping among children and adolescents. *Developmental Psychology, 21,* 534-541.

Midlarsky, E., & Hannah, M. (1989). The generous elderly. *Psychology and Aging, 4,* 346-351.

Midlarsky, E., & Suda, W. (1978). Some antecedents of altruism in children. *Psychological Reports, 43,* 187-208.

Murphy, L. (1937). *Social behavior and child personality.* New York: Columbia University Press.

Nissen, H., & Crawford, M. (1936). A preliminary study of food-sharing behavior in young chimpanzees. *Journal of Comparative Psychology, 22,* 383-419.

Oliner, P., Oliner, S., Baron, L., Krebs, D., & Smolenska, Z. (Eds.). (1992). *Embracing the other: Philosophical, psychological, and historical perspectives on heroic altruism.* New York: New York University Press.

O'Rand, A., & Kriecker, M. (1990). Concepts of the life cycle. *Annual Review of Sociology, 16,* 241-262.

Pepler, D., Corter, C., & Abramovitch, R. (1982). Social relations among children. In K. Rubin & H. Ross (Eds.), *Peer relationships and social skills in childhood* (pp. 209-222). New York: Springer Verlag.

94   PARADIGMS FOR CAREGIVING

Power, C., Higgins, A., & Kohlberg, L. (1989). *Lawrence Kohlberg's approach to moral education.* New York: Columbia University Press.

Rheingold, H. L., & Emery, G. N. (1986). The nurturant acts of very young children. In D. Olweus, J. Block, & M. Radke-Yarrow (Eds.), *Development of antisocial and prosocial behavior* (pp. 75-96). New York: Academic Press.

Riley, M., & Foner, A. (Eds.). (1968). *Aging and society.* New York: Russell Sage.

Rockstein, M., Cheskyi, J., & Sussman, M. (1977). Comparative biology and evolution of aging. In C. Finch & L. Hayflick (Eds.), *Handbook of the biology of aging* (pp. 60-72). New York: Van Nostrand Reinhold.

Rushton, J. P. (1980). *Altruism, socialization, and society.* Englewood Cliffs, NJ: Prentice Hall.

Rushton, J. P., Fuller, D., Neale, M., Nias, D., & Eysenck, J. (1986). Altruism and aggression. *Journal of Personality and Social Psychology, 50,* 1192-1198.

Sagi, A., & Hoffman, M. (1976). Empathic distress in the newborn. *Developmental Psychology, 12,* 175-176.

Sawin, D. (1980). *A field study of children's reactions to distress in their peers.* Unpublished manuscript, University of Texas, Austin.

Schaie, K., & Parham, I. (1976). Stability of adult personality traits. *Journal of Personality and Social Psychology, 34,* 146-158.

Schulz, R., Williamson, G., Morycz, R., & Biegel, D. (1992). Costs and benefits of providing care to Alzheimer's patients. In S. Spacapan & S. Oskamp (Eds.), *Helping and being helped* (pp. 153-182). Newbury Park, CA: Sage.

Simner, N. (1971). Newborn's response to the cry of another infant. *Developmental Psychology, 5,* 136-150.

Skinner, B. F. (1971). *Beyond freedom and dignity.* New York: Knopf.

Spacapan, S., & Oskamp, S. (Eds.). (1992). *Helping and being helped.* Newbury Park, CA: Sage.

Staub, E. (1970). A child in distress. *Journal of Personality and Social Psychology, 14,* 130-140.

Staub, E. (1971). A child in distress. *Developmental Psychology, 5,* 124-132.

Stoneman, Z., Brody, G., Davis, G., & Crapps, J. (1988). Childcare responsibilities, peer relationships and sibling conflict. *American Journal of Mental Retardation, 93,* 174-183.

Summers, M., Summers, C., Ascione, F., & Braeger, T. (1989, April). *Observations of siblings' social interactions: Comparing families with and without a handicapped child.* Paper presented at the annual meeting of the Society for Research in Child Development, Kansas City, KS.

Swirean, P. (1976). Effects of the presence of a hearing impaired preschool child in the family on behavior patterns of normal siblings. *American Annals of the Deaf, 121,* 373-380.

Thompson, S., & Pitts, J. (1992). In sickness and in health. In S. Spacapan & S. Oskamp (Eds.), *Helping and being helped* (pp. 153-182). Newbury Park, CA: Sage.

Ugurel-Semin, R. (1952). Moral behavior and moral judgment of children. *Journal of Abnormal and Social Psychology, 47,* 463-474.

Vaillant, G. (1977). *Adaptation to life.* Boston: Little, Brown.

Veroff, J., Douvan, E., & Kulka, R. (1981). *The inner American.* New York: Basic Books.

Wallach, M., & Wallach, L. (1983). *Psychology's sanction for selfishness.* San Francisco: W. H. Freeman.

White, B. (1975). Critical influences in the origins of competence. *Merrill-Palmer Quarterly, 21,* 243-266.

Whiting, J., & Whiting, B. (1973). Altruistic and egoistic behavior in six cultures. In L. Nader & T. Maretzki (Eds.), *Cultural illness and health.* Washington, DC: American Anthropological Association.

Wilson, E. O. (1971). *The insect societies.* Cambridge, MA: Belknap.

Wilson, E. O. (1975). *Sociobiology.* Cambridge, MA: Harvard University Press.

Wilson, E. O. (1978). *On human nature.* Cambridge, MA: Harvard University Press.

Wolman, B. (1973). *Dictionary of behavioral science.* New York: Van Nostrand.

Wright, D. (1971). *The psychology of moral behavior.* Middlesex, UK: Penguin.

Wundheiler, L. (1985-1986). Oskar Schindler's moral development during the Holocaust. *Humboldt Journal of Social Relations, 13,* 333-356.

Yarrow, M., & Waxler, C. (1976). Dimensions and correlates of prosocial behavior in young children. *Child Development, 47,* 118-125.

Zahn-Waxler, C., Cummings, E., McKnew, D., & Radke-Yarrow, M. (1984). Altruism, aggressive, and social interaction in young children with a manic-depressive parent. *Child Development, 55,* 112-122.

Zahn-Waxler, C., & Radke-Yarrow, M. (1982). The development of altruism. In N. Eisenberg-Berg (Ed.), *The development of prosocial behavior.* New York: Academic Press.

4

Optimal Use of Formal and Informal Systems Over the Life Course

EUGENE LITWAK
DOROTHY JONES JESSOP
HEATHER J. MOULTON

In this chapter we discuss how life-course considerations interact with a task-specific theory of social supports to answer the following questions: (a) Which life-course factors lead individuals to seek formal organizations to take over family tasks, (b) which life-course factors lead to which forms of neglect or abuse, and (c) how do life-course considerations affect the composition and use of different types of informal supports? The task-specific theory states that in advanced industrial societies, such as the United States, formal organizations and informal ones optimally deliver different types of caregiving service. Furthermore, the various informal groups, such as marital, kin, friends, and neighbors, each deliver unique services. If any one of these groups is missing from the network of caregiving groups, the individual who is disabled will receive either less help or a poorer quality of help (Litwak, 1985; Penning, 1990). In this chapter we try to show how life-course considerations encourage and discourage the use of the various components of the helping networks and the kinds of problems that arise as a result. The chapter is divided into three sections. The first starts with the theoretical imperative for formal organizations substituting for informal groups. It concludes with a discussion of the life-course variables that accelerate or slow down these theoretical imperatives.

The second section begins by describing the theoretical limitations on quality of services delivered by formal and informal groups. It finishes by showing how life-course variables specify which types of neglect or abuse can potentially arise. The third section commences with the theoretical rationale for different informal groups (i.e., marital, kin, friend, and neighbor) providing different services. It concludes by showing how life-course considerations delineate which informal groups will be most available at each stage of the life course and, consequently, which types of services will be available.

Before we begin the analysis, the underlying philosophy governing the selection of the variables for the life-course analysis should be made explicit. The analysis of life-course considerations in this chapter starts from the premise that we know some of the elements and some of the relationships that go into life-course analysis, but we lack information on many elements and do not have a precise understanding of the relationship between all the variables that have been identified. Given this state of the art, the best course of action is to present a series of ad hoc propositions that deliberately simplify the analysis to concentrate on defining more precisely a few variables and their relationship to each other. The age of the person who is disabled is used as a rough approximation for the life course, and the simplifying assumption is made that other key life-course variables, such as occupational career and marital and parental status, follow a common trajectory throughout the life course. The analysis is limited to the cultural and economic structure of U.S. society. It is recognized that ethnicity in the United States is diverse and does impact the analysis; however, to simplify matters, ethnicity will be held as a constant. Only two specific conditions for caregiving— mental retardation, which is present in infancy, and Alzheimer's disease, which begins later in life—are considered. The assumption is that the task-specific formulation holds for all disabling conditions, but the influence of life-course variables will certainly vary with the type of health condition examined.[1] Consequently task-specific theory would make different predictions for different conditions. The hypotheses we present here are restricted to Alzheimer's and mental retardation, as well as to all other health conditions that have the same consequences for an individual's functional status. The hypotheses on life-course stages from infancy to middle age are based on conditions of mental retardation, whereas the hypotheses on old age are based on Alzheimer's disease. This reflects the empirical patterning of these conditions.[2]

THE USE OF FORMAL ORGANIZATIONS
TO SUBSTITUTE FOR INFORMAL GROUP SERVICES

Task-Specific Theories
of Substitution and Complementarity

The task-specific theory (Litwak, 1985) argues that both groups and services can be classified by the same dimensions of structure. Furthermore, groups optimally can manage those services that match their structure. When that framework is applied to the analysis of formal organizations and informal groups, it becomes apparent that formal organizations differ from informal ones in that they are structured to optimize technical knowledge. In addition, they have greater human resources than the informal groups we consider in this chapter, which are marital units, kin, friends, and neighbors. Consequently the task-specific formulation suggests that formal organizations should be better able to manage those services that require technical knowledge or large-scale human resources. This observation was viewed as so obvious by past researchers that it seemed truistic to state it as a theoretical proposition. Not so obvious were the other conclusions of the task-specific theory: (a) that informal groups would be superior to formal organizations for managing those services that did not require technical knowledge or (b) that marital units, kin, friendship groups, and neighbors each provided unique services so that one could not be easily substituted for the other (Crohan & Antonucci, 1989; Litwak, 1985). The notion that informal groups would be superior to formal organizations for managing nontechnical services was overlooked for two reasons. One, the early researchers assumed that those with technical knowledge should be able to oversee all meaningful services better than those with nontechnical knowledge (Weber, 1947). Second, it was assumed that individuals, in the context of a formal organization, should manage nontechnical tasks as well as these same individuals when they were part of their informal group. Consequently these researchers were continuously surprised when successive studies showed that informal groups seem to play important roles in domains thought to be dominated by formal organizations. Perhaps the most persuasive data on importance of informal groups is the series of longitudinal studies showing that affiliation with informal groups reduced mortality (House, Landis, & Umberson, 1988). Even earlier, Katz and Lazarsfeld (1955) showed how informal groups played key roles in factory production, the army's combat morale, and mass media's efforts to reach the larger public. There were no obvious explanations for these findings, and even today most of the explanations offered by researchers (House et al., 1988) have not uniquely differentiated the role of informal groups from formal ones (Messeri, Litwak, & Silverstein, 1991).

An understanding of the task-specific formulation starts with an examination of the underlying factors associated with the truism that formal organizations can manage technical services better than informal ones. There is a face validity to the notion that services can be characterized by the degree of specialized or technical knowledge they require. Consequently, it only remains to show that the structure of the formal organization emphasizes the role of technical knowledge to demonstrate within the task-specific framework why formal organizations can manage technical tasks better (Weber, 1947). To start, members of formal organizations are recruited on the basis of technical knowledge, whereas members of informal groups are recruited through birth, marriage, or friendship with little reference to technical knowledge. To ensure the preeminence of technical knowledge, formal organizations generally give their members a limited commitment; that is, they can remain only as long as they are able to maintain their technical proficiency. Furthermore, the formal organization seeks to guard the dominant role of technical knowledge by explicitly de-emphasizing the emotional ties between individuals that are likely to lead to favoritism (e.g., nepotism rules) and concentrating on impersonal economic incentives. By contrast, membership in informal groups often is defined as a lifetime (e.g., parent-child) or long-term (e.g., marital) commitment, which makes it difficult to break relationships on the grounds that they are "technically inefficient." Informal groups are more likely to motivate their members through internalized commitments of love and duty that give priority to loyalty rather than to technical knowledge.

Given these generally accepted distinctions (Weber, 1947) between the structure of formal and informal groups, the question now can be addressed as to why informal groups play a significant role in realms thought to be governed by technical knowledge, such as health, factory production, mass media dissemination, and so on. The answer lies in the observation that many services do not require technical knowledge. In such instances, a close examination of the structure of the two groups suggests that the informal one is superior. Some illustrations of tasks that do not require technical knowledge in the field of health are illuminating. Health professionals' technical knowledge and resources give them little advantage over an untrained family member when it comes to removing a lighted cigarette from the hand of the family member who has fallen asleep in bed. Nor would the technical knowledge of the medical profession provide any extra edge when it comes to reminding an individual to take blood pressure pills every morning, assisting in ordering low cholesterol food in a restaurant, providing daily stimulus to maintain a morning exercise regimen, monitoring everyday driving to assure a companion is not too drunk or too sleepy, or calling an ambulance and providing first aid in a home accident. These are all behaviors that can seriously affect an individual's health, yet do not require highly trained professionals.

What might not be obvious is why persons are more effective in managing nontechnical problems when they are members of an informal group as opposed to those times when they are active as members of formal organizations. Three reasons relating to the structural features of informal groups provide an answer. If a service can be managed as well or almost as well by the informal group as by the formal one, then the informal one is less expensive because it does not entail costs of training specialists or setting up formal organizations (Mayhew, 1970). Under these same circumstances, an informal group is also faster because its small size and lack of complex division of labor means it has shorter lines of communication. Finally, where knowledge is based on everyday socialization, then the internalized commitments of love and duty of the informal group will lead to a better motivated individual than the economic incentives used by formal organizations, because internalized commitments motivate individuals to work even when their activities cannot be observed (Warren, 1968). The objection to internalized commitments—that they lead to nepotism—will not result in loss of efficiency when tasks do not require technical knowledge.

The paradox of informal groups continuing to play a significant role in areas thought to be the exclusive arena of formal organizations can be unraveled. First, services of formal organizations requiring technical knowledge often are intertwined with "hidden" services requiring nontechnical knowledge. This is endemic to the nature of a modern industrial society (Litwak, 1985). Second, services that require nontechnical knowledge are optimally managed by informal groups because they have dimensions that match the dimensions of these services more precisely than do formal organizations, and because they are less expensive, faster, and have better motivated people. Consequently, to achieve most goals in our society, it is necessary to have formal organizations and informal ones working in complementary relations to each other (Litwak, 1985).

The task-specific formulation also provides an understanding of the pressures for informal groups to turn over some of their services to formal ones or to seek paid help when individuals become chronically unable to manage everyday household and personal grooming activities. Commonsense observation, as well as the just established principles of group structure, suggests that the informal group is less expensive, is faster, and provides better motivated people to manage these nontechnical services. Why, then, is there accelerating growth of formal organizations in these areas? The answer, in part, lies in the emergence of modern science, which has led to the survival of individuals with severe chronic ailments (Strauss & Corbin, 1988). For instance, the fastest growing segment of the population are those 85 and older, with approximately 70% requiring some form of assistance (Bould, Sandborn, & Reif, 1989; Longino, 1988), and children with previously fatal conditions who now are living to adulthood (cf. leukemia).

The chief reason society is forced to call on formal organizations for household and grooming services is that informal groups simply lack the human resources to provide 24-hour care for people with serious chronic conditions. Attempts by informal groups to carry out such care on their own can lead to severe psychological, social, and economic impairments to caregivers and their families (Anderson, 1977; Chiriboga, Weiler, & Nielsen, 1990; Zarit, Todd, & Zarit, 1986) as well as abuse to the disabled brought about by overextended family caregivers. The reason formal organizations can take over the burden is apparent: They have more human resources. This arises from two dimensions of formal organizations: (a) their use of economic incentives and (b) their ability to standardize services and make use of a detailed division of labor.

The advantage of economic incentives over the internalized commitments of informal groups as a motivator is obvious. It permits formal organizations to draw on a substantial labor pool of people willing to commit themselves to 8 hours of work daily. This contrasts with the very small labor pool generated by internalized commitments of duty and love, which motivates informal group members. In advanced industrial societies, the labor pool for household services is generally limited to spouses, parents, or adult children. It is further reduced by those members of the informal groups who are in the external labor force or have caregiving duties to other members of their group.

The second reason that formal organizations have a human resources advantage over informal groups is that the former can make use of a detailed division of labor and standardization of services. This permits staff members to handle a larger volume of work than members of an informal system. For instance, one person can cook for 100 if it is a full-time job and it is simplified by standardization, that is, limiting the choice of food, the way it is cooked, the time people will eat, the place they will eat, and with whom they will eat.[3]

Some Life-Course Considerations in the Choice of Formal Organizations

The above analysis suggests the respective roles that informal and formal groups can play and why it is that formal groups take over many caregiving services from families. Now we consider life-course factors that further direct families to turn their services over to the formal organization.

Table 4.1 provides a systematic framework for comparing life-course factors. Listed on the vertical axis are the factors that increase the probability of choosing formal organizations. On the horizontal axis are seven age periods as rough approximations of the stages of the life course: early childhood, from age 1 to 5; childhood, 6 to 11; adolescence, 12 to 18; young adulthood, 19 to 39; middle age, 40 to 64; young-old, 65 to 74; and old-old, 75 or older.

Physical Maturity

One life-course factor that would directly affect the burden of the caregiver is the physical maturation of the person with a disability. If caregiving services such as bathing, toileting, feeding, dressing, and assistance in transporting must be delivered, it is apparent, all other things being equal, that a caregiver of a 10-pound infant with moderate-to-severe mental retardation has a far easier physical job in providing these services than does the caregiver of a 180-pound male suffering from moderate-to-severe Alzheimer's disease. The problem of dressing or lifting a recalcitrant 180-pound Alzheimer male generally requires more than one caregiver, whereas this is seldom the case for managing a recalcitrant 10-pound infant. It is our hypothesis that there would be a gradual increase in the physical burden of providing basic personal grooming and household services to the caregiver that peaks when the

TABLE 4.1 Life-Course Determinants of Choosing Formal Organizations

Hypothesis	Early Childhood, 1-5 years	Childhood, 6-11 years	Adolescence, 12-18 years	Young Adult, 19-39 years	Middle-aged, 40-64 years	Young-Old, 65-74 years	Old-Old, 75+ years
				Age of Persons With a Disability			
		Motivation to Choose Formal Organization to Substitute for Primary Groups					
Physical maturation	Low to moderate	Low	High	Highest	Highest	Highest	Highest
Incest and privacy norms	Low	Low to moderate	High	High	High	High	High
Parenting norms	Low	Low to moderate	Moderate	High	Low	Low	Low
Gender role reversal	Low	Low	Low	Moderate	Moderate	High	High
Parent/child role reversals	Low	Low	Low	Low	Moderate	High	High
Grandparent overload	Low	Moderate	High	Moderate	Low	Low	Low
Female overload	High	Moderate	Low	Low	Moderate	Moderate	High
Sibling overload	Low	Moderate	High	High	Moderate	Low	High
Spousal overload	High	Moderate	Low	Low	Moderate	Low	Moderate

child reaches full physical maturity and continues at that level for all subsequent age groups. Consequently, we would suggest that, with increasing physical maturity, there is increased pressure to turn to paid help or formal organizations. The hypothesis on the life-course variable of physical maturity is depicted in Table 4.1, row 1.

Incest and Privacy Norms

There are a series of norms that increase the probability of choosing a formal organization by suggesting it is inappropriate for caregivers who are members of the informal support groups to provide some types of services. Two such instances are incest norms and privacy norms. The incest norm indirectly mandates that parents of one gender not be in contact with physically mature children of the opposite gender when they are nude. That means mothers who dress, bathe, or toilet physically mature sons, or fathers who provide such services to their daughters, would have to breach this normative barrier. It is also the case that norms on adult privacy often mean that spouses should not provide toileting services to their mates. Insofar as these norms hold, it would be our hypothesis that pressures to turn to formal organizations would peak for caregivers whose children reach young adulthood and remain at this high state for all subsequent age groups as indicated in row 2 of Table 4.1.[4]

Parenting Norms and Stigmatization of Disability

Closely associated with these norms are social standards on parenting that suggest that, as children age, parents should give increasing autonomy to children to dress, toilet themselves, visit friends, and so on. These socialization norms work in conjunction with our society's tendency to stigmatize mental retardation so as to confront parents of a child who is retarded with the alternative of providing increasingly inappropriate services or acknowledging their child's stigmatized condition (Farber, 1959). Based on these considerations, the hypothesis is advanced that each stage of the life course increases the burden of caregiving because it violates normal expectations concerning parenting and makes more explicit the stigmatized condition of the child. This increase in burden causes caregivers to turn to formal organizations for relief. The burden is hypothesized to peak at young adulthood and then decline because, after this point, the person who is disabled is not seen as a child, and the norms of incest or adult privacy are likely to take over. These hypotheses are formalized in row 3 in Table 4.1.

Gender Role-Reversal Norms

Past studies suggest very strong gender differences in provision of caregiving services (Litwak, 1985; Nathanson, 1977; Umberson, 1987; Waldron, 1982). Where the caregiver has to violate these norms in order to provide services to the disabled person, the additional burden is a motivation to turn to formal organizations for help. For instance, a husband who is asked to cook, shop, clean the house, and provide personal grooming for a wife with Alzheimer's disease might see these activities as a gender role violation and turn to formal organizations for help (Noelker & Bass, 1989). A wife who has to do the household repairs, take care of the car, and provide personal hygiene for an Alzheimer's spouse might have similar feelings of role violation and turn to formal organizations for help. Life-course variables suggest that problems of gender role reversals are problems of the older age groups, but not the younger ones. In almost all cases society has mandated that mothers take care of infants and young children or, if the mother is not available, the alternatives, such as foster care, almost always give responsibilities to women. At this point in the life course, the father has no role that the mother has to take over because of the child's disability. By contrast, among older people, spouses and adult children generally are viewed as the prime caregivers. Consequently, when older people become sick, there is often a situation in which male spouses or children are asked to take over female family roles or females are asked to take over male roles. Following these considerations, we predict that problems of gender role violations are likely to commence among the middle-aged group and peak at the oldest groups, as indicated in row 4 of Table 4.1.

Parent/Child Role Reversals

Yet another normative mandate arises when adult children (e.g., daughters) are asked to provide household management and other household services to their disabled parent (e.g., mother). The tension arises because this reverses the relationship that has previously existed between parents and children. For some children and some parents, the idea is so unbearable that they turn to formal organizations for help.

This problem typically arises where children have grown to adult status. Consequently we suggest role-reversal pressures are likely to reach their height in the last two stages of the life course. This pattern is displayed in row 5 of Table 4.1.

Grandparent Role Overload

For those with infants and younger children, the child's grandparent is often the key kin who provides supplementary help to the parents. Grandparents as a source of extra help become increasingly problematic as the child grows older because the grandparents are entering the period of aging that is accompanied by physical frailty and illness. Many grandparents die as the child with a disability reaches young adulthood. It therefore would be our hypothesis that the problem of grandparent role overload occurs when the children reach adolescence, that is, the time grandparents are older and more frail but have not as yet died. That speculation is developed in row 6 of Table 4.1.

Female Caregiving Role Overload

It has been pointed out that one aspect of the female gender role is that of caregiver for the functionally impaired (Litwak, 1985; Nathanson, 1977; Umberson, 1987; Waldron, 1982). Where women must simultaneously take care of two or more needy people, it often leads to role overload. Two life-course stages are hypothesized to lead to peaks of gender overload. Women who have an older child who is disabled and, at the same time, have children who are in the 1 to 5 age group might find themselves in a situation of caregiving overload. This hypothesis is generated by the assumption that healthy children between the ages of 1 and 5 are most demanding in terms of the amount of direct supervision they require. In contrast, the child with a moderate or severe disability might require more effort as he or she physically matures (e.g., peaking at adolescence). The conjunction of these factors produces female caregiving overload in the early middle stage of the life course. The second point at which female caregiving leads to overload occurs when the person with a disability is age 75 years or older. In this case, the adult daughter is often chief caregiver, yet the daughter herself can be 65 to 75 or older and often has a spouse who is even older. Typically that means the daughter is taking care of her spouse and her parent while she, herself, is also frail. This will lead to role overload.

The demographics of aging implies this will be a growing problem. This hypothesis with its bimodal imperatives to seek help from formal organizations is shown in row 7 of Table 4.1.

Sibling Overload

The sibling who lives at home often is asked by parents to pick up many caregiving tasks for the child with retardation. The older the sibling becomes, the greater the public stigmatization of the child with a disability, and the more the caregiving tasks conflict with the socially mandated need for role separation between adolescent and parental family. When the healthy sibling moves to young adulthood and leaves the parental household, the parent generally is deprived of his or her daily help. We therefore would speculate that where the sibling of the child with retardation reaches late adolescence and the child with retardation reaches early adolescence, sibling overload pressures are likely to contribute to parental motivation to seek out formal organizational assistance. Pressure for sibling involvement is likely to increase again when the parents develop chronic disabilities or die at the later stages of the life course. The conflux of life-course factors would suggest that sibling overload may be highest at late adolescence and early adulthood, drop immediately after that, and then increase again in the last two stages of the life course. This pattern is shown in row 8 in Table 4.1.

Spousal Overload

All other things being equal, we think the impact of disability on spousal relations is related to several life-course factors. The length of time people are married is a rough indicator of the bonds of reciprocity that have been built up, in other words, the strength of the tie. Spouses at the first stage of the life course have less commitment to the marriage than those at later stages. The length of caregiving time that the spouses face is also an indicator of the burden of caregiving. A young couple having an infant with retardation, or having a mate who has a disability, must face the prospect of caregiving over the major part of their life course. A person in the last or next-to-last stage of the life course whose spouse has become disabled faces the burden of care for only one or two stages of the life course. It is our hypothesis that this conflux of events leads to higher rates of divorce and abandonment at the initial stages of the life course. The problem of spousal overload also will arise among very old people (85 and older) who are married (Wilson, 1990). In this case it will be a function of the physical frailty of the caregiving spouse, which makes it difficult to provide daily household services to a mate with a disability. These considerations lead to a speculation that spousal overload will arise during the first and last stages of the life course. The pattern is shown in row 9 of Table 4.1.

If Table 4.1 is now examined, two factors become clear. First, the pressures for using formal organizations to substitute for informal ones are very different at different stages of the life course. During the infancy period the major pressures are female caregiver and spousal overload. During the adolescent period the pressures come from burdens produced by physical maturation, violations of incest and child socialization norms, and sibling and grandparent caregiving-role overload. For the last stages of the life course, the pressures continue from physical maturation and violations of incest norms, while spousal caregiving, female caregiving, and sibling role overload reemerge even as pressures from gender role reversals and/or parent/child role reversals emerge for the first time. The analysis of differential pressures for use of formal organizations at different stages of the life course would have great relevance for agencies seeking to moderate these pressures because different pressures are likely to require different interventions.

The second factor that becomes clear is establishing at which stage of the life course there will be the most pressure for use of formal organizations, which requires research on the relative strength of the various life-course burdens. If we were to assume all pressures had equal magnitude, then Table 4.1 would imply that pressures would sharply increase to the young adult stage, drop to a slightly lower plateau, and then peak at the last stage of the life course.[5] Such an assumption would be consistent with the findings of Birenbaum (1971), Farber (1959), Seltzer and Krauss (1989), and Winik, Zetlin, and Kaufman (1985), who suggest that the burdens for caregivers of children with mental retardation increase with the age of the children. They do not, however, consider the problems of Alzheimer's patients and, consequently, do not spell out the complete life-course pattern suggested in Table 4.1. The sharp growth in agency-supervised community residences for retarded adults and a decline of formal institutions for children also would be consistent with this hypothesis.

Others (e.g., Blacher, Nihira, & Meyers, 1987) suggest that the mildly retarded, especially, may be more independent with age and consequently less demanding. These speculations would be more consistent with a hypothesis that pressures at an earlier age should be given far greater weight than those at a later stage of the life course. Donovan (1988) and Bristol (1979), finding that family stress levels vary across the age of the handicapped child, suggest a more complex weight of life-course factors. The taxonomy presented herein has made apparent the need for research that systematically compares these life-course factors.

INTRINSIC PROBLEMS IN
THE USE OF FORMAL AND INFORMAL
ORGANIZATIONS FOR HOUSEHOLD AND
GROOMING SERVICES[6]

To state what life-course factors lead individuals to turn to formal organizations is the first step in our analysis. To understand the types of risks involved in this substitution and how they might be affected by life-course factors is the next step. This analysis takes place against the overall finding that the disabled are more likely to suffer abuse or neglect from their caregivers than are nondisabled children or adults (Groce, 1988). In the analysis on abuse, we do not want the discussion to be misinterpreted as an assertion that abuse is common among any of the groups; however, abuse does occur at times to varying degrees. We feel that to ignore this issue, uncomfortable as it may be, would not do justice to a thorough analysis of the potential structural problems of formal organizations and informal groups. Therefore, we attempt to show three things: (a) how a task-specific approach suggests which forms of abuse are associated with the structure of the formal organizations, (b) which forms of abuse are associated with the structure of the informal groups, and (c) how life-course factors relate to each type of abuse. The focus of the analysis is on the structural limitations of groups that lead to problems. It must be understood that other factors can play a more important role in abuse, such as the personality of the caregiver, the history of the caregiver and the disabled person, the cultural ties of the caregiver and the disabled, the income of the caregiver and the disabled, the gender of the caregiver and the disabled person, the availability of organizations designed to police abuse, and so on. These factors are treated as constants in order to highlight the problem of group structural limitations that lead to abuse.

Types of Abuse Associated With Formal Organizations

The two dimensions of formal organizations that give them the added resources for managing activities of daily living for severely disabled individuals also define the characteristic forms that abuse can take in formal organizations.[7]

Standardization and Loss of Autonomy— Problems of Nursing Homes

It will be recalled that one dimension of the formal organization is the detailed division of labor coupled with the standardization of services that permit staff of formal organizations to deliver a higher volume of household and personal grooming services. We now propose that this same dimension also can lead to the loss of self-esteem and a feeling of humiliation among the disabled. It is true that 1 person can cook for 100 if the meal process is standardized, but it is also true that standardization limits individual autonomy in choice of food, when to eat, and with whom to eat. The loss of autonomy and potential for humiliation become even clearer when personal grooming activities are considered. For instance, 1 staff member can dress and groom 10 residents if the 10 are awakened and put to sleep at a fixed time rather than when they choose, if their hair is cut short (or in the case of women, pulled back and held in place with a rubber band) to minimize combing, if no makeup is applied, and if teeth are not brushed. The reduced night staffs of nursing homes can still manage to take care of the toileting needs of the same number of bedridden patients if toileting is standardized by putting diapers on patients and changing the diapers at fixed intervals. The staff can standardize the eating habits of patients who must be hand fed by lining them up in the hallway and spooning the food into the patients' mouths, one after another, very much like an assembly line. In such institutional contexts, we hypothesize that the humiliating loss of autonomy may be the form of abuse that is significantly associated with the use of formal organizations (Bowers, 1988; Freeman, 1990; Kane, Caplan, Freeman, Aroskar, & Urv-Wong, 1990; Litwak, 1985).[8] Physical restraint use is an excellent example of how structure can lead to abusive situations and result in public policy to address the problem. In the past, well-intentioned staff have managed at-risk residents by restraining them to chairs or beds. In essence this was standardizing residents' behavior so the relatively low number of staff could more easily provide care. At-risk residents were identified as those who had the potential to fall, who wandered due to cognitive impairments, or who imposed harm on other residents or staff due to violent behavior. In addition, restraints were used to maintain body alignment, to prevent people from pulling out their feeding tubes or intravenous lines, and also out of fear of litigation for any harm that might occur to a resident (Blakeslee, Hunt, Thankachan, & Torell, 1986; Francis, 1989; McHutchion & Morse, 1989). A growing public awareness, supported by an emerging body of research of the physical and emotional adverse effects that restraints caused, resulted in a federal mandate via the Omnibus Budget Reconciliation Act (OBRA) of 1987, stating that residents have the right to remain free of restraints (United States Code Annotated, 1992).

Staff Abuse and Economic Incentives—
The Problems of Home-Care Agencies
and Communal Living Arrangements

One characteristic response to this criticism that yet seeks to retain formal organizational resources is to suggest that nursing homes be eliminated and society turn to home-care agencies or some form of communal living that provides more of a one-to-one relationship between staff and resident. Such a staff/resident ratio clearly offers the opportunity for more individual treatment.[9] This highlights the second dimension of formal organizations, economic incentives, which permits them to provide services long after the informal group has run out of resources. We hypothesize that the problems of abuse characterized as slack services and economic crimes arise from motivating staff economically to handle services that cannot be easily supervised (i.e., observed).[10]

Central to this hypothesis is the fact that home-care and personal grooming services are intrinsically difficult to observe. In addition, many of these services do not have objective outcomes that can be easily assessed (e.g., emotional support). A worker may provide a high quality of care when an observer is present, but there is no guarantee that the same quality of care will be provided in the observer's absence. This difference in the quality of care may be subtle. For example, the time it takes to bathe a person may be reduced enough to compromise thoroughness. On the other hand, the care may be delivered adequately, but the worker may be rude or disrespectful to the client. Even if someone is present, the service is often so idiosyncratic that it is hard to evaluate unless the supervisor has a lengthy acquaintance with the disabled person (Bowers, 1988; Litwak, 1985). Without this knowledge of the disabled person, a supervisor may not be able to tell whether the staff person is not performing appropriate care to the client, or whether the client is being irrational and difficult. Cognitively limited individuals often cannot provide such information.

Caregiver Burden and Physical Abuse—
The Problems of Informal Groups

By contrast to the formal organizations, the informal group has small size and internalized commitments. These dimensions in turn suggest which forms of abuse are associated with informal groups. The limited resources mean that the informal group on its own cannot manage the services necessary for the seriously disabled. We suggest two alternative hypotheses depending on the personality of the informal caregiver. Our first hypothesis is that *because of their internalized commitment, members of informal groups are more likely than those of formal ones to make great personal sacrifices to maintain services, that is, to suffer from caregiver burden* (Anderson, 1977; Chiriboga et al., 1990; Zarit et al., 1986).[11]

Our second hypothesis is that *the great personal sacrifices demanded of the caregiver, coupled with the emotional feelings expected from the internalized norms of duty and affection, could cause another group caregiver to turn in anger against the disabled person.* The anger would be manifested in physical and verbal abuse rather than the more impersonal neglect or theft that we hypothesize characterizes the staff of formal organizations.

In summary, we speculate that the distinctive problems in quality of services delivered by formal organizations will be social humiliation, based on loss of autonomy, or impersonal rational neglect and economic exploitation based on the use of economic incentives. The special problems of informal groups will be caregiver burden and emotionally based physical abuse associated with limited resources and internalized commitments. The task-specific theory suggests that problems of abuse will be minimized if the formal and informal groups work in close collaboration with each other, for example, if the formal group provides standardized meals and the informal provides nonstandardized supplements, special food treats, and so on (Litwak, 1985).

Life-Course Considerations and Types of Abuse

In this section we speculate on life-course factors that relate to types of abuse or neglect. We consider the following types of abuse: economic exploitation, social humiliation, and physical abuse. To understand how life-course factors operate, two questions should be addressed: What life-course factors increase the incentives for abuse, and what factors increase the ability of the disabled to resist abuse? In this analysis, like all the others in this chapter, other elements—such as the personality makeup of the abuser, economic resources, family history of the abuser, and society's provision of organizations to guard against abuse—are assumed to be constant so the life-course elements can be specified clearly. Table 4.2 systematically presents our hypotheses. On the horizontal axis are stages in the life course, and the vertical axis contains the types of abuse. In each cell we indicate the level of abuse according to our hypotheses. Two forms of abuse can be readily related to life-course factors.

Economic Exploitation

The incentive for economic exploitation rises with the size of the disabled person's economic resources. It would be our speculation that children rarely have independent economic resources, whereas older people tend to have a range of resources until those resources are dissipated by health costs at the last stage of the life course. The ability to resist economic exploitation would be minimal among the very old, who often are physically frail. Though infants and children also are least able to resist, they typically are guarded by parents who are still vigorous and have the least incentives to exploit the child (Zelizer, 1985). Consequently the hypothesis is advanced that *attempts at economic exploitation will increase with age until the last stage of the life course, when they will drop*. This speculation is reflected in row 1 of Table 4.2.

Social Humiliation

Social humiliation as a form of caregiving abuse also can be clearly related to life-course factors. It occurs when the caregiver takes away an individual's management of his or her everyday activities. The humiliation arises from the fact that the adult is treated like an infant.

TABLE 4.2 Life-Course Determinants of Abusing or Neglecting Care Receivers

Type of Abuse or Neglect	Age of Persons With a Disability						
	Early Childhood, 1-5 years	Childhood, 6-11 years	Adolescence, 12-18 years	Young Adult, 19-39 years	Middle-aged, 40-64 years	Young-Old, 65-74 years	Old-Old, 75+ years
Economic exploitation	Low	Low	Low	Low	High	High	Low
Social humiliation	Low	Low	Low	Moderate	High	High	High
Physical abuse for males	High	Moderate	Moderate	Moderate	Moderate	High	Highest
Physical abuse for females	High	Moderate	High	Moderate	Moderate	High	Highest

By definition such abuse is rare among infants and young children. We would speculate that social humiliation reaches its peak among middle-aged clients and retains that level among older people, as indicated in row 2, Table 4.2.

Physical Violence

Physical abuse will reflect the difficulty the caregiver has in taking care of persons with disabilities at different stages of the life course, plus age-related social norms of prejudice, and the ability of the person with a disability to actively defend him- or herself. Several life-course factors suggest that older persons might be at greater risk for abuse on all counts. As indicated above, it is far more difficult for caregivers to provide the same basic activities of daily living to physically mature but very cognitively limited people than to similarly limited small children and infants. This may be further reinforced by social norms of ageism that see the behavior of older people with cognitive limitations much more negatively than that of young babies and children with similar disabilities, including behaviors such as nudity, mindless sexuality, incontinence, and profanity (Butler, 1975; Ford & Sbordone, 1980; Haug, 1988; Kosberg, 1983). All of these factors predispose the caregiver who is inclined to use violence to use it against older people, rather than younger ones, with a peak being reached among care recipients who are 75 and older.

If other stages of the life course are examined, we hypothesize that caregiver frustration may arise at two other stages: adolescence and infancy. Anger might arise toward infants because their needs can be expressed only through crying and they require 24-hour attention. In addition, they are least able physically to resist abuse or neglect. Adolescence is thought to be a stage of high friction, because social norms mandate a need for the autonomy of children from parents without clear guidelines as to how this is to be accomplished. Adolescent males are generally too formidable physically to be abused and, furthermore, traditional gender norms discourage females from physical resistance (Kaplan, 1988). These life-course and gender factors would lead to the hypothesis that *abuse for females will peak during adolescence whereas for males it will be while they are younger* (Straus, 1988).[12]

These considerations lead us to suggest that physical abuse for males will have a curvilinear relation, with highest violence against young children and very old people as indicated in row 3, Table 4.2. For females we hypothesize three peaks, at infancy, adolescence, and old age, with valleys in between as indicated in row 4, Table 4.2.

In summary our hypotheses are that *life-course variables will lead to economic exploitation and social humiliation among those who are old, whereas physical abuse will peak at either extreme for males and for women it will reach a height when they are very young, adolescents, and very old.*

AVAILABILITY OF INFORMAL GROUPS AND THEIR SERVICES

Theory of Optimal Tasks for Differing Informal Groups

Problems in caregiving services by informal groups to severe or moderately cognitively limited individuals must be understood in two ways: (a) drops in the quality of life for caregivers as they try to deliver services with inadequate human resources and (b) loss of services as informal caregivers can no longer deliver services after they collapse. Task-specific theory provides a rationale for understanding which services will be lost or what quality lowered when an informal caregiver no longer is able to function. The introduction of life-course factors specifies the life-course stage where these losses will arise.

Task-specific theory has been used so far simply to state that when informal groups fail there will be a loss in amount or quality of informal services. The key to understanding the unique loss of services for each type of informal group is the proposition that different informal groups typically have different structures in an advanced industrial society (Crohan & Antonucci, 1989; Litwak, 1985). If they have different structures than the logic of the task-specific principles suggests, they will have different services; that is, a group can optimally manage services that match its structure. For instance, marital units typically have smallest size, continuous face-to-face proximity, long-term commitment, and common lifestyle. Kin groups typically have larger size and do not live in the same household or even neighborhood, nor do they necessarily have the same lifestyle. What they share with the marital unit is long-term commitment. Neighbors, by contrast, share with the marital unit continuous proximity, but typically do not have long-term commitments or common lifestyle, and they also tend to have larger size. Friendship groups do not necessarily have continuous face-to-face contact or long-term commitments, and they also are larger than the marital unit. What friends share in common with the marital unit is a lifestyle. The task-specific theory suggests that services can be divided by these same dimensions. Some services (e.g., regular bathing, toileting, feeding, etc.) normally require long-term commitment and continuous proximity, but not large size. They match the structure of the marital unit and consequently the task-specific theory states they can be managed optimally by members of the marital household. Other services require long-term commitments and large size, but not necessarily continuous proximity or common lifestyle, such as providing temporary financial help when the household unit is suffering from a cash flow problem, or temporary household help to supplement a spouse when acute illness disables a mate. These are services that match the typical kin structure. Some services are more suited to the neighborhood structure, because they require continuous proximity, as does the marital unit, but also require larger size and not necessarily long-term commitment or common lifestyle. Services typically having these dimensions are providing daily surveillance for young children playing outside the house, spotting potential burglars when residents are out of their home, spotting fires when residents are asleep, and providing emergency first aid for home accidents (Fischer, 1982; Litwak, 1985). Still other services require common lifestyles but not necessarily long-term commitments or continuous proximity, such as providing new retirees information on the "nitty gritty" of daily living or companions for leisure-time activities (Hanlon, 1982; Litwak, 1985; Rosow, 1967). These services share the same dimensions as friendship structures.

Life-Course Considerations in Use of Informal Groups

In this section we consider how life-course factors affect the availability of each informal group.

Availability of a Spouse

We hypothesized a curvilinear relationship between life course and the availability of a spouse. In the earliest stage the spouse is less likely to be available because the marriage bond has not had time to mature and the caregiving has to take place over the full range of life-course stages, whereas in the last stage the physical frailty of the spouse makes it difficult for him or her to provide help. Consequently we would predict that caregiving services, such as personal grooming and household services, will suffer more during these life course stages. Our hypotheses are presented in row 1, Table 4.3.

Availability of Key Kin

As indicated above, in the first stage of the life course the key kin helper tends to be the grandparent of the child. In the next stage the kin resources will be other children in the household and a lesser reliance on grandparents. When the child with a disability moves to the next stage, adolescence, other children in the household tend to back away from the helping role insofar as it conflicts with the social mandate that adult children should separate from the parental household. The grandparents bow out almost completely because of their increasing physical fragility and need to help their own spouse. As we move to people who become disabled at middle age and older, there is the beginning of a shift to adult children as caregivers. It is not strong because the spouses, typically, can manage at this stage. However, as we move to the older groups, the adult children become more and more the primary caregivers, and the key tensions arise from role reversals and aging of the grown child helpers. This analysis suggests gaps in the availability of kin when the disabled person reaches adolescence because the chief helpers, the grandparents and siblings, are not available. For those with Alzheimer's, the chief kin helpers tend to be adult children, and we hypothesize that kin will be least available for them in the oldest group. Because need increases among the very old, services delivered by kin, such as supplemental or temporary help in cooking and personal grooming, or financial help for cash flow problems, will rise on an absolute level but decline relative to need if our hypotheses are correct. As suggested in the first section of this chapter, *very different kin are hypothesized to be of help at different stages; consequently the types of stresses that must be addressed to ensure optimal kin services vary considerably.* Our hypotheses on kin are shown in row 2 in Table 4.3.

Friends

As indicated above, task-specific theory suggests friends in our society optimally provide services that require common lifestyles. Friendships can be based on different aspects of lifestyle that typically derive from occupation, gender, marital and parental status, ethnicity, and, in our analysis, chronic disabilities (Allan & Adams, 1989; Blau, 1961; Jackson, 1977). These in turn have complex relationships to life course that are beyond the scope of this chapter. [13] Consequently, to demonstrate the role of friendship groups, we simplify our analysis by considering only friends of primary caregivers who are also caregivers.

Life-course factors highlight the following: (a) the size of the potential human pool from which friends can be drawn, (b) the length of time given to locate friends, and (c) the robustness of the friends. It is our hypothesis that those at the beginning of the life course (e.g., parents who have an infant with disability) and those at the last stage of the life course (e.g., those 75 and older) are least likely to have friends who are providing similar caregiving services. The reasoning for the lack in the first stage is that the pool of potential friends is very small, and a person looking for friends, who are also caregivers has had little time to search for them. For those who are very old, the key caregiver—the spouse—is also old and his or her friends generally will be old as well (Blau, 1961; Litwak, 1985; Rosow, 1967). The pool of older people with health problems is large, but the people in it are very frail and cannot provide services that require physical resources. The number of personal friends with common caregiving problems is likely to be very small because of the high rates of mortality in this age bracket. The time the older person has to look for new friends is very short. Given the task-specific framework, the hypothesis is also advanced that *caregivers at both extremes of the life course are least likely to get information, advice, or instrumental help on the everyday nitty gritty of dealing with a cognitively limited person.* These hypotheses are shown in row 3 of Table 4.3.

Neighbors

We speculate that larger social norms make neighbors most available in the first and last phases of the life course. Because young children are so dependent, there normally are strong incentives to develop solid neighborhood ties so as to encourage neighbors to provide additional child surveillance. For the oldest groups, similar incentives arise because increasing physical frailty leads older people to limit their activities to the local neighborhood (Rosow, 1967). This makes them sensitive to the need to provide daily surveillance for each other. If these speculations are correct, then the task-specific framework suggests that caregivers

TABLE 4.3 Life-Course Determinants of the Availability of Informal Helping Groups

Type of Informal Group	Age of Persons With a Disability						
	Early Childhood, 1-5 years	Childhood, 6-11 years	Adolescence, 12-18 years	Young Adult, 19-39 years	Middle-aged, 40-64 years	Young-Old, 65-74 years	Old-Old, 75+ years
	The Probability of Various Informal Helping Groups Being Available and Type of Service						
Spouse: length of reciprocity and caregiving duration	Moderate probability of availability (high divorce rates); low probability of getting ADL[a] and IADL[b] services	Moderate to high probability of helping (low divorce rates); moderate to high ADL and IADL services	Moderate to high probability of helping; moderate to high ADL and IADL services	High probability of helping; high probability of ADL and IADL services	High probability of helping; high probability of ADL and IADL services	Moderate to high probability of helping (widowhood begins); moderate probability of ADL and IADL services	Low probability of helping (widowhood substantial); low probability of ADL and IADL services
Kin	Mental retardation: high probability of grandparent; high probability of getting supplemental ADL and IADL, financing for cash-flow problem	Mental retardation: high probability of grandparent plus other child in household; high probability of getting supplemental ADL and IADL plus financing for cash-flow problem	Mental retardation: beginning grandparent loss by overload and loss of other child by role separation conflict; moderate probability of getting supplemental ADL and IADL plus financing for cash-flow problems	Mental retardation: major loss of grandparent by role overload and major loss of sibling through role separation; low probability of getting supplemental ADL and IADL plus financing for cash flow	Early Alzheimer's: high probability of adult child availability with minor parent/child role reversal; high probability of supplemental ADL and IADL plus financing for cash-flow problem	Moderate Alzheimer's: moderate probability of adult child availability because of age with minor parent/child role reversal; high probability of supplemental ADL and IADL plus financing for cash-flow problem	Advanced Alzheimer's: moderate to low probability of adult child availability because of age with major parent/child role reversal; moderate to low probability of supplemental ADL and IADL plus financing for cash-flow problems

Friends: time to locate, size of pool, and robustness	Low availability; size of pool small and little time; low probability of advice on daily care	Moderate availability; moderate probability of advice on daily care	High availability; long time and robust group; high probability of advice on daily care	High availability; long time and robust group; high probability of advice on daily care	Moderate availability; short time but robust group; moderate probability of advice on daily care	Moderate availability; short time but robust group and larger pool; moderate to high probability of advice on daily care	Low availability; short time, large pool, but frail group; low probability of advice on daily care
Neighbors: norms on helping	High availability because high norms for helping; high probability of emergency first aid and safety against crime	High availability because high norms for helping; high probability of emergency first aid and safety against crime	Moderate availability because moderate norms for helping; moderate probability of emergency first aid and safety against crime	Low availability because low norms for helping; moderate probability of emergency first aid and safety against crime	Low availability because low norms for helping; moderate probability of emergency first aid and safety against crime	High availability because high norms for helping; high probability of emergency first aid and safety against crime	High availability because high norms for helping; high probability of emergency first aid and safety against crime

[a] ADL stands for activities of daily living and include such basic things as bathing, toileting, eating, grooming hair, and walking. In this and the other cells in this table the services are illustrative of the type of services managed by this informal group but are not exhaustive.

[b] IADL stands for instrumental activities of daily living and includes daily household activities such as cooking, housecleaning, laundry, shopping, and taking care of minor household services such as lawn mowing, replacing light bulbs, and so on.

in these two stages are more likely to have resources available for household emergencies, such as accidents or emergency shopping, as well as for greater protection against crime and household fires. Those in the middle stages of the life course are least likely to have these services. This hypothesis is represented in Table 4.3, row 4.

To summarize, though task-specific theory suggests that each type of social support is necessary, life-course factors suggest the types vary in their availability and services during the life course. If the hypotheses in Table 4.3 are correct, life-course factors make spouses and friends most available during the middle phases of the life course, but make neighbors least available during these periods. Kin for children with retardation are most likely to be available in the first stages and least available in adolescence and later periods. For those with Alzheimer's, kin are most likely to be available in the middle age and young-old periods and least available in the old-old period.

Underlying Dimensions of Chronic and Disabling Conditions

This analysis has looked at life-course factors with only two conditions of disability in mind: mental retardation and Alzheimer's disease. The complex nature of these conditions and the extreme differences in their manifestations in different individuals have not been taken into account for simplicity of presentation. In addition, the two conditions are taken as prototypical of conditions with similar characteristics: Alzheimer's as a progressive disease of the later years of the life course and mental retardation as a chronic and ongoing condition arising in the developmental period and lasting over the whole life course. As Pless and Pinkerton (1975) indicated a generation ago, and others have demonstrated (Hamburg, Eliott, & Parron, 1982; Jessop & Stein, 1985; Stein & Jessop, 1984), the underlying characteristics (or dimensions) of illness (i.e., the degree to which function is limited; whether the illness is progressive, static, or remitting; whether it is episodic or constant; whether it is associated with cognitive impairment or not; whether it is characterized by hospitalization or not; whether it is visible or invisible; whether it is stigmatized or not; etc.) are what affect the caregiving provided. Because different illnesses and disabilities may have different underlying characteristics, they may interact with life-course variables in different ways.

Consequently an analysis of the generic underlying categories of disability and illness for all conditions would supply a general solution to life-course effects on caregiving, but that is beyond the scope of this chapter. One quick illustration with the two conditions we have examined can highlight the need for future investigators to undertake such an effort. The above analysis suggests two very different caregiving paths for those who are born with mental retardation and those who suffer from dementia in old age. The child who is retarded typically will be devoid of spouse and children when he or she reaches old age and typically will have to rely on siblings who also are aging. By contrast, individuals who suffer from Alzheimer's in old age typically will have all of these support groups. The task-specific framework suggests two consequences: (a) that the mentally retarded who reach old age will be more deprived of informal household and personal services than those with Alzheimer's and (b) that the mentally retarded also are more likely to suffer from economic exploitation, social humiliation, and physical abuse.

SUMMARY AND CONCLUSION

The task-specific theory provides a bedrock proposition that, in advanced industrial societies such as the United States, formal organizations and informal ones play distinctive roles in the provision of services to the disabled. Furthermore, it states that different types of informal groups (that is, the spouse, kin, friends, neighbors, etc.) each provide distinct services. If care to disabled individuals is to be optimized, it is necessary to have a network that includes all of these groups because substitution leads to loss of services as well as reduced quality of care. What the analysis of life course suggests is that the social pressures to turn to these different caregiving groups, the tensions that arise from their use, and the resources available to these helping groups vary by stage in the life course. The life-course variables that encourage the use of formal organizations in the first stage are spousal and female role overload. The life-course variables that influence the use of formal organizations in the middle stages are physical maturation of the disabled, norms on child socialization and incest, and role overload of siblings and grandparents. By contrast, the life-course factors that lead to formal organizational help among disabled elderly are norms on adult privacy, parent/child role reversals, gender role reversals, and reemergence of spousal and female caregiving role overload, as well as continuing effects of physical maturation incest and privacy norms. The distinctive character of these life-course factors would be highlighted if the treatment modality necessary to deal with each of these tensions were considered. For example, the problem of treating spousal overload in the first phase would differ enormously from the problems of treating gender role reversals and violation of norms of privacy in the last stage. These hypotheses suggest that there are differential stresses on caregivers at different stages of the life course, leading to two major research questions. One is a systematic study to examine whether the hypothesized differential stresses on caregivers at each stage of the life course do in fact empirically occur. The other is to measure the comparative magnitude of these stresses so as to understand at what stage of the life course the greatest pressures arise for use of formal organizations. For instance, we have hypothesized that during the first stages of the life course the chief stresses and strains for caregivers of retarded individuals will come from spousal overload and female gender-role overload. The second question asks, which of these is most important?

The task-specific theory also suggests that use of formal organizations to substitute for informal groups will lead to an increase of the risks of social humiliation, staff neglect, and economic crimes. By contrast, reliance on informal caregivers will increase the risks of caregiver burden and physical abuse. The analysis of life-course factors further suggests that economic exploitation and social humiliation are more likely to arise in the later stages of the life course, whereas physical abuse for males may be more prevalent among infants and old people. Physical abuse for females is hypothesized to peak at three points: infancy, adolescence, and old age. Our hypotheses suggest the need for a research program that systematically compares the differential prevalence of economic, physical, social humiliation, and other types of abuse/neglect across the life course and their special ties to formal and informal groups.

In addition, it was pointed out that the task-specific theory generated hypotheses on the unique contribution of different types of informal groups at each stage of the life course. For instance, life-course factors are likely to weaken the role of the spouse and friends at the beginning and end of the life course and, consequently, lead to the loss of personal grooming and household services as well as the loss of knowledge and advice on everyday care of the disabled. The analysis of neighbors suggests a reverse pattern, with neighbors being most available in the first and last stages of the life course, which means, in the middle period, a loss of services characterized by emergency first aid and safety from crime. Kin are thought to be available during the first stages of the life course and drop off after adolescence, pick up again at middle age, and then drop off again among the old-old. This means that services such as supplemental household help for limited periods of time and short-term cash flow problems can best be provided during the first and late-middle stages of the life course. These hypotheses suggest a research program that examines the unique contributions of each type of informal group at each stage of the life course.

Finally, we have suggested the need to look at a variety of conditions aside from mental retardation and Alzheimer's so the underlying behavior problems that relate to caregiving can be identified and a more general statement of caregiving over the life course can be made.

The hypotheses we have presented are in some instances built on available evidence from cross-sectional studies. In some instances they are based on face validity propositions. In other cases they simply represent our best bets. We see the introduction of a task specific framework as providing a research agenda that elaborates past efforts to understand caregiving over the life course (Antonucci & Akiyama, 1987; Kahn & Antonucci, 1980).

NOTES

1. For instance, there is less chance for those whose onset of mental retardation is at infancy to get married and have children than for those whose cognitive disorder arises in old age. Consequently, Alzheimer's patients typically have both spouses and children available for caregiving in their old age. But mentally retarded children who reach old age typically do not have either spouses or children and at best must rely on siblings and secondary relatives. When people with mental retardation do get married and have children, they often require caregiving help in rearing their children that is not typical of those who are not mentally retarded.

2. Children who are mentally retarded appear to age earlier than the general public and therefore have a shorter lifespan (Eyman et al., 1987). Consequently policy makers will be less likely to have to deal with their distinctive pattern of caregiving in old age. But policy makers must confront the fact that there is an increasing lifespan among those with mental retardation, and their unique problems of caregiving are at the frontiers of research attention.

3. The prior analysis of structure suggests that although these dimensions provide extra resources, they are not optimal for the delivery of nontechnical services and still require supplemental help from informal groups (Litwak, 1985). Before considering those negative consequences, we examine the life-course variables that increase the caregiver's burden.

4. In this chapter we ignore what happens when norms conflict. For instance, the editors of this book pointed out that there is a potential conflict between incest/privacy norms and gender norms that dictate that daughters should help their chronically ill fathers

with bathing and toileting. The analysis of such conflicts and how they are resolved is worthy of further investigation.

5. This estimate is made by assigning a number rating of 1 to low, 2 to moderate, and 3 to high. The resulting sums for each stage of the life course (i.e., column) going from infancy to those 75 and older would be 13, 14.5, 18, 19, 17, 18, and 22.

6. The authors of this chapter do not agree on this section on abuse. The views in this section are reflective of Eugene Litwak and Heather J. Moulton and not their coauthor, Dorothy Jones Jessop.

7. We hypothesize that another dimension of formal organizations, limited commitment, which permits formal organizations to optimize services that require technical knowledge, tends to have a negative impact when a formal organization seeks to manage typical family services, the rationale being that some family services require long-term commitments by a single individual. This is very clear when infants are being socialized and cared for. It is also clear for people with mental retardation who live in community residences. Although the need for long-term commitments of an individual are not as obvious for older people who need family services, it is nevertheless true for them as well (Litwak, 1985). Consequently the hypothesis is advanced that the high turnover rates of staff of community residences and nursing homes do not simply reflect low wage scales and arduous work, but also are a structural feature of formal organizations. In addition, the training and administrative costs are not the only costs of this high rate of turnover, as there is also a loss in the quality of those services that require long-term commitments.

8. Not emphasized in studies of older people, but a very important topic in socialization of children, are the consequences of losing the nonstandardized elements of services. A notable series of studies suggested that standardized care of infants in hospital settings leads to lower I.Q. and higher emotional problems (Kahn & Antonucci, 1980). Presently hospital programs address these issues through child life programs. Litwak (1985) and Bowers (1988) also suggest significant losses in quality of services arising from standardized care, but for the most part researchers in the field of aging do not really differentiate between standardized and nonstandardized care and provide no data on this issue.

9. The traditional objection to the extensive use of such solutions has been cost, another critical dimension of formal organizations. This has raised a heated debate that has yet to be resolved.

10. This hypothesis would not deny that low pay also will lead to slack service. It simply notes that all things being equal, informal group members, motivated by internalized commitments of duty or affection, are less likely to express these forms of abuse. The hypothesis that staff of formal organizations are a major source of slack service seems to fly in the face of empirical reality for children and infants, where most of the cases of neglect arise from family members. The seeming paradox is quickly unraveled once it is understood that there are relatively few instances in which staff of formal organizations take over daily supervision of children and infants. If one were, however, to examine areas of life in which formal organizations play a more substantial role (e.g., young adults with retardation or older Alzheimer's patients) or look at the historical situations in which formal organizations played a larger role in caring for children with mental retardation, then we hypothesize that the percentage of cases of neglect would be higher among staff of formal organizations. To some extent the historical shift in the philosophy of placement of children with retardation from formal organizations to family settings (Janiecki & Wisniewski, 1985) was motivated by an understanding of the damage produced by the standardized care and neglect of economically motivated staff.

11. It is also possible that informal members who lack resources may react as the formal organizational individual might, that is, to simply reduce services, which will lead to neglect (Anderson, 1977). We hypothesize that this form of neglect will be different from that of the formal organizations in two respects: (a) It will be associated with limited resources rather than plentiful resources and economic incentives, and (b) it will be identified with greater feelings of guilt or caregiver burden. Formal organizations also have caregiver burden, but use somewhat different terminology: staff burnout. Our hypothesis suggests that members of the informal group are more likely to exhibit either problems of burden or physical agression than are staff of formal organizations.

12. If, however, we are thinking of adolescents with cognitive limitations so that their mental age is 4 or 5, questions can be raised about this hypothesis: Will the cognitively limited be treated more by their mental or their biological age?

13. We would see the following kinds of tensions and complexities arising between caregivers and friends based on noncaregiving roles, such as friends based on occupation, marital status, gender, ethnicity, and so on. First, the more time-consuming the caregiving tasks, the greater the tension in maintaining friendship ties with noncaregivers. Second, the dynamics of lifestyles based on other criteria have their own unique relationship to life course so that the tension between caregivers and friends who are not caregivers would alter depending on which lifestyle formed the basis for friendship. For instance, tensions in marital states might take place during the first years of marriage when the couples are learning to accommodate one another; during the birth of the first child, which radically alters the marital ties; at the empty nest period; if there is a divorce; and so on. The tensions that arise from occupation may or may not coincide with these marital tensions; that is, tensions may be produced by economic downturns that lead to unemployment. Alternatively, tensions may reflect career phases in which one is competing for better jobs, and this in turn may vary by occupation so factory workers see this as a phase in the early stages of the life course whereas professionals in bureaucracies may see it as lasting until middle age.

REFERENCES

Allan, G. A., & Adams, R. G. (1989). Aging and the structure of friendship. In R. Adams & R. Blieszner (Eds.), *Older adult friendship: Structure and process* (pp. 45-64). Newbury Park, CA: Sage.

Anderson, M. (1977). The impact on family relations for the elderly of changes since Victorian times in government income-maintenance provision. In E. Shanas & M. B. Sussman (Eds.), *Family, bureaucracy, and the elderly* (pp. 36-59). Durham, NC: Duke University Press.

Antonucci, T. C., & Akiyama, H. (1987). Social networks in adult life and a preliminary examination of the convoy model. *Journal of Gerontology, 42*(5), 519-527.

Birenbaum, A. (1971). The mentally retarded child in the home and family life cycle. *Journal of Health and Social Behavior, 12,* 196-205.

Blacher, J., Nihira, K., & Meyers, C. (1987). Characteristics of home environment of families with mentally retarded children: Comparison across levels of retardation. *American Journal of Mental Deficiency, 91,* 313-320.

Blakeslee, J. A., Hunt, A. R., Thankachan, G., & Torell, G. A. (1986). *Physical restraints: A dilemma in long-term care* (Symposium proceedings). Presented at the American Association of Homes for the Aging Annual Conference, New York, and Gerontological Society of America Annual Conference, Chicago.

Blau, Z. (1961). Structural constraints of friendships in old age. *American Sociological Review, 26,* 428-438.

Bould, S., Sandborn, B., & Reif, L. (1989). *Eighty-five plus: The oldest old.* Belmont, CA: Wadsworth.

Bowers, B. J. (1988). Family perceptions of care in a nursing home. *The Gerontologist, 28,* 361-368.

Bristol, M. (1979). Maternal coping with autistic children: The effect of child characteristics and interpersonal support (Doctoral dissertation, University of North Carolina at Chapel Hill). *Dissertation Abstracts International, 40,* 3943A-3944A.

Butler, R. N. (1975). *Why survive? Being old in America.* New York: Harper & Row.

Chiriboga, D. A., Weiler, P. G., & Nielsen, K. (1990). The stress of caregivers. In D. E. Biegel & A. Blum (Eds.), *Aging and caregivers: Theory, research, and policy* (pp. 121-138). Newbury Park, CA: Sage.

Crohan, S. E., & Antonucci, T. C. (1989). Friends as a source of social support in old age. In R. G. Adams & R. Blieszner (Eds.), *Older adult friendships: Structure and process* (pp. 129-146). Newbury Park, CA: Sage.

Donovan, A. (1988). Family stress and ways of coping with adolescents who have handicaps: Maternal perceptions. *American Journal on Mental Retardation, 92,* 502-509.

Farber, B. (1959). *Effects of a severely retarded child on family integration.* Monographs of the Society for Research in Child Development, Vol. 24, No. 2. Lafayette, IN: Society for Research in Child Development.

Fischer, C. S. (1982). *To dwell among friends: Personal networks in town and city.* Chicago: University of Chicago Press.

Ford, C. V., & Sbordone, R. J. (1980). Attitudes of psychiatrists toward elderly patients. *American Journal of Psychiatry, 1237,* 571-575.

Francis, J. (1989). Using restraints in the elderly because of fear of litigation. *New England Journal of Medicine, 320,* 870-871.

Freeman, I. C. (1990). Developing systems that promote autonomy. In R. A. Kane & A. L. Caplan (Eds.), *Everyday ethics: Resolving dilemmas in nursing home life* (pp. 291-305). New York: Springer.

Groce, N. E. (1988). In M. B. Straus (Ed.), *Abuse and victimization across the life span* (pp. 223-239). Baltimore, MD: Johns Hopkins University Press.

Hamburg, D. A., Eliott, G. R., & Parron, D. J. (1982). *Health and behavior: Frontiers of research in the biobehavioral sciences.* Washington, DC: National Academy Press.

Hanlon, M. D. (1982). Primary group assistance during unemployment. *Human Organizations, 41,* 156-161.

Haug, M. R. (1988). Professional client relationships and the older patient. In S. K. Steinmetz (Ed.), *Family and support systems across the life span* (pp. 225-242). New York: Plenum.

House, J., Landis, K. R., & Umberson, D. (1988). Social relationships and health. *Science, 241,* 540-545.

Jackson, R. M. (1977). Social structure and friendship choice. In C. S. Fischer, R. M. Jackson, C. A. Stueve, K. Gerson, & L. M. Jones with M. Baldassare (Eds.),

Networks and places: Social relations in the urban setting (pp. 39-58). New York: Free Press.

Jessop, D. J., & Stein, R. E. K. (1985). Uncertainty and its relation to the psychological and social correlates of chronic illness in children. *Social Science and Medicine,* *20*(10), 993-999.

Kahn, R., & Antonucci, T. C. (1980). Convoys over the life course: Attachment, roles and social support. In P. B. Baltes & O. R. Brim (Eds.), *Life span development and behavior* (pp. 253-286). New York: Academic Press.

Kane, R. A., Caplan, A. L., Freeman, I. C., Aroskar, M. A., & Urv-Wong, E. K. (1990). Avenues to appropriate autonomy: What next? In R. A. Kane & A. L. Caplan (Eds.), *Everyday ethics: Resolving dilemmas in nursing home life* (pp. 306-318). New York: Springer.

Kaplan, A. G. (1988). How normal is normal development? Some connections between adult development and the roots of abuse and victimization. In M. B. Straus (Ed.), *Abuse and victimization across the life span* (pp. 127-139). Baltimore, MD: Johns Hopkins University Press.

Katz, E., & Lazarsfeld, P. F. (1955). *Personal influence.* Glencoe, IL: Free Press.

Kosberg, J. I. (1983). The importance of attitudes on the interaction between health care providers and geriatric populations. *Interdisciplinary Topics in Gerontology, 17,* 132-143.

Litwak, E. (1985). *Helping the elderly: Complementary roles of informal networks and formal systems.* New York: Guilford.

Longino, C. (1988). Who are the oldest Americans? *The Gerontologist, 28,* 515-523.

Mayhew, L. (1970). Ascription in modern societies. In E. O. Laumann, P. M. Siegel, & R. W. Hodge (Eds.), *Logic of social hierarchies* (pp. 308-323). Chicago: Markham.

McHutchion, E., & Morse, J. (1989). Releasing restraints: A nursing dilemma. *Journal of Gerontological Nursing, 15*(2), 16-21.

Messeri, P., Litwak, E., & Silverstein, M. (1993, June). Choosing optimal support groups: A review and reformulation. *Journal of Health and Social Behavior 34(22),* 122-137.

Nathanson, C. A. (1977). Sex roles as variables in preventive health behavior. *Journal of Community Health, 3,* 142-155.

Noelker, L. S., & Bass, D. M. (1989). Home care for elderly persons: Linkages between formal and informal caregivers. *Journals of Gerontology, 44,* S63-S70.

Penning, M. J. (1990). Receipt of assistance by elderly people: Hierarchical selection and task specificity. *The Gerontologist, 30,* 220-227.

Pless, I. B., & Pinkerton, P. (1975). *Chronic childhood disorder: Promoting patterns of adjustment.* Chicago: Yearbook Medical Publishers.

Rosow, I. (1967). *The social integration of the aged.* New York: Free Press.

Seltzer, M., & Krauss, M. (1989). Aging parents with adult mentally retarded children: Family risk factors and sources of support. *American Journal on Mental Retardation, 94,* 303-312.

Stein, R. E. K., & Jessop, D. J. (1984). Does pediatric home care make a difference for children with chronic illness? Findings from the pediatric ambulatory care treatment study. *Pediatrics, 73*(6), 845-853.

Straus, M. B. (1988). Abused adolescents. In M. B. Straus (Ed.), *Abuse and victimization across the life span* (pp. 107-126). Baltimore, MD: Johns Hopkins University Press.

Strauss, A., & Corbin, J. M. (1988). *Shaping a new health care system*. San Francisco: Jossey-Bass.

Umberson, D. (1987). Family status and health behaviors: Social control as a dimension of social integration. *Journal of Health and Social Behavior, 28*, 306-319.

United States Code Annotated. (1992). *The public health and welfare: Title 42 USCA 139r (c)(1)(A)(ii)*. St. Paul, MN: West Publishing.

Waldron, I. (1982). An analysis of cause of sex differences in morbidity and mortality. In W. R. Gove & G. R. Carpenter (Eds.), *The fundamental connection between nature and nurture* (pp. 69-116). Lexington, MA: D. C. Heath.

Warren, D. I. (1968). Power, visibility, and conformity in formal organizations. *American Sociological Review, 33*, 951-970.

Weber, M. (1947). *The theory of social and economic organization* (A. M. Henderson & T. Parsons, Eds. & Trans.). New York: Oxford University Press.

Wilson, V. (1990). The consequences of elderly wives caring for disabled husbands: Implications for practice. *Social Work, 35*(5), 417-421.

Winik, L., Zetlin, A., & Kaufman, S. (1985). Adult mildly retarded persons and their parents: The relationship between involvement and adjustment. *Applied Research on Mental Retardation, 6*, 409-419.

Zarit, S. H., Todd, P. A., & Zarit, J. M. (1986). Subjective burden of husbands and wives as caregivers: A longitudinal study. *The Gerontologist, 26*, 260-266.

Zelizer, V. (1985). *Pricing the priceless child: The changing social value of children*. New York: Basic Books.

PART II

Illness and Life Stage: Challenges for Caregiving

5

Caregiving and Children

JOAN M. PATTERSON
BARBARA J. LEONARD

Families caring for children with special medical needs are normal families in a nonnormal situation. Tension between normality (trying to achieve it, determining what it is) and nonnormality (the special challenges and extra demands that are chronic) is one of the many polarities creating a struggle for these families. And like life struggles generally faced by individuals and families, it strengthens and enhances some, and it overwhelms and undermines others. The challenge to health professionals is, first, to identify and describe those factors associated with competence and resilience in children with illness and in their parents and families. Second, there is a need to promote those factors through education of health providers, through prevention programs and clinical interventions with families, and through public policies, all of which provide the supports these families and their children need to develop competently.

When we consider caregiving across the lifespan, one aspect unique to children as the recipients of care is that there are few, if any, alternatives other than care by parents at home. U.S. society needs and expects parents to care for their children and to socialize them for adult roles. This is the family's responsibility—whether children are sick or well, whether their needs are normative, catastrophic, or chronic. Divorcing children is not an option (although sometimes one parent may

AUTHORS' NOTE: Preparation of this chapter was supported by the National Institute on Disability and Rehabilitation Research (Grant #H133890012) and special project funds from the University of Minnesota School of Public Health. The authors thank Janet Titus and Gayle Geber for their contributions in the preparation of this chapter.

leave and not have contact); there is no expectation that children can live independently, and there is a strong movement away from institutional care. If parents cannot provide care at home, even with help, termination of parental rights so the child can be placed in alternative living facilities is often the only option. Very few parents opt for this extreme legal severance of family ties and, instead, continue providing care, often when the care needs are extensive and the sources of formal and informal help are inadequate, unpredictable, or, worse, a source of added strain for them.

The purpose of this chapter is to examine issues associated with providing home care for children with chronic illnesses and disabilities. First, the impacts on parents, siblings, and family well-being of providing home care at the child-rearing stage of the life cycle are discussed. Second, the unique challenges and hardships of this kind of home care are emphasized. Finally, *mediating factors* (resources and coping behaviors), which help buffer this added strain and burden for families, are presented.

These three themes are discussed by drawing on the findings from a study conducted at the University of Minnesota, in which the impact on families of caring for medically fragile children at home has been examined. An effort is made in this chapter to provide an in-depth discussion of the qualitative findings of this study. Quantitative results have been reported elsewhere (see citations below).

Medically fragile children are at the extreme end of the continuum of children with chronic conditions because their care needs are more extensive, usually very specialized, and often require complex medical equipment to sustain life. Although this population is unique, especially as recipients of home care, social scientists have found that studying the extreme case often calls attention to factors overlooked with those experiencing less severe conditions. If our understanding is increased, the relevance of such findings for less critically ill populations of children can be tested.

WHO ARE MEDICALLY FRAGILE CHILDREN?

The definition of "medically fragile" used in this study included children who (a) needed a medical device to compensate for the loss of a vital body function and who required substantial daily skilled nursing care to avert death or further disability (Office of Technology Assessment [OTA], 1987) or (b) did not need technological equipment but required skilled nursing care. During the past decade there has been a dramatic increase in the number of these children being discharged from hospitals to home care (Office of Technology Assessment, 1987). This trend is due to several factors:

1. Advances in medicine have saved the lives of children who formerly would have died and now live but require long-term care.
2. Improvements in the miniaturization of medical equipment have made it possible to transfer many of these children home.
3. A competitive health-care climate has led to cost-containment policies encouraging or requiring parents to provide care at home to save money for third-party payers.
4. There has been increasing recognition and advocacy for children to live in the least restrictive environment to optimize developmental outcomes.
5. Parents themselves want their children at home (Bock, Lierman, Ahmann, & Weinstock, 1983; Burr, Guyer, Tordes, Abrahams, & Chiodo, 1983; Frates, Splaingard, Smith, & Harrison, 1985; Goldberg, Faure, Vaughn, Snarski, & Seleny, 1984).

Although estimates of prevalence are lacking or very crude, OTA estimated in 1987 that there were between 2,300 and 17,000 such children in the United States (Office of Technology Assessment, 1987). However, based on a census conducted in Massachusetts, it was estimated that there may be at least twice that number (Palfrey et al., 1991). Although the numbers may be small relative to the total population of chronically ill children in the United States, the cost of their care is very high. In 1987, estimates of direct costs of care provided in hospitals ranged from $15,000 to $52,000 per month, compared to $389 to $7,425 per month when care is provided at home (Office of Technology Assessment, 1987). The savings for home care are due largely to the substitution of parental nursing care for some or all of professional nursing care. However, not reflected in these dollar savings are the potential costs to families—the social and lost-opportunity costs, the costs to the health of parents and siblings, and family financial costs.

Although early clinical reports have suggested that medically fragile children do as well or better at home (Burr et al., 1983; Frates et al., 1985; Goldberg et al., 1984), reports on the impact on the family from providing this level of care are only beginning to emerge. Aday, Aitken, and Wegener (1988), in an evaluation of three home-care programs for ventilator-assisted children, reported moderate levels of caregiver distress.

In our earlier reports of the impact on parents of caring for technology-assisted children at home, high levels of psychological distress were found (Leonard, Brust, & Nelson, 1993). Quint, Chesterman, and Crain (1990), in a study of ventilator-supported children, suggest that parent coping (especially for mothers) may decline over time. These early findings raise concern about the *long-term* impact on families of providing this level of care.

STUDY PROCEDURES

Study Participants

The study was comprised of 48 families in two midwestern states with a medically fragile child living at home. The parents were surveyed by interview and self-report questionnaires at two different times: initially in 1986-1987 (Time 1) and again 2.5 years later (Time 2). At Time 1, 75 families were invited to participate in the study. These families were identified in two ways. First, all families of medically fragile children whose home-care services were funded by the model Waiver Program in these two states were invited to participate. The model Waiver Program is a federal Medicaid program that waives parental income in determining eligibility and is administered through the states by state-determined criteria. Second, 16 additional families caring for medically fragile children were identified through equipment vendors and a support group. Of the 75 invited to participate, 14 declined. Reasons for nonparticipation were impossible to determine because of the agencies' desire to maintain confidentiality of families served. The response rate at Time 1 was 81%.

At Time 2, 48 families (78.7% of the original 61) agreed to participate in the follow-up study. For the 13 families who did not respond to our letter inviting participation in the follow-up, the agencies coordinating their care helped us determine that 5 of these children had died, 1 was terminal, 1 had a parent who was terminally ill, 1 parent could not speak English (and no interpreter was available), and 5 were from families described as less stable because they frequently missed clinic visits and were hard to contact. The sample described here is the 48 families for whom there was data at both Time 1 and Time 2.

The characteristics of the children and their families are presented in Table 5.1. The children's average age was 6.25 years at Time 2; 62.5%

were female. Their diagnoses were varied and included multiple congenital anomalies, bronchopulmonary dysplasia, and central nervous system diseases. Seventy percent of these children fit one of OTA's defined levels of technology dependence, with 25% on ventilators, 6.2% on prolonged nutritional or drug IVs, and 37.5% needing other respiratory or nutritional support. Twenty-nine percent did not need technological equipment, but required skilled nursing care. The long-term prognosis for 43.7% of the children was hopeful; for another half, the prognosis was uncertain. The average length of time families had been providing care was 4.7 years.

The median family income was $30,001-$40,000. Twenty-five percent of the mothers and 36.5% of the fathers had completed college or more. All fathers but one were employed, and 65% of the mothers were employed. Eighty-five percent of the parents in this sample were in their first marriage. The representativeness of this sample was impossible to determine because state and national data on the size and characteristics of this population of children are only beginning to emerge. However, it appears that the present sample may be more representative of stable, functional families, given their education, income, and marital status.

Theoretical Framework

The theoretical basis for the follow-up study was the Family Adjustment and Adaptation Response Model (Patterson, 1988), in which systems and developmental concepts are integrated with family stress theory. The outcome of the stress process is family adaptation, conceptualized as the health and role functioning of individual members and the health and functioning of the family unit. The level of adaptation is based on the degree to which the family system can balance the demands it faces (e.g., from stressor events, chronic hardships, and ongoing role strains) with capabilities for meeting the demands. Capabilities include resources of the individual, the family, and the community and coping behaviors of family members. The meanings attributed to both demands and capabilities help to mediate this balance.

Although this study was not a test of the full model, it guided the identification of which critical child, family, and community variables influence a family's adaptation to chronic stress. Parents' psychological health status and the aggregated physical health status of all family members each were used as partial indicators of adaptation. Independent variables included demands such as functional dependence of the

TABLE 5.1 Characteristics of Medically Fragile Children and Their Parents
            (*N* = 48)

Child		
Age	Mean = 6.25 years (range, 3-19.8 years)	
Gender	Female = 62.5%, male = 37.5%	
Time on home care	Mean = 4.77 years (range, 2.33-17.67 years)	
Primary diagnosis	Syndromes	28.0%
	Central nervous system disease	28.0%
	Multiple anomalies	22.0%
	Bronchopulmonary dysplasia	12.0%
	Spinal cord injury	5.0%
	Degenerative hereditary disease	5.0%
Technology level	I Ventilator	25.0%
	II Total parenteral nutrition	6.2%
	III Oxygen/gastrostomy	37.5%
	IV Apnea monitor/catheter	2.1%
	V None	29.2%
Prognosis	Hope for survival	43.7%
	Not sure	50.0%
	No hope for survival	6.2%
Parents		
Marital status	Married once	85.1%
	Remarried	11.5%
	Widowed/divorced	3.4%
Family income	<$20,000	15.2%
	$20,001-30,000	28.3%
	$30,001-40,000	23.9%
	$40,001-50,000	17.4%
	>$50,001	15.2%

child, caregiver burden, financial burden, hardships of home care, and
strain with home-care providers. Capabilities included family resources
of cohesion, organization, and lack of conflict; parents' sense of mastery of illness demands; social support; and hours of home-care ser-

TABLE 5.1 Continued

		Mothers	Fathers
Employment	Not employed	35.4%	2.4%
	Employed	64.5%	97.6%
Education	<High school	2.1%	2.4%
	High school graduate	31.3%	19.5%
	Some college or voc-tech	41.7%	36.6%
	College graduate	14.6%	19.2%
	>College graduate	10.4%	22.0%

vices. We expected that families who had more perceived capabilities relative to their perceived demands would show better adaptation.

Data Sources

Both quantitative and qualitative methods were used in this study. The use of standardized scales for assessing several of these variables allowed for comparison of study families' scores with reported norms using t test analyses. In addition, given the relative newness of home care for medically fragile children, we used qualitative methods to inductively determine the nature of this experience for families. Parents' responses to open-ended questions asking them to describe these variables were analyzed qualitatively by identifying cross-cutting themes and then tabulating the frequency each theme was reported across all families. In addition to answering the mailed questionnaires for the above data, each parent was interviewed separately by telephone (audio-recorded) to obtain additional subjective impressions of the impact of home care on their family. In addition to the qualitative analyses, results using the scales described below are reported in this chapter.

Functional status of the medically fragile child was assessed by mother's report of the child's ability to perform 14 self-care tasks (such as dressing, feeding, toileting, etc.). Mother's reports of the degree of dependency (on a Likert scale of 4 to 1) were summed across the 14 tasks. Because mothers had completed this scale regarding their child at Time 1, change in functional status could be calculated.

Parents' psychological distress was assessed using the Brief Symptom Inventory (BSI) (Derogatis & Spencer, 1982). The BSI has 53 Likert-scaled items for assessing nine aspects of psychological distress (e.g., depression, anxiety, hostility). The global score has good reliability and validity, and there are male and female nonpsychiatric norms available.

Sibling functioning was assessed by asking one parent to report on a 5-point Likert scale (from excellent to very poor) the quality of each sibling's social relationships, school performance, coping ability, and overall happiness.

Impact on the family scales (Stein & Reissman, 1980) were used to assess four types of impact of caring for a chronically ill child: financial burden, relationship disruption, personal strain, and mastery of illness demands. These scales have good internal reliabilities (alphas range from .60 to .86) and normative data are available.

HOW ARE THESE CHILDREN
AND THEIR FAMILIES DOING?

The Medically Fragile Child

When parents were asked to report how well their child was doing now, compared to 2.5 years ago, two thirds (66.7%) reported "better," and only 6.2% reported "worse" (27.1% were the same; see Table 5.2). In examining their level of functional status, that is, the help they needed for activities of daily living, there was improvement for more than half (56.9%), with 25% showing considerable improvement. Thirty percent stayed the same, and only 14% became more functionally dependent than they were at Time 1. Thus, for the sample retained at follow-up, the children appeared to be doing as well or better when studied 2.5 years later.

Parents

What about their parents? How did providing this level of care affect parents' mental health, their physical health, and their ability to function in their work roles? One of the primary concerns prompting interest in this follow-up study was the level of parental distress assessed at

TABLE 5.2 Parent-Reported Changes in Medically Fragile Child's Health Status (*N* = 48)

In past 2 years, is child:	Worse	6.2%
	Same	27.1%
	Better	66.7%
Functional status*	Time 1: Mean = 32.09 (range 17-39)	
	Time 2: Mean = 28.23 (range 13-39)	
Change in functional status*	Got a lot worse	2.3%
(from Time 1 to Time 2)	Got worse	11.3%
	Stayed same	29.5%
	Got better	31.9%
	Got a lot better	25.0%

*Functional status was measured as the amount of help (on a scale of 1-4) needed by the child for activities of daily living. High score means more help was needed.

Time 1. We used the BSI (Derogatis & Spencer, 1982) to measure symptoms of psychological distress. Fifty-eight percent of the mothers and 67% of the fathers in the 61 families studied at Time 1 scored in the "case" range on the BSI, which is a criterion cutoff suggesting that their level of distress symptoms warrants psychiatric intervention (Leonard, Brust, & Patterson, 1991; Leonard et al., 1993). When examined by family, 75% of families had one or both parents seriously distressed. It was our expectation that parents' distress would lessen over time as they adapted to the chronic demands of home care. Or, if distress remained high for some, we expected there would be additional negative consequences, such as physical illness or diminished work functioning.

In the follow-up study 2.5 years later, half of the parents (40% of the fathers and 55% of the mothers) showed some improvement in distress scores (Leonard, Patterson, Nelson, Titus, & Sielaff, 1991). However, when examined by the "case" definition of distress, less than 20% of mothers or fathers improved enough to move out of the Time 1 "case" range (see Table 5.3). Primarily, 75% of parents did not change in their case classification. Thirty-seven percent of mothers and 50% of fathers were cases at both times, and 37% of mothers and 27% of fathers were not a case at either time. Although approximately half of the parents showed higher distress scores over time, only 3 mothers and 2 fathers

TABLE 5.3 Two-Year Changes in Number of Parents Classified in Case
Range on Psychological Distress

	Time 2 No Case	Time 2 Case*
Fathers		
Time 1, no case	9 (26.5%)	2 (5.9%)
Time 1, case*	6 (17.6%)	17 (50.0%)
Mothers		
Time 1, no case	16 (37.2%)	3 (7.0%)
Time 1, case*	8 (18.6%)	16 (37.2%)

*Case means above the 90th percentile on the Brief Symptom Inventory (Derogatis & Spencer, 1982).

got enough worse to be classified as "case" at Time 2. When mothers' scores and fathers' scores were paired, 69% of the families had one or both parents in the case range at Time 2.

Given that half of these parents were in the distressed "case" range at Time 2, we expected an associated negative impact on physical health and work functioning. However, only for mothers was there a statistically significant relationship between symptoms of distress and changes in physical health (Patterson, Leonard, & Titus, 1992). Twenty percent of mothers and 25% of fathers did report their physical health to be worse in the past year; one third said it was the same; and approximately 40% said it had improved. Regarding work impact, only for fathers were symptoms of distress associated with a decline in perceived quality of performance at work ($r = -.37, p < .05$). Thirty-nine percent of fathers reported that the major way having a medically fragile child impacted their work was in decreased ability to concentrate. It is interesting to note that for fathers, greater distress also was associated with missing *fewer* days of work ($r = -.32, p < .05$). Working more hours was reported by 32% of fathers, usually because of the added financial burdens associated with the child's needs and because mothers often stopped working or worked part-time because of needing to care for the child.

Based on these findings, it would appear that more than half of these parents are seriously distressed after several years of providing home care ($X = 4.8$ years, range 2.3 years − 17.7 years), but this distress is not associated with physical illness and it only moderately has impacted work performancè for fathers. This would suggest that there may be important mediators of this chronic distress for parents.

Siblings

There were 59 siblings represented in these 48 families. From the qualitative analyses, parents described in about equal proportion the positive and negative impacts on siblings (Leonard, Titus, & Patterson, 1991). On the positive side, parents emphasized that their other children developed increased understanding, compassion, and tolerance for children with disabilities as well as for people in general. In addition, the added demands at home necessitated their helping out more and resulted in a greater sense of responsibility, maturity, and competence. Many parents were very emotional talking about how much they appreciated their other children, especially their positive attitudes, emotional support, and tangible help.

On the negative side, some parents reported that their other children experienced social isolation because they had to help at home more, the family couldn't go places with them, there was less money, or their peers teased them about the disability. Some siblings were jealous of the attention given to the special-needs child and the fact that they got less. Other parents reported that their child's emotional well-being suffered due to greater apprehension, worry, and sadness. From a small number of parents (less than 10%) there were reports of school and behavior problems among siblings.

When parents were asked to rate their other children's social relationships, school performance, coping ability, and happiness, less than 9% rated any of these dimensions as "poor" (see Table 5.4). Sixty percent to 85% saw their children as good to excellent in these areas. In many ways, these positive, high ratings were not consistent with the anxiety, concern, and worry about their children's well-being expressed by these parents through the open-ended questions. These conflicting findings raise an interesting methodological question about the meaning of standardized quantitative ratings relative to qualitative data. Perhaps parents are willing to volunteer information about their children's problems but much less willing to transfer those concerns into lower ratings about their child's well-being when they are provided with a structured item that may seem like a label to them.

Overwhelmingly, parents were concerned about the lack of time to spend with other children and the loss of normalcy in family life.

TABLE 5.4 Parents' Rating of Siblings' Functioning (*N* = 59)

Area of Functioning	Good to Excellent Percentage	Okay Percentage	Poor Percentage
Social relationships	83.1	11.8	5.1
School performance	84.1	11.4	4.5
Coping ability	61.0	30.5	8.5
Happiness	62.7	30.5	6.8

Parents calculated an average of 5 hours per day caring for their special-needs child and 2.2 hours caring for their other children individually (Leonard, Titus, & Patterson, 1991). They reported sometimes doing compensatory things to make up for these losses, and they worried that these things might spoil their children. Parents seemed to grieve most for what their children were missing, long before they acknowledged the burden on themselves. The overall impression that remains, however, is that most of these children were coping quite well, and were resilient and strong, but that the family climate was heavy with burdens, making for sadness and worry.

Impact on the Marriage and Family

Similar to the ways parents described the impact on siblings, there were about equal numbers of positive and negative descriptions of the impact on the marriage and family. How the marriage was affected seemed to go in tandem with how the parents described family impact. The most consistent positive descriptions made by parents were that their child's condition had brought them closer together as a couple and a family, had created a stronger bond, and had built a stronger sense of family. They emphasized that they appreciated each other more, especially regarding little things, but also regarding the skills and competence of other members of the family. Working together to share the tasks and responsibilities also was emphasized. For some, communication and shared decision-making skills improved. Because they had less time to do things together, they valued more that which they did have. Many were careful to schedule and plan time for each other and the family because otherwise it would not happen.

In contrast, there were nearly as many comments describing the negative side—the ways in which caring for a medically fragile child had taken its toll on their marriages and families. The intense, chronic demands for care led to exhaustion, tension, irritability, and little or no time together. There were more arguments, conflicts about who should provide care, about making decisions, about dealing with professionals, and so on. A couple's different styles of grieving and coping sometimes caused resentment. In many families the high care demands necessitated greater role specialization within the family, especially due to mothers being unable to work outside the home and fathers having to work more because of the financial burdens. The more traditional role structure in these families was, of course, counter to the present trend toward egalitarian marriages with greater role sharing. Because the care needs were so intense, some mothers focused all of their energy on the special-needs child while fathers tried to attend to other children in the family. Although many mothers acknowledged their husbands' support and help, mothers were the ones primarily responsible for child care. Some greatly resented this, and others saw no alternative. As parents described this role structure, they did not necessarily prefer it, but saw little choice.

In addition to these qualitative analyses of family impact, parents' scores on the Impact on Family Scales (Stein & Reissman, 1980) were examined. These scales assess four kinds of impact: financial burden; the negative impact on and disruption of social and family relationships; personal strain; and, on the positive side, the parents' sense of mastery of illness demands. The scores of parents in the sample were compared to reported scale norms. On all of these scales the parents in this sample scored higher (see Table 5.5), indicating a greater impact. Particularly noteworthy is the significant difference on the mastery scale, suggesting that the parents in this study were coping very well. In the interviews parents talked about this positive impact on themselves. Many described changes such as becoming more assertive, compassionate, optimistic, tolerant, and interested in disability issues. Learning the technical care their child needed; dealing with agencies, insurers, and providers; and keeping track of schedules, bills, and reimbursements were all challenges many parents mastered. The result was increased competence and a sense of mastery.

WHAT ARE THE HARDSHIPS OF HOME CARE?

In addition to being tested on standardized scales, parents were asked to describe the hardships in their own words. The qualitative analyses resulted

TABLE 5.5 *T*-Tests of Means for Impact on Family Scales

Scale	Normative Mean	Mothers Mean (SD)	T-Test	Fathers Mean (SD)	T-Test
Economic impact	10.4	11.6 (2.53)	2.91*	10.7 (1.92)	0.73
Relationship disruption	22.1	24.4 (3.39)	2.92*	24.4 (3.25)	2.76*
Personal strain	16.6	18.4 (2.69)	3.04*	16.8 (2.80)	0.22
Mastery of illness	9.9	15.2 (2.50)	13.61**	15.1 (1.97)	13.98**

*p < .01
**p < .001

in four major categories of hardships: losses, problems with services, care and parenting strains, and added family strains (see Table 5.6).

Losses

The loss of family privacy was the number one hardship, identified by more than one third of this sample. This loss emerged from the presence of paid providers caring for the child in the home—nurses, nursing assistants, and home health aides. For the most part families wanted and needed this help, but they lost something most people take for granted. Although no parent used these words, this loss of privacy can be viewed as family boundary invasion (Boss, 1987). The degree of invasion varied depending on the skill and personality of the providers, the number of hours they were present in the home, parents' assertiveness, the size of the house, and so on. There was also boundary ambiguity depending upon the relationship developed with providers— were they "part of the family" as some parents warmly described?

The issue of privacy or boundary invasion is critical for understanding family functioning and the parent-professional relationship—whether the context is home care or any other service setting. It is important to remember that a boundary is what sets a system apart from its context, making it a separate entity. Well-functioning family systems have semipermeable boundaries, allowing for a flow of persons, goods, and information in and out. Normatively, each family sets the rules governing its boundaries. However, vulnerable families, who have greater needs than their internal resources can meet, often lose some or all control of their boundaries when they seek assistance from public programs. If a family's boundaries become too eroded, the family loses

TABLE 5.6 Frequency of Parent-Reported Hardships Associated With Caring for a Medically Fragile Child (in percentages)

	Mothers (N = 46)	*Fathers (N = 40)*
Losses		
Loss of privacy	35	20
Loss of spontaneity, normal family life	35	33
Loss of time for other family members, spouse, self, friends	39	43
Lost work opportunities	17	5
Problems with services		
Problems with care providers in the home	26	18
Problems finding services, determining eligibility, hassles with payers	33	20
Problems with school programs, staff	13	5
Problems with technical equipment	17	8
Care and parenting strains		
Strains of constant care needs, making decisions	17	45
Worry about future of child and family	9	15
Grief regarding child's disability, suffering, losses	24	18
Family strains		
Strain in marriage and family	20	3
Personal symptoms of distress	17	13
Strain in finances	28	28

its identity, integrity, and sense of itself and ultimately disintegrates. This, then, is a major challenge for providers of care: how to provide service, help, and care for the family *without* destroying their boundaries—or stated another way, without destroying their integrity, their identity, and their ability to control their own destiny. Families should be empowered to remain in control. Many providers of care, particularly home care, do not recognize this. They act on the belief that they are professionally responsible for that child (even if this is the home instead of the hospital) and sometimes get into control battles with parents about who should do what or how it should be done. Some even go beyond the child and try to manage others in the family, believing this is in the child's best interest. Perhaps they are right, and it would be better for the child, but the issue of who is in charge is the transcending issue and must be attended to if parents and professionals are genuinely going to work collaboratively in providing care to the child. In addition to developing the requisite skills for providing competent care, this is the most critical training issue for home care providers today. In many ways, the ramifications go beyond home care and have relevance for all helping relationships.

The other losses parents identified included the loss of spontaneity and normal family life. They couldn't pick up and go; complicated arrangements had to be made—either to take the child along, which may have been a greater hassle than it was worth for small outings, or to arrange respite care or babysitting, which, if available, often had to be done weeks in advance. Because the care needs were constant, time-consuming, and demanding, there was little time for oneself, for the rest of the family, or for any social life with friends or relatives. One was left with a strong sense of social isolation in these families. Not only were they confined to their homes more than they desired, but further, the home domain was not totally their own because of the presence of equipment and providers. Finally, recurrent grieving for the loss of a normal life for their special-needs child was a strain for many parents. In contrast to grief experienced in other life-cycle stages, this grief may be a greater hardship for the caregiver when children are being cared for because they are so young and their whole life has been inextricably altered.

Problems With Services

Accessing and managing the care their child needed was fraught with problems for these parents. Finding the services and providers, determining eligibility, worrying about spending all insurance limits or being cut from publicly funded programs, working with the schools to receive appropriate services, and having problems with the equipment the child needed created a chronic set of hassles and burden for parents. Sometimes, care providers in the home created problems by their undesirable personal habits, inattentiveness to the child, and, especially, unreliability in showing up. Parents knew they were the only back-up when someone did not show up, and this had implications for their jobs as well as for their physical and emotional exhaustion.

Care and Parenting Strains

In addition to problems with other people and equipment, there were a host of added strains within the family. The direct care itself could be exhausting—whether it was because the child was getting bigger and harder to manage, because equipment malfunctions placed the child at risk for dying, or because the child required constant monitoring to prevent an accident or to respond to a medical emergency. The number and complexity of decisions placed a strain on parents.

Parenting a medically fragile child posed its own set of challenges. Primarily, parents expressed concern about trying to do what was right and appropriate. Developing competence as a parent is an important developmental task at this stage of life and a major source of identity and self-esteem for adults who choose to have children. Having a child with complex health-care needs greatly exacerbates successful accomplishment of this task. Limitations imposed by the child's condition create uncertainty for parents about appropriate parenting. How much normalcy is okay? How much independence is safe? What are appropriate expectations? And when the disability precludes a child from achieving developmental milestones, how is a parent to know whether she or he is doing a good job? The feedback or cues parents generally get from their child that sustain good parent-child interaction often are hard to interpret and may be very different from those of nondisabled children. Many parents need special education and need to change their expectations—not just once but often at each developmental stage of the child. For parents who are able to develop appropriate skills and expectations, there can be a great sense of mastery and competence, contributing to their development as an adult. Most parents require assistance in learning what is appropriate, in processing strong emotional reactions, and in obtaining feedback on how they are doing. These interventions must be provided in a way that does not undermine parents' competence, a complication that seemed to happen with some home care providers in this sample.

Added Family Stressors and Strains

Added strains in the marriage and family were reported by significantly more mothers (20%) than fathers (3%), suggesting that mothers felt this tension more. Fathers (see below) had a greater tendency to focus their attention away from the family and on work and hobbies, whereas mothers seemed to focus more on the child, the family, and even on themselves as they reflected about the situation. Both mothers and fathers reported greater work-related strains, but for mothers this was primarily in terms of lost opportunities to work, and for fathers it was greater pressure to retain a job or work more hours.

Normatively at the child-rearing stage of the life cycle, parents are advancing in their careers, gaining job experience, and pursuing new opportunities that contribute to their own development. This normative task is exacerbated by the presence of a child with serious medical problems. About 30% of the mothers in this sample had to leave the workforce partially or completely to care for their child. Their career aspirations were put on hold, and perhaps given up indefinitely. For those parents who continued to work, choices were more restricted. Relocations and promotions often were turned down because they needed to stay close to trusted medical care, or they could not take on new demands that would reduce the flexibility needed to respond to unpredictable changes in their child's condition. Fear of losing insurance coverage restricted job changes or prompted some parents to work extra hours or jobs.

It is important to remember that the care requirements of the medically fragile child are not the only needs these families had. Other life stressors and strains continued to affect them, too, aggravating the overall pile-up of demands. In some instances such stressors seemed to be totally independent events, and in other instances they may have been consequences of having a medically fragile child. Normative life stressors, such as having more children or career changes or strains, were cited. The illnesses or deaths of relatives and moving or remodeling also were identified by a number of families.

WHAT HELPS THESE FAMILIES
MANAGE THE SITUATION?

As a way of trying to identify the mediators of the chronic demands these families faced, the families were asked to describe the personal, family, and community resources they drew on and the coping behaviors they used. In other words, they were asked, "What do you *have* that helps, and what do you *do* that helps?" Again, what is presented here is the result of qualitative analyses versus statistical mediators.

Resources of Other Individuals

Primarily parents focused on different aspects of social support they received from others, with their spouse being the primary source, followed by their other children, relatives, and professionals. Emotional support, that is, someone to listen, understand, and show they care, was most important. Providing tangible help in caring for the child can be considered instrumental support. Attitudes often are taken for granted in persons who provide support. But these parents identified it so often that it may be an important prerequisite in the giving of emotional and instrumental support. Being caring, committed, positive, and hopeful were components of this attitude.

Family Resources

At the family system level, emotional support or cohesion of the group and shared responsibility for meeting the demands were recognized. Time spent together and good communication helped families maintain these resources. Many families acknowledged the importance of shared beliefs and values, particularly spiritual beliefs, as an important resource. For many, these beliefs had become more important and more shared as a result of the experience of having a medically fragile child.

Community Resources

About half of the parents mentioned receiving emotional and tangible support from friends and/or relatives. Notably, the absence of this kind of support was another source of strain for these families. When the absence of this support was due to lack of time to spend together, there was one kind of sadness. But when its absence was due to friends and relatives turning away from them, being afraid of their child, or feeling overwhelmed by the circumstances, there was a much deeper loss and pain for these families. Despite the reported problems with accessing services, such as Waiver, family subsidy, and so on, more than half of the parents mentioned publicly funded programs as a critically important resource for them. A small number of parents found time for and benefitted from parent groups.

Clearly, although parents had many problems with home care providers generally and with certain ones in particular, there were as many positive comments about them as negative ones. In addition to appreciating competence and skill, parents valued home care providers who showed genuine caring for their child, were supportive to the parent, and showed respect for the family.

Coping Strategies Parents Use

The resources just identified were not just dormant in these families. Families were proactive in obtaining and/or maintaining them. This is called coping. Coping is an effort to restore balance to the family by direct action to reduce demands and/or increase resources, by managing emotions and tensions, and finally and importantly by changing the way one thinks about a situation (Patterson, 1988). All these strategies were identified, and families varied in how many they used (see Table 5.7). Primarily, these were the coping efforts of parents, but as is noted below, they appeared to function on behalf of the family. Many times it was the parent getting other family members to work together. Some families increased personal, family, and community resources. In some families, closeness was increased through communication and doing things together, especially little things. Some worked to maintain normalcy in routine and activities so their home would not become a hospital, and the special medical needs would not take all of their energy. Some shared responsibility with their spouses and became better organized.

Some families coped by turning to the community to get more help and services—more hours of nursing care, more respite care, more financial resources, and better insurance benefits. In these later instances, working with a parent group can be more effective, and a few parents used collective group action. As busy as they were, some parents found time to volunteer to help other families. This strategy, in some ways, gave added meaning to the child's special needs and the family's lifestyle, and this meaning appeared to be a cause that transcended their own situation. For fathers especially, turning to work and investing more time and energy there was a means of coping. This may have been a way to escape the tension, a kind of sublimation, but often it was to ensure financial security for the family—to advance their position or to earn more money.

Parents wisely directed some of their coping efforts toward taking care of themselves. Taking time to be alone was especially important for mothers (24%). Fathers were more likely to take time for hobbies and recreation (33%). Talking to friends and relatives to release emotions and solve problems was used primarily by mothers (15%). Working to be healthy through adequate rest, good nutrition, exercise, and counseling was another way parents took care of themselves.

TABLE 5.7 Parent-Reported Coping Strategies Used When Caring for a Medically Fragile Child (in percentages)

	Mothers (N = 46)	Fathers (N = 40)
Take one day at a time	17	13
Have faith in God; pray	9	13
Recognize priorities; make positive attributions	20	13
Stay calm, patient, accepting; don't worry	13	10
Take time to be alone; reflect	24	5
Hobbies, projects, recreation	13	33
Humor	4	—
Rest, exercise, nutrition, counseling	13	8
Discuss things with friends, relatives	15	3
Do things as normal family; build closeness	11	6
Share responsibility with spouse	9	13
Be organized; get more help	9	10
Invest in job/work	11	18
Invest in volunteer groups; advocacy	7	3

By far the most important coping strategy used by these parents was positive appraisal—they changed the way they thought about their situation. The importance of this strategy cannot be overstated in view of the overwhelming chronic demands they faced that they could not get rid of, as well as in light of the serious limitations they often experienced in trying to get additional resources for their situation. They managed by "taking one day at a time," which was one way to reduce the perception of demands and challenges by breaking them down into smaller units. By not focusing on the future and on what might be, they could meet the challenges of the present. This, of course, is an important strategy used effectively by many self-help groups to build confidence and courage and to reduce anxiety. Putting faith in God or some higher power was another appraisal strategy to share responsibility and thereby reduce the burden. Clarifying values and priorities not only reduced the time that might have been spent on other pursuits but also allowed parents to value and invest in what they did have, especially their child and their family. And regarding their child and family, they described appreciating them more, making positive attributions about even the smallest things. Parents managed their emotions by accepting their situation, trying not to worry, and staying calm and patient in the face of the demands.

CHANGE IN WORLDVIEW

One of the most potent impacts of this level of chronic stress on these families appeared to be their changed orientation to life or a change in worldview. Cutting across and through all of the hardships, resources, and ways of coping was a sense that life had taken on a new meaning for these families. They approached things differently now. Many used the phrase "life is fragile" and emphasized that we should never take anything for granted. They expressed the view that one should value and appreciate what one has, especially the little things and other people. Keep these as priorities and let the rest go. For the most part, they did not sound embittered or angry about life. But they did sound sad and burdened.

This chronic burden contributed to a kind of demoralization for these parents and was reflected in their high distress scores. Although these scores fell in the "case range" of the norms established for the BSI, it is important to note that the meaning of high symptom levels most probably does not indicate these parents have diagnosable psychopathology because they were simultaneously coping and managing quite well. Breslau and Davis (1986) have reported that most of the parents with children with chronic illness in their sample, who scored in the clinical case range on a standardized self-report depression inventory, did not meet the DSM-III criteria for a diagnosis of clinical depression based on a clinical interview. They and others (Link & Dohrenwend, 1989) have referred to this as "demoralization" rather than clinical depression. The fact that so many parents (and their children) were able to develop strong coping repertoires was most likely what protected them from the negative sequelae. Particularly important in this coping repertoire were the appraisal strategies. This draws attention to the important psychological construct introduced by Aaron Antonovsky (1979) to describe survivors of the Holocaust—a sense of coherence. Coherence is an abiding belief that life is meaningful, comprehensible, and manageable and that things will work out the best that they can under the circumstances. In contrast to our Western preference for persons with a high internal locus of control, a sense of coherence is a balance between internal and external control. These parents accepted what they could not change and even came to appreciate it, while simultaneously working to make life the best they could for their child and their whole family. It must be remembered, however, that, as noted above, this sample of parents may not be representative of all families caring for chronically ill children. Those on whom we report here may be the most resilient families, those who were able to carry on and, yes, even grow from their situation.

IMPLICATIONS AND CONCLUSIONS

Families caring for medically fragile children experience some hardships that are unique to them and others that more generically affect all families caring for chronically ill children. Having providers in the home is atypical and invades privacy more and disrupts family routine more. However, we would argue that whenever families must interface with service delivery systems because of a child's special needs, both privacy and routine are affected. The issues related to boundary invasion discussed above are important for *all* service providers to keep in mind.

The costs of providing care for medically fragile children represent the high end of the cost continuum, and the strain families feel about who will continue to pay and their own financial security is intensified for those with a medically fragile child. However, the growing crisis in the financing of high cost health-care services makes this issue of financing care relevant for increasing numbers of families with chronically ill children.

The disruption to family, marital, and sibling relationships, the difficulty in maintaining informal support networks, and the problems of gaining respect and collaboration from the formal service delivery system are generic issues experienced by many families with children with special needs. As providers of health care, education, and social services; as policy makers; as parents; and as concerned human beings, we need to ask, "Is this level of chronic stress necessary? Do these families really need to live with this much burden?" When listening to them, it is possible to hear ways of lessening the stress. At several levels the capability exists to provide better supports to families caring for special-needs children.

Generally, our interventions and policies should flow from a philosophy that we, as citizens and human beings, share a responsibility to care for our children. This means supporting parents in this important work rather than blaming them when they struggle, expecting from them what they do not have to give. Professional training, public policies, and direct interventions should be the targets of our efforts.

In training professionals, we need to place greater emphasis on empowerment strategies (Dunst, Trivette, & Deal, 1988). Professionals need to (a) understand their own boundaries, aspirations, and goals; (b) understand family variability in structure and functioning and learn respect for a wide array of strengths; and (c) learn strategies for empowering those with whom they work so family integrity and parental self-esteem can be enhanced.

Public policies that provide more secure funding for the programs needed by these children and their families should be carefully articulated. The sources of funding should be multiple and should involve some kind of shared pool from both the public and private sectors. Few families can absorb these added costs, especially for any extended period. Worrying about losing benefits and the family's financial future are major hardships endured over and above providing the care. In addition, policies that allow families to have more choices about the specific services they receive, from which providers, and at which times of the day, week, or year would help reduce the loss of control they find so overwhelming.

Interventions need to be more coordinated and more timely. To prevent negative psychosocial sequelae, we need primary interventions that promote competence and adaptive ability at the time of diagnosis and at other critical transitions in the life cycle or in the course of the illness (Patterson & Geber, 1991). At the secondary level we need to respond to families in crisis when the demands of the medical condition plus other life challenges have exceeded their ability to manage. Finally, there are some families who, at the time their child is diagnosed with special care needs, already exhibit dysfunctional patterns of family interaction. These families should be referred for therapy, preferably therapy that is coordinated with other providers of care for the child.

Finally, we need more research to evaluate training programs and to test the effectiveness of family systems care with carefully controlled studies. Just as biomedical research has improved treatment, saving and extending the lives of many children with chronic illness conditions, so, too, research testing models of psychosocial care will improve the *quality of life* for these children and their families.

REFERENCES

Aday, L. A., Aitken, M. I., & Wegener, D. H. (1988). *Pediatric home care. Results of a national evaluation of programs for ventilator-assisted children.* Chicago: Pluribus.

Antonovsky, A. (1979). *Health, stress & coping.* San Francisco: Jossey-Bass.

Bock, R. H., Lierman, C., Ahmann, E., & Weinstock, N. (1983). There's no place like home. *Children's Health Care, 12,* 93-96.

Boss, P. (1987). Family stress. In M. Sussman & S. Steinmetz (Eds.), *Handbook of marriage and the family* (pp. 695-723). New York: Plenum.

Breslau, N., & Davis, G. C. (1986). Chronic stress and major depression. *Archives of General Psychiatry, 43*(4), 309-314.

Burr, B. H., Guyer, B., Tordes, I. D., Abrahams, B., & Chiodo, T. (1983). Home care for children on respirators. *New England Journal of Medicine, 309,* 1319-1323.

Derogatis, L. R., & Spencer, P. M. (1982). *Administration and procedures: BSI manual-I.* Baltimore, MD: Johns Hopkins University Press.

Dunst, C., Trivette, C., & Deal, A. (1988). *Enabling and empowering families: Principles and guidelines for practice.* Cambridge, MA: Brookline.

Frates, R. C., Splaingard, M. L., Smith, E. O., & Harrison, G. M. (1985). Outcome of home mechanical ventilation in children. *Journal of Pediatrics, 106,* 850-856.

Goldberg, A. I., Faure, E. A. M., Vaughn, C. J., Snarski, R., & Seleny, F. L. (1984). Home care for life-supported persons: An approach to program development. *Journal of Pediatrics, 104,* 785-795.

Leonard, B., Brust, J., & Nelson, R. (1993). Parental distress: Caring for medically fragile children. *Journal of Pediatric Nursing, 8*(1), 22-30.

Leonard, B., Brust, J., & Patterson, J. (1991). Home care reimbursement for technology-dependent children: Its impact on parental distress. *Lifestyles: Family and Economic Issues.*

Leonard, B., Patterson, J., Nelson, R., Titus, J., & Sielaff, B. (1991). *A longitudinal study of the impact of caring for medically fragile children on parent distress.* Unpublished manuscript.

Leonard, B., Titus, J., & Patterson, J. (1991). *The impact on siblings of home care for medically fragile children.* Unpublished manuscript.

Link, B., & Dohrenwend, B. P. (1989). Formulation of hypotheses about the true prevalence of demoralization in the United States. In B. P. Dohrenwend, B. S. Dohrenwend, M. S. Gould, B. Link, R. Newgebauer, & R. Wunsch-Hitzig (Eds.), *Mental illness in the United States: Epidemiologic estimates* (pp. 114-132). New York: Praeger.

Office of Technology Assessment. (1987). *Technology-dependent children: Hospital vs. home care—A technical memorandum* (OTA-TM-H-38). Washington, DC: Government Printing Office.

Palfrey, J. S., Walker, D. K., Haynie, M., Singer, J. D., Porter, S., & Bushey, B. (1991). Technology's children: Report of a statewide census of children dependent on medical supports. *Pediatrics, 87,* 611-618.

Patterson, J. (1988). Families experiencing stress. The family adjustment and adaptation response model. *Family Systems Medicine, 6*(2), 202-239.

Patterson, J., & Geber, G. (1991). Preventing mental health problems in children with chronic illness or disability. *Children's Health Care, 20*(3), 150-161.

Patterson, J., Leonard, B., & Titus, J. (1992). Home care for medically fragile children: Impact on family health and well-being. *Journal of Developmental and Behavioral Pediatrics, 13*(4), 248-255.

Quint, R. D., Chesterman, E., & Crain, L. S. (1990). Home care for ventilator-dependent children. *American Journal of Diseases of Children, 144,* 1238-1241.

Stein, R. E., & Reissman, C. K. (1980). The development of an impact-on-family scale: Preliminary findings. *Medical Care, 18*(4), 465-472.

6

Caregivers of Persons Living With AIDS

PATRICIA FLATLEY BRENNAN
SHIRLEY M. MOORE

Since 1981, more than 200,000 American men, women, and children have received the diagnosis of Acquired Immune Deficiency Syndrome (AIDS). More than 12,000 cases were diagnosed in the first quarter of 1992 alone (*Morbidity and Mortality Weekly Report,* 1992). Ten years' experience with a catastrophic illness on par with polio or plague revealed few truths about the illness: AIDS is a communicable disease that follows an unpredictable course of persistent physical decline interrupted by periods of bizarre and unusual clinical manifestations including cancers and multi-organ failure, and it is always fatal. For most of the period from infection through diagnosis and death, the individual faces challenges of living with a chronic, fatal disease; the dying takes only a short time. The emerging social picture of AIDS suggests a commonality shared by all persons living with AIDS: informal caregivers, including friends, family members, and volunteers, provide most of the care required by the person living with AIDS (PLWA). Understanding these caregivers is important, but traditional models of caregiving are insufficient to characterize and understand the AIDS caregiving experience. Features particular to AIDS and its social context herald distinctive caregiving challenges.

AUTHORS' NOTE: Support for this work was provided by *Self Care Nursing for AIDS/ARC via Computer Networks* (NR2001), National Center for Nursing Research, and *Supporting Home Care via Community Computer Networks* (AG8619), National Institute of Aging, Patricia Flatley Brennan, Principal Investigator.

As compared to better understood caregiving situations, such as elder caregiving in which physical and behavioral problems predominate, PLWA caregiving appears less formal and more diffuse. Persons who provide care for PLWAs are caregivers in the sense of Olesen (1989), in that they provide routine monitoring of health and household concerns as well as management of specific health problems. However, the unique characteristics of the AIDS illness itself and the social response to it result in a less overt, hidden nature of caregiving than that found in caregiving for persons with Alzheimer's disease or cancer. Illumination of the PLWA caregiving experience is enhanced by an understanding of the AIDS illness.

AIDS: A COLLECTION OF ILLS

AIDS is not a single disease but a syndrome, a collection of symptoms characteristic of a disease process. In AIDS, the disease process is immunodeficiency brought about by a virus (human immunodeficiency virus, or HIV) that interferes with the body's ability to ward off infection. Persons living with AIDS become ill from two sources: primary infection by HIV, and secondary infections, known as opportunistic infections, that take hold in the body because of a weakened immune function.

HIV infection follows through four main stages defined by the Center for Disease Classification as Stage I, Stage II, Stage III, and Stage IV. These stages constitute the HIV spectrum. Stage I occurs immediately after exposure to HIV and is measured in days or weeks since exposure. It is during this period that an individual develops antibodies (seroconversion) to the human immunodeficiency virus. Stage II, occurring months to years after the initial infection, involves inflammation of the lymph glands (lymphadenopathy). Stage III AIDS is defined by the appearance of one or more warning symptoms such as fatigue, weight loss, or confusion. During this stage the primary HIV infection results in progressive destruction of the immune system. Once an individual develops one or more diseases characteristic of AIDS illnesses, including *Pneumocystis carinii* pneumonia and Kaposi's sarcoma, Stage IV has begun. Stage IV symptoms may appear as soon as several months after infection, or as long as 10 years after infection. Stage IV is characterized by periods of severe illnesses interspersed with longer periods of a stable, though progressively weakened, state.

In addition to the progressive physical decline evident in the AIDS illness, there are profound changes in the relationships in the life of the person living with AIDS. Blood tests can determine that an individual has been infected with HIV. The antibodies to the human immunodeficiency virus can be detected in the blood once seroconversion has occurred, long before any symptoms appear. Recent developments in clinical treatment argue positively for early testing and prophylactic treatment. Early testing permits individuals infected with HIV to learn of their illness before the manifestation of any symptoms. If these results are disclosed, family members and friends may begin the monitoring and observing aspects of caregiving before any physical care is needed.

In 1994 AIDS remains an incurable, fatal disease. Contemporary treatment for HIV infection includes prophylaxis and symptom management. Routine treatment for infected, asymptomatic individuals includes Zidovudine (AZT) alone or in combination with other antiviral drugs. This therapy is believed to slow the progression of the illness, not change the ultimate outcome. Persons living with AIDS generally live at home, requiring hospitalization for about 30 days per year (Andrews, Keyes, Fanning, & Kizer, 1991).

Caregiving for persons living with AIDS begins as insidiously as do the symptoms of HIV infection. Early signs of AIDS include difficulties in mentation, particularly short-term memory problems, and difficulties structuring abstract thought (Price & Brew, 1988). Family members and friends who observe the early, subtle cognitive problems of HIV infection may slowly take on caregiving responsibilities. As the illness progresses, caregiving responsibilities expand to include greater physical and psychosocial assistance. It is these others, whose efforts serve to preserve normal function for the infected individual, who are the focus of this chapter: the caregivers of persons living with AIDS. Because the fundamental thesis of this chapter is that caregiving is but one manifestation of a larger relationship, a model of intimate relationships guides the discussion.

THEORETICAL PREMISES

Common conceptualizations of caregiving arose from examination of the activities conducted by one in the service of another (Noelker & Bass, 1989). Examples of these activities included bathing, meal preparation, and simple medical treatments. In AIDS caregiving, however, the activities differ, requiring fewer physical care functions and centering, rather, on monitoring and promotion of normal function. Although caregiving generally occurs within families, AIDS caregiving imposes unique challenges on the extant family as well as the emergent family. Emergent families consist of individuals bound by choice or circumstance who share intimate relations. Therefore, general models of family function provide a better framework for examining the AIDS caregiving experience than general caregiving models that focus on physical and/or behavioral dysfunction. For this chapter a broad conceptualization of family is used, advanced by Tiblier, Walker, and Rolland (1989): "[It] includes family of origin, family of procreation, cohabiting couples, friendship networks, and the 'emergent family' of caregivers which often evolves following an AIDS diagnosis" (p. 83).

Although persons living with AIDS range from infants to elders, AIDS is primarily a disease of children and young to middle-year adults. The structures of family systems of these groups are variable, including traditionally shaped nuclear families, emancipated young men and women, and adults who have formed new families. Primarily afflicting those from 20 to 35 years old, AIDS becomes an additional family crisis to those attempting to establish new family structures or redefine relations with the family of origin.

Family theory models provide appropriate guides for understanding caregiving in AIDS, for caregiving occurs in the context of others who assume or resume roles found in family systems. The Circumplex Model of Family Functioning, as formulated by Olson, Spenkle, and Russel (1979), serves as an apt model for the discussion. This model posits two characteristics of families—cohesion and adaptability—that determine the family's ability to accomplish developmental tasks and cope with stressors. Cohesion refers to the degree of bonding within a family group; adaptability represents the degree of flexibility demonstrated by the family. A variety of stressors are associated with AIDS caregiving, such as social stigma, cognitive and physical changes in the PLWA, lack of financial resources to meet medical costs, and fears about impending death. The family unit's level of cohesion and degree of adaptability in part determine its ability to manage stressors.

Family cohesion represents the emotional bonding that family members have toward one another, such as how much family members engage in shared activities or respond to each other's needs. Family adaptability is the extent to which the family system is flexible and is characterized as the ability of the family system to change its power structure, role relationships, and relationship rules. In the circumplex model, families that have balanced levels of cohesion and adaptability are better able to manage stressful situations. One member's diagnosis of AIDS presents a specific stressor to the family, demanding a response in terms of new roles, new communication patterns, and new conceptualizations of members. The nature of cohesion and adaptability among family members both aid and interfere with the PLWA caregiving relationship.

This chapter examines caregiving in AIDS from the perspective of the circumplex model concepts of cohesion and adaptability. In addition, an exploration of the social and physiological dimensions of AIDS is presented. Certain characteristics of the illness, including communicability, social stigma and fear, and the trajectory of decline, present specific stressors to the family relationship and the caregiving experience itself. To engender a sense of the stressors faced by PLWA caregivers, the next section provides an overview of the AIDS caregiving challenges along the HIV spectrum.

CAREGIVING ALONG THE HIV SPECTRUM

The trajectory of illness, from initial infection to death, is commonly referred to as the HIV spectrum. Based on interviews with PLWA caregivers (Moore & Moore, 1989), the types of information requested—such as caring for the household (i.e., dealing with the mood changes of the PLWA, diet information, care options for the future), signs and symptoms of acute health threats, and disease progression—indicated that they were assuming a monitoring-type role with a patient. These health-monitoring activities often represent role changes for the caregiver and the patient. The degree of adaptability that characterized the underlying relationship between parent, lover, or friend and the PLWA may well determine the success with which these new roles are adopted by both parties in the caregiving relationship.

PLWAs, persons living with AIDS, is the term used to refer to one who has experienced a definitive symptom of the illness. The acronym denotes the focus of caregiving: assisting another to live while infected. Persons living with AIDS require caregivers who can help promote as normal a lifestyle as possible. The psychological ramifications of diagnosis with a fatal disease before adulthood, coupled with the relatively gradual decline during which the ill person remains capable of taking an interest in life for long episodes, place strong emphasis on the need for psychological support. Therefore, caregivers who can help a PLWA maintain an interest in life play a large role in AIDS caregiving. AIDS is a disease that evokes social reactions, including stigma. The impact of the stigma of the disease leaves the PLWA alone and isolated. Stigmatized individuals perceive that others, including professionals, do not really accept them and are not ready to make contact on equal grounds (Goffman, 1963). Adequate levels of cohesion between the caregiver and the PLWA provide a well-functioning relationship within which the caregiver can maintain social contact and support. Diagnosis with a fatal illness evokes a host of psychological reactions in all persons, but may be particularly strong in a young person (Lewis, 1988). Prevalent feelings include fears about the future, anger, and bewilderment. Early in the illness PLWAs display psychological stress responses similar to those experienced by other individuals diagnosed with a fatal illness. In addition to providing support to the PLWA, the caregiver also must assume a role of guidance and monitoring to help the PLWA cope with feelings of immobility, confusion, and difficulty with abstract thought. Rarely is physical care needed for persons early in the illness.

The diagnosis of AIDS forces a recognition of serious life threat. The focus of caregiving is the promotion of normal life (Lewis, 1988). This focus is congruent with contemporary thinking about management of all chronic illnesses. As such, then, caregiving activities focus on conserving the PLWA's strength, ensuring an adequate balance of activity and rest, and promotion of positive life attitudes. Although the importance of positive attitudes, hope, and healing energies assumes a larger role in the treatment of numerous illnesses, for the person living with AIDS these factors have become central (Tilleraas, 1990). Guidance for these strategies comes from the works of Louise Hay and those of Bernie Siegel (1988), popular authors advocating hope, mobilizing little-understood strategies such as visualization and imaging, and encouraging personal participation in the fight against AIDS.

A diminished immune response leaves the PLWA vulnerable to numerous opportunistic infections and generalized fatigue. As the illness progresses the caregiver incorporates more physical care support into the caregiving repertoire. Meal preparation, supervision of household tasks, and assistance with heavy activities such as lifting constitute an additional set of caregiving activities. The success of this incorporation depends on the flexibility in the caregiver-care recipient relationship. As a subsystem of the family system, the caregiver-care recipient unit must clarify its boundaries, that is, who are the members in this caregiving subsystem and how well are the designated lines of responsibility defined. Family relationships that have rigid boundaries are said to be disengaged or to have too little cohesion. Family systems that have relationships that are diffuse and too close are considered enmeshed or possessing high levels of cohesion. When cohesion is particularly low or very high, the needed adaptations to the stresses of caregiving are more likely to occur with dysfunctional behaviors (Minuchin, 1974).

Throughout most of AIDS caregiving, traditional caregiving activities are not the focus. The unstable trajectory of the illness demands extensive physical care one week followed by several weeks during which little physical care is demanded. Sometimes the caregiver must take the initiative for future planning regarding estate concerns and funeral arrangements. The caregivers must respond and adapt to this variable, ever-changing need. Often the absence of legal ties between caregivers and persons living with AIDS necessitates the intrusion of legal counsel into this very private experience.

Bouts of serious illness and debility forebear the terminal experience of AIDS. During the illness periods the caregiver provides help in all aspects of the activities of daily living. Bathing, toileting, and feeding consume the caregiver's focus. Cognitive problems, many times severe, require vigilance and understanding on the part of the caregiver. Ongoing psychological support remains an ever-present challenge to the caregiver. The greater the accommodation of the caregiver and care recipient to a changing relationship, the easier it is for the caregiver to assume these new and often demanding roles.

In the end, caregiving consists of watchful monitoring as the illness plays out its eventual and unavoidable course. The disease causes a gradual wasting of muscles and an eventual failure of all organ systems. Caregivers face the final period called upon for physical comfort measures, psychological support, and household maintenance. As with other caregivers who provide intimate care to persons near death, AIDS caregivers must determine the appropriate level of emotional closeness that comprises psychological support along with providing personal care. Too little or too much cohesion in the relationship may exacerbate the stress of this period as the members of the family unit are called upon to continually renegotiate their boundaries and modify their caregiving roles.

In this final period of the disease, AIDS caregiving becomes most similar to other types of caregiving, demanding the functional caregiving activities found in any caregiving situation. The caregiver must be vigilant to intercede as needed and to pull back from the caregiving role as the functional status of the person permits. Household maintenance and psychological support are the major tasks of caregiving during all phases of the illness. However, physical care and comfort measures assume predominant importance during the end stages of the disease. Although persons living with AIDS who have caregivers are likely to have a single caregiver, it is just as likely that a caregiving team of friends or even anonymous volunteers may serve the PLWA.

To help family caregivers meet the demands of AIDS caregiving, many community health agencies provide courses. The American Red Cross of Greater New York developed a six-session course targeting the home caregiver (Rose & Catanzaro, 1989). During the first session of the course participants view a film, *Beyond Fear,* designed to sensitize caregivers to their new roles and to dispel common myths. In subsequent sessions class leaders address such topics as the aspects of the physical care of the person living with AIDS (hygiene, nutrition), available community resources, and psychological dimensions of care. As PLWA caregivers come together in these teaching and support groups, both traditional caregiving concerns and concerns unique to AIDS caregiving are discussed.

CAREGIVERS OF PERSONS LIVING WITH AIDS

Caregivers With a Relationship

It is useful to examine the AIDS caregiving relationship in the context of the whole relationship shared between the PLWA and the caregiver. The caregiver-PLWA relationship is the primary, although not exclusive, family structure of interest. It is insufficient to focus solely on this relationship, nor is it possible to generalize about the entire family structure simply by focusing on this relationship. For example, some parents of children with AIDS also are infected; in these families, caregiving responsibilities also may be assumed by a grandparent. Among gay men with AIDS, parental caregivers are as likely to be found as are lovers and friends. The family caregiving constellation is complicated, too; sometimes rejection by the family of origin adds additional burden to the caregiving family. Other times members of the family of origin provide additional meaningful support to the caregiving family. As in most caregiving situations, PLWA caregivers usually share a relationship of some type with the ill person before the manifestation of the illness. These relationships include lover, friend, parent, or concerned other. Much of what is known about the PLWA caregiving experience has emerged during interviews with the caregivers.

Relationship challenges comprised the major stressors operating in the caregiving situations. In interviews with the intimate friends and lovers of gay AIDS patients, three relationship problems emerged: (a) the magnitude of the caregiver role, (b) uncertainties of the care partners regarding their own futures, and (c) conflicts with other life roles (Pearlin, Semple, & Turner, 1988). PLWA caregivers in gay relationships were accustomed to being in a relationship based on interdependence, autonomy, and egalitarianism that, during the illness experience, became altered as the PLWA became increasingly dependent (Flaskerud, 1987). This flexibility in role responsibilities in the relationship may be helpful as the caregiver is required to take on new caregiving role responsibilities as the disease progresses.

Handling the multiple relationship changes experienced by both PLWAs and their caregivers was reported as a great stressor by both kin and non-kin PLWA caregivers. Many PLWA parent caregivers were resolving feelings about rejection of the PLWA's lifestyle at the same time they were assuming care responsibilities for the PLWA (Chekryn, 1989). In addition, issues of dependence/independence arose as parental caregiving responsibilities were assumed during a life phase when there is normally independence between children and parents. Adapting to new roles became necessary for both the PLWAs and their parents. The lovers of PLWAs expressed that they were struggling with the need to build or maintain changing relationships between PLWAs and their families who were estranged previously (Chachkes, 1986; Cowles & Rodgers, 1991). Relationships with greater flexibility or adaptability among members are more likely to promote successful assumption of these required role changes. Another stressor reported by many kin and non-kin caregivers was the reluctance to disclose the true diagnosis of AIDS to close friends or even family. Keeping this secret meant that caregivers were not able to reach out to their own friends for support for themselves at a time when they needed it the most (Cowles & Rodgers, 1991).

Reports of the bereavement experiences of PLWA caregivers indicated that despite the lack of kinship, the intensity of the caregiver-PLWA relationship contributed to difficult bereavement and the need for support. The absence of a blood or legal relationship did not diminish the intensity of the bereavement experience (Govoni, 1988; Lennon, Martin, & Dean, 1990; Murphy & Perry, 1988). The influence of social support on AIDS-related grief among gay men showed that the simple availability of social support did not alter the level of grief, but the perceived adequacy of social support was strongly related to level of grief (Lennon et al., 1990).

Within the circumplex model the essential elements are the family and its cohesion and adaptability. Therefore, the discussion of the AIDS caregivers focuses on the nature of the caregiving unit, conceptualizing this unit as a type of family. This perspective departs from the public conceptualization of AIDS as a disease of subgroups and reframes the caregiving situation as a family experience.

One half of 1% of the U.S. population is infected with HIV. Few individuals will remain untouched by the epidemic. Any individual may be called upon to give care to or know a caregiver of a person living with AIDS. The caregivers of persons living with AIDS include lovers, intimate friends, parents, and caring strangers. Sometimes the caregiver also is infected with HIV. The characteristic these individuals share is their willingness to assume some responsibility for an individual infected with HIV. AIDS care partners come primarily from one of two groups of individuals sharing intimate relationships with persons living with AIDS: lovers and friends.

Lovers and Friends

Intimate friends and lovers provide much of the care for the person living with AIDS. This relationship is best, although not exclusively, exemplified in a gay couple, involving two adults sharing intimacy and family-like bonds. In a study of 21 PLWA caregivers by Moore (1989), 65% of the caregivers defined themselves as lovers or friends. These caregivers were predominantly male and had an average age of 43 years. This is in contrast to other commonly known caregiving situations, such as Alzheimer's disease, in which spouses or adult children are the primary caregivers (Stone, Cafferata, & Sangl, 1987).

Whatever the gender and sexual preferences of the dyad, however, certain features remain constant. The dyad remains together by choice, loyalty, or other psychological motivation rather than by a legal or financial arrangement. Caregiving activities and responsibilities are intertwined with affiliation and bonding. These relationships may be as enduring and stable as found in traditional family structure. A challenge to the caregivers is preserving the desired relationship without the legal protection afforded biological families or marital dyads. In their descriptive study of the stress of PLWA caregivers, Pearlin and colleagues (1988) point out the element of identification that the AIDS caregiver may have with the care recipient, as the caregiver frequently has shared the same risk factors as those of the PLWA. Such identification may support the denial of the caregiving situation by both caregiver and care recipient. These investigators also point out the burden of guilt that caregivers of PLWAs may have due to their own relative good health. This guilt about one's present advantage in health may be another reason for the less overt assumption of a caregiver role.

Parents

Parental caregivers fall generally into two groups: elder parents of adult children and young parents of juveniles. As parents and as caregivers, these two groups face unique challenges. Families with adult children, and their members, are at different developmental stages than families with juvenile children. The interpersonal dynamics among family members differ, and the developmental status of each member is also different.

Parents caring for an adult child with AIDS face multiple challenges. The diagnosis of AIDS, and subsequent need for care, initiates a return to home and family left years before. Instead of the usual family developmental tasks at this phase of family life that center on personal identity development among members, key developmental tasks focus on renewing and revising the cohesion issues of bonding and attachment. Concomitantly, adaptability may be taxed as parental PLWA caregivers experience the added stressors of initial acknowledgment of the homosexuality or the drug abuse of their adult child (Chachkes, 1986; Garrett, 1988). Elder parents caring for adult children with AIDS experience a disruption of the natural order of families (O'Donnel & Bernier, 1990). The elder parent may find herself or himself resuming a long-discarded role as the guardian and decision maker for a child (Allers, 1990). Resumption of these roles is most successful in families who previously have demonstrated role flexibility among their members.

Health problems common to other elder caregivers (Stone et al., 1987) are also evident among the older parental caregivers of PLWAs.

Health problems reported by these older PLWA caregivers include hypertension, congestive heart failure, arthritis, and cataracts (Moore, 1989).

Grossman (1991) recognized the dual stigma experienced by gay AIDS patients: (a) realization that the idealized child had adopted a lifestyle foreign to the parent and (b) awareness that this child now had a fatal, contagious illness. Thus the family faces stress from multiple sources: lifestyle conflicts, unrealized role expectations, and loss. It is plausible that family members' skills in role adaptability and satisfaction with the level of cohesion determine the quality of coping with this experience.

The experience of mothers reconnecting with sons separated by differences in life choices, only to give up the child to death by AIDS, was documented in the stories of Judi in Reider and Ruppelt's (1988) exploration of the female caregivers of AIDS patients. Judi's son Michael was diagnosed with AIDS when he was 19 years old and died 3 years later in 1984. The family consisted of Judi, her husband of 24 years, Ralph, and another son and had well-established roles and family loyalties. Judi initially recognized her son and mediated his reconnection with the family. The family experienced disruption and lack of adaptability in reaction to the disclosure of Michael's gay lifestyle and the terminal nature of his illness. Ralph began drinking, and Judi served as the sole advocate for her son. The family's history of healthy functioning enabled them eventually to adopt new roles and establish cohesive bonds as a redefined family unit.

It is estimated that less than 2% of all AIDS patients are children under the age of 15 (Chu, Buehler, Oxtoby, & Kilbourne, 1991). In the case of many but not all of these children, a parent serves as the primary informal caregiver. Young parents with juvenile children afflicted with AIDS also experience stressors as a family. The stressors arise from the child's illness, in part because of the terminal nature of AIDS and in part because of social response to the contagious nature of AIDS. Families planning for an open-ended future with a child now must revise not only their horizon but also their hopes and dreams for the child. Fears of contagion experienced by those outside of the family system reduce the nurturing behaviors frequently offered to ill children (Nelson & Album, 1987), thereby increasing demands within the family system to become self-sufficient. The potential for emotional enmeshment between these parental caregivers and their infected children is great. This enmeshment may hamper the parents' ability to effectively cope with the declining health of their child.

In some situations, both the parents and the child are infected with HIV. Parents who may have passed the virus to the child grapple with additional problems, including guilt at having infected the child and fears of their own illness. The parents' own HIV infection diminishes their ability to maintain a cohesive family structure and cope with the child's needs. The complexity of these situations interferes with family adaptability, potentially interfering with the parents' ability to adapt to the caregiving role demands.

Many other configurations of caregiving relationships are found in the AIDS caregiving environment. Lifestyles that led to estrangement from one's family of origin; living situations remote from one's birth town; and the absence of intact, nuclear families all contribute to the situation in which caregivers of PLWAs are less likely than other caregivers to be related by blood or marriage to the ill person. A strong sense of community among the members of groups in which AIDS first appeared has resulted in an unusual network of caring strangers: buddies.

The Buddy Caregiver

In the early days of the epidemic, before the acronym AIDS appeared, members of gay communities in large U.S. cities experienced a sudden increase in unusual skin cancers and wasting diseases. Known first as GRID, gay-related immune disease, the syndrome appeared to result from some unique aspect of the gay male lifestyle. Members of the gay community mobilized against the disease, forming networks of formal and informal activists. The Gay Men's Health Crisis emerged as a social policy and fund-raising coalition. The most famous of all AIDS caregiving organizations is the Shanti Project, begun in the Castro district of San Francisco during the early days of the epidemic (Salyer, Waters, & Yow, 1987). Shanti served to meet the daily living needs of PLWAs, providing food, housing, companionship, and assistance. An important legacy of the early days is a unique community social support system known as the "buddy system." Buddy systems have been organized in communities throughout the United States.

AIDS buddies are volunteers, frequently strangers to the PLWA, whose purpose is to establish a relationship and socialize with the infected person. Buddies may help with routine household tasks, but their primary role is to visit with the PLWA, spend time together in social outings, and convey a sense of interested caring. Buddies do not take the place of professional caregivers and seldom assume all the responsibilities of family caregivers. Yet their place, as social supports directly for the PLWA, assumes prime importance during the long course of the illness. The circumplex model generally depicts family as individuals sharing an enduring commitment. To apply this model to understand the buddy caregiver relationship, one must consider two manifestations of relationships between buddies and the family structure. The AIDS buddy was an important social support for the PLWAs interviewed by Moore (1989). Buddies sometimes replaced absent, unavailable, or rejecting family members. In other families, buddies served in a supportive role, never becoming central to the family role structure. The concept of buddy caregivers is similar to church visitors and other extended caregiving networks and warrants consideration with the circumplex model.

WHAT IS UNIQUE ABOUT AIDS CAREGIVING?

Contagion, Manifestation, and Stigma

As an illness, AIDS possesses two unique characteristics: infectivity and selective manifestation that distinguishes its victims from other illnesses requiring caregiving. Infectivity denotes AIDS as a contagious illness, transmission occurring from person to person. Selective manifestation refers to the fact that AIDS disproportionately affects certain population groups such as ethnic minorities, women, and gay men. Unlike most other disease states that present the need for caregiving, AIDS is a contagious disease. One needs to look back almost 40 years to the polio and tuberculosis epidemics to find a contagious illness that necessitated such extensive caregiving on the part of family members and friends. Caregiving for a person with a contagious disease may evoke in the caregiver a sense of vulnerability to the same illness afflicting the patient. The emotional bonding in such a relationship may be highly susceptible to extremes in separateness or enmeshment. This sense of vulnerability may prohibit caregivers from engaging in the emotional intimacy that may be desired by PLWAs during this stressful time. Alternatively, caregivers who feel particularly threatened by their vulnerability may seek emotional support from the PLWA. Either of these extremes in emotional bonding can potentially threaten the quality of the caregiving relationship.

These two dimensions, infectivity and selective manifestation, complicate the caregiving situation. First, the traditional concept of caregiving, a service offered altruistically to another deemed worthy of care, now is required by an individual whose lifestyle choices may have contributed to the illness. Second, the afflicted individuals belong to cultural groups that are sufficiently different from the mainstream of society as to be unaffected by the common social sympathy offered toward other ill persons. The experience of selective manifestation in part contributes to the unique nature of AIDS caregiving, in which caregivers, likely to come from the same group as the individual with AIDS, also may be subject to similar social pressures. Furthermore, because the bond among nondominate group members is likely to be stronger than *traditional* family or legal ties (Shilts, 1987), many of the caregivers may assume their role out of loyalty to the group and not other motivations, such as family responsibility or interpersonal choice.

Stigma represents a sociological phenomena attaching blame, guilt, shame, or other negative dimensions to a life state (Grossman, 1991). Stigmatized individuals are separated from society and believed to be different and undesirable because of their life condition. The person living with AIDS experiences stigma as a result of lifestyle factors and in anticipation of the fear of contagion brought about because of the disease. Afflicted individuals are separated from society; this stigma extends to involve the caregivers, now stigmatized because of their relationship to the ill person. This shared stigmatization may lead to an emotional enmeshment between the caregiver and the PLWA. Thus social issues of the AIDS experience are intertwined with the complexity of AIDS as an illness.

The traditional caregiving role requires formal acknowledgment by both parties: the caregiver and the care recipient. However, this overt acknowledgment does not always exist in the PLWA caregiving station. Olesen (1989) argues that even in the absence of its acknowledgment, caregiving activities do occur. Within relationships in which balanced levels of adaptability are present, family and friends may take on many aspects of the role of promoting the PLWA's self-care long before this role is recognized by either the caregivers themselves or the care recipient.

Many times both the ill person and the caregiver engage in an unspoken collusion to not acknowledge the extent to which caregiving occurs. Two factors within the PLWA-care partner situation contribute to an appearance of noncaregiving in the midst of a well-established caregiving system. First, an attitude of wellness, and a focus on positive thought and health by PLWAs, their caregivers, and many involved in the formal caregiving system, places great importance on not acknowledging the illness. A prevailing holistic philosophy espoused by PLWAs emphasizes positive thinking and the ability to alter physical health status through maintaining healthful attitudes (Tenney, 1986). As in cardiac patients, an attitude of denial may, in fact, help the PLWA maintain an aura of health and well-being while living with a potentially fatal disease (Croog, Shapiro, & Levine, 1971; Dinsdale & Hackett, 1982). However, this denial contributes to the obscuring of the caregiver, who still must attend to the health and well-being of the household while not having the role acknowledged.

In addition to the pervasive attitude of wellness, a second factor contributes to the hidden nature of AIDS caregiving. Caregiver activities focus on home maintenance activities that foster a sense of maintenance of a normal lifestyle. In other, better studied examples of caregiving, the caregiving relationship is evidenced in the physical care provided by the caregiver to the identified patient (Stone et al., 1987). For example, caregivers of cancer patients focus on the maintenance of skin integrity, adequate nutritional intake, and wound management early in the caregiving process (Hileman & Lackey, 1990). Several possible explanations for the less overt nature of the PLWA caregiving experience exist. A prevailing concern regarding the care of PLWAs and their caregivers is that AIDS is a social disease, exposing both the patient and the caregiver to the effects of stigmatization in the community. This stigmatization potentially reduces the participation of caregivers in the neighborhood networks of support open to patients with less controversial illnesses (Goffman, 1963); thus these caregivers are left on their own to cope with the problems associated with AIDS caregiving.

An understanding of the hidden nature of the PLWA caregiving relationship also can be facilitated using the circumplex model relationship dimensions of cohesion and adaptability. Cohesion or emotional bonding in the PLWA caregiving relationship may be excessively strong because of subgroup membership, stigma of the disease, or shared risk. In addition, the highly egalitarian, autonomous relationship that characterizes many gay relationships may lead to denial of the newly needed, more overt caregiving roles. However, these egalitarian relationships may provide the flexibility needed as roles in the relationship change as greater dependence on the caregiver evolves. As the PLWA and the caregiver strive to maintain normalcy and positive life attitudes, there is a cautious assumption of the new role responsibilities of care recipient and caregiver. The hidden caregiving role in AIDS has both positive and negative implications. A positive aspect of this less overt caregiving role is that an environment of normalcy can be maintained. A negative consequence of a less overt assumption of the caregiver role is that support from outside the caregiving relationship is less likely to occur.

SUMMARY

Treatment for the PLWA and prevention of disease consumed the attention of clinicians and researchers during the first 10 years of the AIDS epidemic. The handful of studies that examined caregiver issues demonstrated both similarities and differences between AIDS caregiving and other caregiving situations. Caregiving is characterized by aspects of stigma, contagion, a hidden nature, short episodes of physical caring, and a disproportionate demand for support to maintain normal function of the PLWA.

Very little firsthand information about the AIDS caregiving relationship is known due to the relative newness of the disease, the social concerns focusing on discovery of a cure, and the unique and varied natures of the AIDS caregiving relationships. Understanding the unique features of the PLWA caregiving experience encompasses a grasp of the illness, the phases of the caregiving relationship, and the nature of the PLWA-caregiver relationship. The challenges presented in the AIDS caregiving experience are being navigated successfully as these caregivers help PLWAs live and die in the community. Existing and emergent families form the context of AIDS caregiving, and the diverse and ever-changing demographics of these families further attests to the uniqueness of AIDS caregiving.

Future research is needed that will broadly characterize both the wide range of AIDS caregiving and the multiple manifestations of AIDS caregiving. Work also is needed to determine the extent to which the hidden nature of caregiving is beneficial and/or detrimental to the family. Novel strategies of identifying caregivers and comprehending their experiences will better illuminate the situation.

REFERENCES

Allers, C. T. (1990). AIDS and the older adult. *The Gerontologist, 30,* 405-407.

Andrews, R., Keyes, M., Fanning, T., & Kizer, K. (1991). Lifetime Medicaid service utilization and expenditures for AIDS in New York and California. *Journal of Acquired Immune Deficiency Syndromes, 4,* 1046-1058.

Chachkes, E. (1986, Spring). AIDS aftermath: Patients and families. *Discharge Planning Update, 6,* 8-10.

Chekryn, J. (1989). Families of people with AIDS. *The Canadian Nurse, 85*(8), 30-32.

Chu, S. Y., Buehler, J. W., Oxtoby, M. J., & Kilbourne, B. W. (1991). Impact of the human immunodeficiency epidemic on mortality in children, United States. *Pediatrics, 87*(6), 806-810.

Cowles, K. V., & Rodgers, B. L. (1991). When a loved one has AIDS: Care for the significant other. *Journal of Psychosocial Nursing, 29*(4), 7-12.

Croog, S., Shapiro, D., & Levine, S. (1971). Denial among male heart patients. *Psychosomatic Medicine, 33*(5), 385-397.

Dinsdale, J., & Hackett, T. (1982). Effect of denial on cardiac health and psychological assessment. *American Journal of Psychiatry, 139*(11), 1477-1480.

Flaskerud, J. H. (1987). AIDS: Psychosocial aspects. *Journal of Psychosocial Nursing, 25*(12), 9-16.

Garrett, J. (1988, September). The AIDS patient: Helping him and his parents cope. *Nursing, 88,* 50-52.

Goffman, E. (1963). *Stigma: Notes on the management of spoiled identity.* Englewood Cliffs, NJ: Prentice Hall.

Govoni, L. (1988). Psychosocial issues of AIDS in the nursing care of homosexual men and their significant others. *Nursing Clinics of North America, 23*(4), 749-764.

Grossman, A. H. (1991). Gay men and HIV/AIDS: Understanding the double stigma. *Journal of Association of Nurses in AIDS Care, 2*(4), 28-32.

Hileman, J. W., & Lackey, N. R. (1990). Self-identified needs of patients with cancer at home and their home caregivers: A descriptive study. *Oncology Nursing Forum, 17*(6), 907-913.

Lennon, M. C., Martin, J. L., & Dean, L. (1990). The influence of social support on AIDS-related grief reaction among gay men. *Social Science Medicine, 31*(4), 477-484.

Lewis, A. (1988). *Nursing care of the person with AIDS/ARC.* Rockville, MD: Aspen Publishers.

Minuchin, S. (1974). *Families and family therapy.* Cambridge, MA: Harvard University Press.

Moore, S. M. (1989). *Caregivers of persons with AIDS/ARC.* Paper presented at the Sigma Theta Tau International Scientific Sessions.

Morbidity and Mortality Weekly Report. (1992, April 3). P. 217, Table 2.

Murphy, P., & Perry, K. (1988). Hidden grievers. *Death Studies, 12,* 451-462.

Nelson, L. P., & Album, M. M. (1987). AIDS: Children wth HIV infection and their families. *Journal of Dentistry for Children, 54*(5), 353-358.

Noelker, L. S., & Bass, D. M. (1989). Home care for elderly persons: Linkages between formal and informal caregivers. *Journal of Gerontology Social Studies, 44*(2)S, 63-70.

O'Donnel, T. G., & Bernier, S. L. (1990). Parents as caregivers: When a son has AIDS. *Journal of Psychosocial Nursing, 28*(6), 14-17.

Olesen, V. (1989). Caregiving, ethical and informal: Emerging challenges in the sociology of health and illness. *Journal of Health and Social Behavior, 30,* 1-10.

Olson, D. H., Spenkle, D. H., & Russel, C. S. (1979). Circumplex model of marital and family systems: Cohesion and adaptability dimensions, family types, and clinical applications. *Family Process, 18,* 3-28.

Pearlin, L., Semple, S., & Turner, H. (1988). Stress of AIDS caregiving: A preliminary overview of the issues. *Death Studies, 12,* 501-517.

Price, R. W., & Brew, B. J. (1988). The AIDS dementia complex. *The Journal of Infectious Diseases, 158*(5), 1079-1083.

Reider, I., & Ruppelt, P. (Eds.). (1988). *AIDS: The women.* San Francisco: Cleis.

Rose, M., & Catanzaro, A. M. (1989). AIDS caregiving crisis: A proactive approach. *Holistic Nursing Practice, 3*(2), 39-45.

Salyer, J., Waters, H., & Yow, P. (1987). Shanti project: Service organization for persons with AIDS. *Caring, 6,* 24-27.

Shilts, R. (1987). *And the band played on: Politics, people, and the AIDS epidemic.* New York: St. Martin's.

Siegel, B. (1988). *Love, medicine, and miracles: Lessons learned about self-healing.* New York: Harper & Row.

Stone, R., Cafferata, G., & Sangl, J. (1987). Caregivers of the frail elderly: A national profile. *The Gerontologist, 27*(5), 616-626.

Tenney, L. (1986). *AIDS: A nutritional approach.* Provo, UT: Woodland.

Tiblier, K., Walker, G., & Rolland, J. (1989). Therapeutic issues when working with families of persons with AIDS. In E. Macklin (Ed.), *AIDS and families* (pp. 81-128). New York: Haworth.

Tilleraas, P. (1990). *Circle of hope: Our stories of AIDS, addiction, and recovery.* San Francisco: Harper & Row.

7

Predictors of Caregiver Burden Among Support Group Members of Persons With Chronic Mental Illness

DAVID E. BIEGEL
LI-YU SONG
VENKATESAN CHAKRAVARTHY

Chronic mental illness has significant effects on patients, families, and the larger society. For the person with chronic mental illness, such as a young adult with schizophrenia, living with chronic mental illness means having a mental disorder that is severe and long-lasting. Schizophrenia interferes with one's ability to form and maintain interpersonal relationships, care for oneself, complete one's education, or obtain and maintain employment. Data from the National Institutes of Mental Health (NIMH) Epidemiological Catchment Area Study indicate that for persons with schizophrenia, symptoms last an average of 9 years before remission (Robins & Regier, 1991).

AUTHORS' NOTE: Research for this paper was supported by grant #89-1022 from the Office of Program Evaluation and Research, Ohio Department of Mental Health, and by grants from the Cuyahoga County Community Mental Health Board, and the Center for Practice Innovations, Mandel School of Applied Social Sciences, Case Western Reserve University. The authors acknowledge the support of, and express appreciation to, the Alliance for the Mentally Ill of Metro Cleveland, which cosponsored this research and provided access to its membership for this study.

The onset of schizophrenia is often late adolescence or young adulthood and thus the disease strikes individuals at the stage of their lifespan when they soon would be expected to become emancipated and form their own households. Instead, these individuals often become dependent upon their families and require continued assistance to maintain themselves in the community. Persons with schizophrenia often experience relapses that require frequent hospitalizations. Of those affected by schizophrenia, approximately 50% will experience some form of disability with residual impairment on an intermittent basis through their lifetime; an additional 25% will never recover from their initial illness episode and will require care for the rest of their lives. During the first few years of the disorder, residual impairment often increases between episodes (American Psychiatric Association, 1987; Carpenter, 1987; Keith & Matthews, 1984).

Chronic mental illness, like other chronic illnesses, affects not just the patient but also the entire family system. Chronic illness often is very disruptive of family life and may lead to reassignments of tasks and roles assumed by particular family members. The stress of chronic illness on families also can lead to family conflicts and can affect the health of individual family members (Bruhn, 1977; Leventhal, Leventhal, & Nguyen, 1985). Providing care to a chronically ill person especially affects family caregivers, those individuals within families who provide the most support and assistance to their ill family member. Across chronic illnesses, many family caregivers report experiencing moderate to high levels of burden and some caregivers experience moderate to high levels of depression as well (Biegel, Sales, & Schulz, 1991; Bruhn, 1977; Leventhal et al., 1985).

A significant number of families are affected by chronic mental illness, although no accurate information is available concerning the number of persons with mental illness living in the community and living with families. However, estimates by Goldman and colleagues that have been used in planning by NIMH indicate that there are between 1.7 and 2.4 million individuals in the United States with chronic mental illness, more than 60% of whom live in the community (Goldman, 1984; Goldman, Gattozzi, & Taube, 1981). It is estimated that approximately 150,000 to 170,000 individuals with chronic mental illness return to their family homes on an annual basis.

Family caregivers of persons with chronic mental illness are affected by both the illness of their family member, contextual problems (based upon changes in treatment for persons with mental illness over the past

25 years), and the current inadequacies of the mental health treatment system. Studies of the problems and needs of family caregivers of persons with chronic mental illness indicate that caregiving burdens are long-standing and pervasive and that families often experience feelings of worry, guilt, resentment, and grief. Among the major problems and needs of these caregivers, as cited in the literature, are the following:

- Coping with behavioral problems of their ill relative
- Feeling isolated with no one to talk to
- Not having enough help in providing care for their relative with mental illness, even for those caregivers having a strong overall social network
- Interference with household routines and with the personal needs of family members
- Not getting adequate information about the family member's illness
- Needing assistance when the family member refuses to take medication regularly or is unable to regulate medication use
- Inability of the ill family member to carry out the tasks of daily living and to participate in family life
- Lack of a respite from caregiving responsibilities
- Insufficient help from mental health professionals (Biegel et al., 1991; Biegel & Yamatani, 1986; Grad & Sainsbury, 1963; Lamb, 1982; Leff, 1983; Spaniol & Jung, 1983; Thompson & Doll, 1982)

The burdens of family caregivers also are affected by contextual variables. For example, the policy of deinstitutionalization has meant that many clients are now treated in community programs instead of being hospitalized. However, enhanced civil rights for clients means that clients usually are not mandated to utilize community services and therefore may not actually use them. For those clients experiencing hospitalization, hospital stays are shorter and clients are returning to the community and to their families with more severe emotional problems than in the past (Pepper & Ryglewicz, 1984).

Further contributing to the strains experienced by the families is the fact that caseload sizes are high in many parts of the country and mental health case managers often are not able to assist their clients to widen their social networks and thus decrease clients' dependency on their families. For example, despite the promise of the NIMH Community Support Program, the development of comprehensive, community-based systems of social support for persons with chronic mental illness remains an unfulfilled goal, with many barriers to care still remaining

(Biegel, Tracy, & Corvo, in press; Gerhart, 1990). In addition, many of the ancillary services needed by clients, such as housing, job training, or social skills training, are available in only a limited fashion. A number of researchers believe the combination of these factors has caused greater strains on families today than in the past, with families having to make up for gaps and inadequacies of the service delivery system (Pepper & Ryglewicz, 1984).

The above literature clearly demonstrates that caring for a family member with mental illness can be burdensome for the caregiver; in fact these burdens often are unpredictable and can last for a considerable number of years. Although there is now substantial documentation concerning the existence and extent of caregiver burden, there is much less knowledge in the mental health field concerning the factors leading to higher levels of caregiver burden. The generation of such knowledge is essential to better understand the caregiving experience and to assist mental health professionals in efforts to address caregiver needs and reduce caregiver burden.

This chapter provides a critical review of the caregiving literature in the mental health field with an emphasis on methodological considerations, gaps, and limitations. Then, in an attempt to address some of the limitations in the literature, the chapter presents findings from an empirical study of family caregivers who are members of support groups for families of persons with mental illness. The study is focused on enhancing our understanding of the predictors of caregiver burden with specific attention to an examination of which variables contribute most to higher levels of burden for caregivers of persons with mental illness. The following sections provide an overview of the nature and extent of caregiver burden and present a conceptual framework for our research. To put our study in perspective, we also review existing knowledge concerning the predictors of caregiver burden, summarize gaps in this literature, and indicate areas in which our study attempts to address these gaps. The following sections then present the study methodology, findings, and implications for practice, policy, and research.

THE NATURE AND
EXTENT OF CAREGIVER BURDEN

The concept of burden is a central feature of virtually all caregiving studies. It has been most frequently treated as a primary outcome measure or as a predictor of other outcomes, such as the decision to hospitalize the client. Similar to caregiving research with other chronic diseases, there has been a lack of consensus as to the conceptualization and measurement of this concept in caregivers of persons with chronic mental illness. Some researchers have attempted to distinguish between objective and subjective aspects of burden (Brown, Bone, Dalison, & Wing, 1966; Thompson & Doll, 1982). Objective burden relates to disruptions of family life caused by the client's illness and/or to the time and effort required for the caregiver to attend to the needs of the ill family member. It thus may include activity restrictions, time spent, types of assistance/tasks provided, financial resources expended, and so on. Subjective burden, on the other hand, pertains to the amount of felt strain experienced by the caregiver in such areas as emotional status, physical status, and financial and work domains.

The first studies focusing, at least in part, on caregiving burdens of family members of persons with mental illness were conducted in England and indicate that families experience considerable amounts of strain (Brown et al., 1966; Grad & Sainsbury, 1963; Hoenig & Hamilton, 1966; Sainsbury & Grad, 1962). Grad and Sainsbury were the first researchers to conceptualize and measure "burden" in caregivers of persons with mental illness (Grad & Sainsbury, 1963; Sainsbury & Grad, 1962). The authors report that more than half of all families studied had suffered some difficulties because of the client's illness, with one fifth of the families reporting severe hardship. More than half of the respondents reported excessive anxiety due to worry about the client, and one third reported restrictions of social and leisure activities and upsets in domestic routine. Client behaviors found to be most upsetting included the client's constant focus on bodily complaints, concern about the possibility of client suicide, and ongoing demands by the client. Children were disturbed in one third of the families, and in one quarter of the families someone had to stay away from work to care for the client.

Studies by Brown and colleagues (1966) and Hoenig and Hamilton (1966) examined the effects on families of having a formerly hospitalized family member return to live with them. The clients studied by Brown and colleagues represented a working-class to lower-class group. Specific problems reported by the caregivers were similar to those in the Grad and Sainsbury study reported above. Almost half of the caregivers reported worry about the client, with more than one third reporting their health to be negatively affected, and the same percentage reported negative effects on children in the family. Almost one third had leisure or entertainment activities curtailed, with financial problems being reported by more than one quarter of the sample. Yet, despite these problems, very few of the respondents reported wanting the client to be hospitalized or to live elsewhere.

Building on the work of Grad and Sainsbury, Hoenig and Hamilton conceptualized caregiving burdens in a more sophisticated manner, distinguishing between objective and subjective components. Objective burden was defined to include certain specific effects on the daily life of the household or the occurrence of certain abnormal behavior in the client.[1] Subjective burden was based upon the respondents' view of whether or not they were carrying a burden during the four years of the study. Findings showed the presence of objective burden in more than half of the households. The degree of subjective burden reported was less than might be expected. In almost one quarter of households in which the client had caused objective burden, there was no reporting of subjective burden. This finding of tolerance of caregivers toward their levels of burden is similar to that reported above in the Brown and colleagues study.

Pasaminick, Scarpetti, and Dinitz (1967) reported on an experimental home care program to treat schizophrenics in the community. Considerable burdens were identified, with more than half of the respondents reporting major burdens pertaining to general worry and concern about the client, odd speech and behavior patterns, and clients being noisy or wandering during the night. Biegel and Yamatani (1986), utilizing the same burden scale as in the above study, report similar findings regarding caregiver burden in a sample of middle-class caregivers who were members of self-help groups for families of the mentally ill.

In a follow-up with the same sample used in the Pasaminick and colleagues' (1967) study, Davis, Dinitz, and Pasaminick (1974) reported finding levels of burden over an eight-year period that demonstrate the continuing problems that families experience in caring for a schizophrenic relative. Families worry about their ill family member, they get upset by the client's bizarre behavior, and they frequently commit the client to state and private treatment facilities. These results become even more significant when one realizes that families had been dealing with these problems, for better or worse, for at least the eight years of the study. This finding demonstrates that cumulative effects of individual components of burden and overall burden levels need to be considered as well as static levels of burden at any single point.

Data from several other more recent studies of lower-class, lower middle-class, and middle-class caregivers are generally consistent with the above reports (Doll, 1975, 1976; Hatfield, 1978, 1979a, 1979b; Kint, 1978; Kreisman & Joy, 1974; Thompson & Doll, 1982).[2] For example, Kreisman, Simmons, and Joy (1979) indicated that four fifths of the caregivers reported worrying about the client and had difficulty finding effective treatment. Three quarters of these caregivers reported disruption of family life, and more than 60% reported financial, employment, or social life problems. Feelings of guilt and stigma were similar to those found in the Kint study, with two fifths of the caregivers reporting feeling guilty and one fifth reporting problems of stigma. Major behavior problems of the client included withdrawal, failure to consider the future, and suicide attempts.

In contrast to the findings concerning burden reported above, Crotty and Kulys (1986) reported low levels of burden by family caregivers of persons with chronic mental illness. The sample was drawn from an urban outpatient community mental health center that served an ethnically mixed working-class community. Burden was assessed using a nine-item scale that measured the impact of the mentally ill relative upon the caregiver and the family. Findings showed that caregivers reported only mild levels of burden, with only two of the nine items registering high levels of burden. One fifth of the respondents reported that the client was not burdensome at all in any of the nine areas.

Comparing the results of the above studies is complicated by the fact that burden was conceptualized and operationalized differently across studies, sometimes without the use of standardized scales, and by the fact that these studies varied widely in their sampling techniques. Nonetheless, findings demonstrate fairly consistently that many family caregivers of persons with mental illness experience moderate to high levels of caregiver burden and that this burden often is experienced for considerable periods of time.

CONCEPTUAL FRAMEWORK
AND LITERATURE REVIEW

The effort to explain caregiving outcomes generally has been framed in terms of the stress-coping paradigm (Pearlin, Mullan, Semple, & Skaff, 1990). Caregiving is seen as the stressor, and burden and diminished subjective well-being are seen as the negative consequences (Biegel et al., 1991; George, 1980; House, 1974). A large number of variables have been included in operational definitions of caregiver stress—first and foremost, characteristics of the illness and illness-related attitudes and behaviors of the care receiver are considered to be primary or objective stressors that have a direct effect on caregiver well-being. Illness stage, functional status/impairment, and illness behaviors, such as disruptiveness, are primarily examples of caregiving stressors. Demographic characteristics of the care receiver also may be included as stressors or they may be defined as control variables. Other variables, known as conditioning variables, also have been included in the paradigm. These variables, at both the individual and the situational level, may have moderating as well as direct effects. For example, caregiving resources, including coping strategies and social supports, have been cited as important conditioning variables. That is, caregiving is expected to have particular negative consequences under conditions in which the caregiver receives little support and has limited coping resources. Demographic characteristics and environmental context of the caregiver also may be included as conditioning variables in the stress paradigm. Caregiving outcomes have included subjective appraisals by caregivers of the burdens posed by caregiving and objective or subjective indicators of psychological distress.

Based on the above, the present study includes a wide range of variables to predict the degree of caregiver distress or burden. These variables can be grouped into two broad classes of variables. The first set of variables relates to the ill family member and can be identified as stressor variables. This set of variables includes such objective illness characteristics as length of illness, hospitalization history, and frequency of client behavioral problems. Illness characteristics are indications of illness severity as well as its resultant care demands. In addition, certain demographic characteristics of the client, such as age and gender, have been identified as predictors of caregiver burden with other chronic illnesses and also are included in our framework as stressor variables.

The second set of predictor variables relates to the status of the caregiver and can be identified as conditioning variables. Demographic characteristics of caregivers (e.g., age, gender, family relationship to client, marital status, and socioeconomic status), caregivers' health status, and caregivers' other caregiving responsibilities may impact caregivers' ability to respond to the demands of the caregiving situation. Additional conditioning variables include the caregiver's involvement with the client (in this study, determined by where the client is living and the caregiver's frequency of contact with the client) and the nature of social supports available to the caregiver, including both the overall support system surrounding the caregiver as well as the specific supports, both informal and formal, available to help fulfill the caregiving role. We examine the direct effect of these conditioning variables on the level of caregiver burden. In addition, the study examines the possible moderating effects of one set of variables, social support, to see whether the effects of the predictor variables on caregiver burden will vary given different levels of overall social support, family support, and agency support.

This study aims to examine the correlation of these individual predictor variables with the level of caregiver burden, as well as the relative contribution of individual predictor variables, while controlling for other individual predictors. It thus is proposed that stressors and resources, such as social support, will have a combined influence on subjective appraisal of burden.

This model expands the stress-coping paradigm in caregiving with persons with mental illness by including a larger than customary set of predictors acknowledging that caregiving outcomes are embedded in the social fabric defining the caregiver-care receiver dyad; that is, these dyads are shaped by their demographic or ascribed status characteristics and interrelationships. This moves beyond just consideration of social support variables that have been considered by traditional caregiving research. In addition, rather than considering burden as a unidimensional construct, our conceptualization acknowledges its multidimensional aspects. Specifically, burden is conceptualized into four components: family disruption, dependency, stigma, and strain.

Table 7.1 presented a summary of previous research findings concerning predictors of burden for caregivers of persons with mental illness. As shown in the table, there are considerable gaps and inconsistencies in the literature. It must be noted that comparisons are limited by the fact that burden was not measured consistently across studies. In some cases there was one overall measure of burden; in other cases burden was divided into objective burden, pertaining to disruptions in family life, or subjective burden, defined as emotional costs of the patient's presence on the caregiver and family.

Beginning with predictor variables concerning client's illness, research studies consistently find that higher levels of client distress and behavioral problems are associated with higher levels of caregiver burden. However, findings concerning the relationship between the number of hospitalizations, length of hospitalizations, length of illness, and caregiver burden are inconsistent. For example, whereas Thompson and Doll (1982) and Brown and colleagues (1966) indicate that caregivers report higher burden with a greater number of hospitalizations, Biegel, Milligan, Putnam, and Song (in press) and Crotty and Kulys (1986) report no relationship between the number of hospitalizations and caregiver burden. There are also inconsistent findings in the literature concerning the relationship between the length of hospitalization and caregiver burden (Herz, Endicott, & Spitzer, 1976; Hoenig & Hamilton, 1966).[3] Several studies did find a relationship between length of illness and caregiver burden, such that the longer the illness, the higher the level of caregiver burden (Brown et al., 1966; Grad & Sainsbury, 1963; Hoenig & Hamilton, 1966). However, other studies did not find such a relationship (Biegel, Milligan, et al., in press).

A number of previous studies found no relationship between client gender or age and caregiver burden (Biegel, Milligan, et al., in press; Crotty & Kulys, 1986; Doll, 1975, 1976; Hoenig & Hamilton, 1966; Noh & Avison, 1988; Thompson & Doll, 1982). However, Grad and Sainsbury (1963) did find that caregivers of elderly clients were more burdened than caregivers of younger clients, and Cook and Pickett (1988) found that caregivers of older clients and female clients had higher levels of burden.

Research findings concerning the relationship between caregiver demographic and socioeconomic characteristics and caregiver burden are inconsistent. Although Doll and colleagues (Doll, 1975, 1976; Thompson & Doll, 1982) report no relationship between caregiver characteristics and caregiver burden, Crotty and Kulys (1986) report a relationship between household size and caregiver burden such that smaller households experienced more caregiver burden. Hoenig and Hamilton (1966) report no significant relationships between caregiver demographic and socioeconomic characteristics and objective burden, but do report a relationship between subjective burden and socioeconomic status of the caregiver such that lower-class caregivers report experiencing less subjective stress. This latter finding concerning the relationship between socioeconomic status and subjective stress was not supported by the work of Noh and Avison (1988), who found no relationship between family income and subjective burden, but is consistent with more recent research by Bulger, Wandersman, and Goldman (1993). Interestingly, Bulger and colleagues (1993) also find that the relationship between social class and burden is different depending on whether one is examining subjective or objective burden. Thus lower-

TABLE 7.1   Predictors of Caregiver Burden—Summary of Previous
              Research

Variable	Pattern Found
Client distress/behavior	Greater client distress, higher caregiver overall burden (Biegel, Milligan, et al., in press; Doll, 1976), higher objective and subjective burden (Biegel, Milligan, et al., in press; Potasznik & Nelson, 1984; Thompson & Doll, 1982), and higher subjective burden (Bulger, Wandersman, & Goldman, 1993; Noh & Avison, 1988)
	Caregiver burden is still present even when clients had few symptoms (Thompson & Doll, 1982)
Hospitalization	The greater the number of client hospitalizations, the higher the caregiver burden (Brown et al., 1966; Thompson & Doll, 1982)
	No relationship between the number of client hospitalizations and the level of caregiver burden (Biegel, Milligan, et al., in press; Crotty & Kulys, 1986)
	Inconsistent findings concerning the relationship between length of hospitalization and caregiver burden (Herz, Endicott, & Spitzer, 1976; Hoenig & Hamilton, 1966)
Length of illness	Inconsistent findings concerning the relationship between the length of illness and caregiver burden (Biegel, Milligan, et al., in press; Brown et al., 1966; Grad & Sainsbury, 1963; Hoenig & Hamilton, 1966)
Client characteristics	No relationship between client age, gender, and caregiver burden (Biegel, Crotty, & Kulys, 1986; Doll, 1975, 1976; Hoenig & Hamilton, 1966; Noh & Avison, 1988; Thompson & Doll, 1982)
	Caregivers of elderly clients have higher levels of burden than caregivers of younger clients (Grad & Sainsbury, 1963); caregivers of older clients and female clients have higher levels of burden (Cook & Pickett, 1988)
Caregiver characteristics	Inconsistent findings concerning the relationship between caregiver demographic and socioeconomic characteristics and caregiver burden (Bulger, Wandersman, & Goldman, 1993; Crotty & Kulys, 1986; Doll, 1975, 1976; Hoenig & Hamilton, 1966; Noh & Avison, 1988; Thompson & Doll, 1982)

TABLE 7.1 Continued

Variable	Pattern Found
Relationship to client	No association between caregiver relationship and caregiver burden (Biegel, Milligan, et al., in press; Gubman, Tessler, & Willis, 1987)
	Spouse caregivers experience more objective burden and less subjective burden than do nonspouse caregivers (Hoenig & Hamilton, 1966)
	Spouse caregivers have higher overall levels of burden than do nonspouse caregivers (Grad & Sainsbury, 1963)
Caregiver health	No relationship between caregiver health and overall caregiver burden; caregivers with poorer self-reported health status have higher levels of family disruption (objective burden) (Biegel, Milligan, et al., in press)
Caregiver-client interaction	Inconsistent findings concerning level of interaction between clients and caregivers and caregiver burden (Anderson & Lynch, 1984; Biegel, Milligan, et al., in press)
	Clients who lived alone but who remained in contact with the family had a severe effect on the family (Grad & Sainsbury, 1963)
Social networks and social support	The lower the perceived satisfaction with the network, the greater the subjective and objective burden (Potasznik & Nelson, 1984)
	The lower the perceived family support, the higher the level of caregiver burden (Biegel, Sales, & Schulz, 1992)
	No relationship between social support and subjective burden (Noh & Avison, 1988)
	No interaction effect between patient symptoms and social support on the level of caregiver burden (Noh & Avison, 1988; Potasznik & Nelson, 1984)

income caregivers report higher levels of objective burden than higher-income caregivers. In one of the few studies to examine race differences, Bulger and colleagues (1993) found that white caregivers had higher levels of subjective burden than black caregivers; however, the authors reported, but did not control for, significant differences in SES status by race. It is thus unclear as to whether this finding represents a true difference by the race of the caregiver.

There is also inconsistency in the findings of previous studies regarding the caregiver's family relationship to the client and caregiver burden. Biegel, Milligan, and colleagues (in press), Thompson and Doll (1982), and Gubman, Tessler, and Willis (1987) report no significant relationships. On the other hand, Hoenig and Hamilton (1966) report finding more objective burden in the conjugal than in the parental home, with the parental home reporting less objective but more subjective burden. The authors interpreted this finding to mean that parents are less able to tolerate family members with mental illness than are other types of caregivers.

There has been little previous research concerning the relationship between caregiver health and burden. Biegel, Milligan, and colleagues (in press) found no relationship between caregiver health and levels of overall caregiver burden. However, they found that caregivers with poorer self-reported health status have higher levels of family disruption or objective burden. Several other studies did not directly examine the relationship between caregiver health and burden but did report on associations between caregiver health and other variables. For example, Grad and Sainsbury (1963) found that one fifth of the caregivers attributed their neurotic symptoms, such as insomnia, headaches, excessive irritability, and depression, to concern about the client's behavior. Brown and colleagues (1966) report an indirect relationship between caregiver health and burden. They indicate that almost half of caregivers of clients with multiple admissions report that the caregivers' health was negatively affected, as compared with one quarter of caregivers of clients with one admission.

There has been little prior research concerning the frequency of caregiver-client interaction and the level of caregiver burden. Findings from the few studies that have conducted examinations in this area are inconsistent. For example, whereas Biegel, Milligan, and colleagues (in press) found no relationship between burden and the level of caregiver interaction with the ill family member, Grad and Sainsbury (1963) found that client living status was related to caregiver burden. Clients who lived alone but who remained in contact with the family had a severe effect on the family. However, clients who lived in lodgings, boardinghouses, or hotels were not a problem, either to those with whom they lived or to their own families. Anderson and Lynch (1984) found that greater levels of interaction between family members and clients were associated with higher stress experienced by family members.

Of particular note is the paucity of research concerning the relationship between social support, both formal and informal, and caregiver burden. Although social support networks of persons with mental illness have been examined in a number of studies during the past decade (Beels, 1978; Crotty & Kulys, 1985), much less attention has been paid to social support systems of caregivers of this population. Previous research has documented caregivers' sense of isolation, lack of intimate relationships, and withdrawal by others, as well as the tendency of relatives and friends to avoid visiting the caregiver's household. Biegel and Yamatani (1986), in a study of predominantly middle-class members of self-help groups for families of persons with mental illness, found that even caregivers who reported strong overall systems of social support identified the lack of social support, or anybody to talk to, concerning the specific problems and needs they experienced as caregivers of persons with mental illness. In a study of caregivers who were members of self-help groups for families of persons with mental illness, Potasznik and Nelson (1984) found that the less caregivers were satisifed with their social support network, the greater their levels of both subjective and objective burden. Similarly, in a more recent study of lower social class caregivers, Biegel, Milligan, and colleagues (in press) found that caregivers who felt they were not getting sufficient help from their families had higher levels of caregiver burden. However, Noh and Avison's (1988) study of spouse caregivers finds no relationship between caregivers' social support and subjective burden.

Research with other caregiving populations had found that agency professionals can play important roles in addressing issues of caregiver burden (Biegel et al., 1991). Given the ambiguous, anxiety-producing, and often difficult to comprehend nature of mental illness, mental health professionals can play a particularly important role in shaping families' responses to caregiving demands and the illness situation. However, the mental health literature has reported consistently over the past decade that caregivers are not satisfied with their relationships with mental health professionals (Francell, Conn, & Gray, 1988; Holden & Lewine, 1982; Spaniol & Jung, 1983). Unfortunately, there has been little empirical analysis of the effects of these relationships upon the levels of caregiver burden.

In conclusion, the literature examining predictors of caregiver distress has identified a number of variables that contribute to caregiver burden. However, as we can see, the present data are far from conclusive and a number of gaps in the mental health literature still remain. Many previous studies are atheoretical and do not take advantage of extant knowledge of caregiving with other chronic illnesses; studies have not examined a wide range of variables that can predict caregiver distress, and the analysis techniques that have been utilized in most studies have not identified which variables make a greater contribution to the level of caregiving distress; studies do not always use standardized scales and even when standardized scales are used, measures do not always capture the multidimensional nature of the constructs examined; and studies do not always identify salient aspects of the caregiver population, including social class, which makes comparisons of findings across studies more difficult.

This chapter attempts to address a number of the above limitations in an examination of family caregiving with persons with mental illness. This study utilizes a stress-coping theoretical framework adapted from use with caregivers of Alzheimer's disease patients. Caregiving research with the elderly in general, and Alzheimer's disease in particular, is more conceptually and methodologically sophisticated than research with caregivers of persons with mental illness. This chapter seeks to build upon research with the former to enhance research with the latter. Second, our analyses examine the combined effects of multiple independent variables upon the level of caregiver burden; the relative contribution of each independent variable is examined while controlling for the effect of other individual variables on burden. Though some studies of caregivers of persons with mental illness have moved beyond simple bivariate analyses (Bulger et al., 1993; Cook & Pickett, 1988; Noh & Avison, 1988; Potasznik & Nelson, 1984), most studies have not taken this approach.

Third, this study includes predictor variables pertaining to caregivers' beliefs about the adequacy of informal support from other family members as well as the adequacy of formal support from mental health professionals. Previous research with family caregivers of persons with mental illness has demonstrated the importance of asking respondents about the specific social support they receive in caring for their family member with mental illness, in addition to examining their overall social support systems. Family caregivers of persons with mental illness have reported significant social support deficits in addressing the burdens of their caregiving, despite positive overall levels of support (Biegel & Yamatani, 1986).

All too often in the past, families were blamed as the causal agent of their ill relatives' disease (Hatfield, 1987). Although this has changed to the point that many mental health centers now facilitate, sponsor, or staff support groups for family members who have a relative with chronic mental illness, we know little about the effect that families' perceptions of the help they are getting from mental health professionals have on their level of perceived burden. Thus, though a number of studies in the past decade have documented families' concerns about their relationships with mental health professionals, previous studies have not examined the effect of perceived support, or lack thereof, from mental health agency professionals on caregiver burden.

Finally, this study takes a multidimensional approach to caregiver burden through the development of subscales that measure specific types of burden. These subscales build upon previous classifications of types of burden, but are more specific in regard to types of subjective burden.

METHOD

Study Sample

All family caregivers who were members of the Alliance for the Mentally Ill of Metro Cleveland (AMI of Metro Cleveland), an organization of caregivers of persons with mental illness, were mailed a self-administered questionnaire, with a stamped return envelope and a cover letter from the president of AMI of Metro Cleveland. Most of the members of this organization are middle-class and white. A follow-up letter was sent to everyone about six weeks later. To facilitate comparisons with the authors' previously obtained sample of white and black lower social class caregivers (Biegel, Milligan, et al., in press), the questionnaire included questions identical to those utilized in the lower social class sample pertaining to caregiver distress, relationship with mental health professionals, and client and caregiver characteristics.

Two hundred and thirty-three questionnaires were mailed out and 117 completed questionnaires were received. This represents a response rate of 50%, which is very high for mail surveys. We believe that cosponsorship by AMI of Metro Cleveland of this survey, and its endorsement through the letter from the AMI of Metro Cleveland president, was instrumental in securing this high response rate.

Of the 117 returned questionnaires, 18 cases were eliminated from the data set because of too much missing data or because the respondent was not a family caregiver. Thus, data from 99 respondents was utilized in this sample.

Data Collection Instrument[4]

Client Behavioral Problems

As noted above, previous research studies have found that the level of client behavioral problems/distress is related to caregiver burden. Caregivers were asked to report the frequency of a wide range of possible client behaviors, such as sleeping problems, taking medication, hallucinations, money management, suspiciousness, or forgetfulness. A 38-item behavioral problems scale was developed for this study that was based on selected items used in research with caregivers of Alzheimer's disease patients (Schulz, Williamson, Morycz, & Biegel, 1992), from selected items in the Family Distress Scale developed by Pasaminick and colleagues (1967) in research with families of persons with mental illness, and from a review of the research literature of behavioral problems identified by caregivers of persons with mental illness. The reliability of this scale was high (Cronbach's alpha = .93). This scale is an improvement upon the Family Distress Scale, which is primarily a measure of caregiver burden, but which confounds client behavior items with caregiver reactions to those behaviors.

Caregiver Burden

A 27-item scale of overall caregiver burden was developed for this study based on items included in the Caregiver Burden Scale (CBS) developed by Zarit, Reever, and Bach-Peterson (1980) for use with caregivers of Alzheimer's disease patients; selected items in the Family Distress Scale developed by Pasaminick and colleagues (1967); and items generated from a review of the research literature on burdens of caregivers with mental illness. The scale measures feelings that caregivers have about their psychological well-being and social life as well as their feelings about their family member with mental illness (e.g., feeling inadequate, resentful, stressed, useful, depended upon, or embarrassed in regard to the care recipient). The reliability of this scale was very good (Cronbach's alpha = .87).

Previous studies with caregivers of persons with mental illness have conceptualized burden into two components, objective burden and subjective burden (Doll, 1975, 1976; Hoenig & Hamilton, 1966; Thompson & Doll, 1982). Objective burden has been defined as disruptions to family life caused by the person with mental illness; subjective burden is the emotional costs of having a person with mental illness in one's family. To better specify the salient dimensions of burden among caregivers, using exploratory factor analysis, four burden subscales were extracted— Family Disruption (11 items), Client Dependency (4 items), Stigma (6 items), and Caregiver Strain (5 items)—from the 26 items in our overall burden scale. The first subscale is very similar to previous measures of objective burden, whereas the remaining three subscales can be said to be components of subjective, or emotional, burden. Each of the four subscales was highly correlated with the overall burden scale, and the subscales were moderately correlated with each other, with correlation coefficients ranging from .34 to .63. Reliability of these four subscales was moderate to good, with Cronbach's standardized alphas as follows: Stigma (.73), Family Disruption (.81), Dependency (.68), and Strain (.59).

Physical Health

Respondents were asked to rate their overall health on a 5-point scale from excellent to poor. This question was developed and validated by the National Center for Health Services Research (Brook et al., 1979) for the Health Insurance Study.

Social Support and Social Networks

Respondents were asked about their overall social support systems as well as their view of the adequacy of help received from family members and agency professionals. As a measure of overall social support, the study used the Index of Socially Supportive Behaviors, which has been well validated in previous research. This 20-item scale asks respondents to indicate, on a 5-point scale (ranging from "not at all" to "about every day"), their opinion concerning items that measure appraisal, belonging, and financial and emotional support. The reliability of this scale was high, with a Cronbach's alpha of .90.

Concerning social support received in connection with their caregiving role, respondents were asked whether they thought the amount of help and support they received from their family members was much less than needed, somewhat less than needed, about enough, somewhat more than needed, or much too much. They also were asked the same question concerning the amount of help they received from mental health professionals.

Client and Caregiver Characteristics

Data was collected on the following demographic and socioeconomic characteristics of caregivers: age, gender, race, marital status, years of education, major occupation, income, household size, and years of education and major occupation for the caregiver's spouse, if applicable. Education and occupation levels of the caregiver (and the caregiver's spouse, if any) were used to calculate the caregiver's family socioeconomic status, using the Hollingshead and Redlich Two-Factor Index of Social Position (Hollingshead & Redlich, 1958). In addition, caregivers were asked whether they provided assistance to other household members having significant physical health, mental health, or substance abuse problems.

The following data about the family member with mental illness were collected from the caregiver: age, gender, length of illness, recent hospitalizations, and place of residence. Caregivers also were asked about their family relationship to, and amount of contact with, their family member with mental illness.

Analysis Plan

The study aims to examine the correlations of 20 individual predictor (or independent) variables with the level of caregiver burden, as well as to assess the relative contribution of individual predictor variables while controlling for other independent variables. To address a gap of many previous research studies, the lack of multivariate analyses of the predictors of caregiver burden, a series of multiple regression analyses were conducted. Because the number of the independent variables was too large to enter in a regression analysis given our sample size, bivariate correlations between each predictor and overall burden and burden subscale were examined first. Variables that were statistically significant in the bivariate analyses then were used as independent variables in the multiple regression analyses for overall burden and for our four burden subscales (family disruption, stigma, strain, and dependency).

In addition, to test the moderating effects of the social support variables on the relationships between other independent variables and caregiver burden, interaction terms were created by multiplying the significant social support variables with other predictor variables found to be significant in the bivariate analyses. To avoid problems of multicolinearity between the interaction terms and the original variables, the original variables were centered (subtracted from the mean) before the interaction terms were created. When multiple regression analyses were performed, the original variables were entered in the first block, and then the interaction terms were entered in the second block. If the interaction terms did not produce significant R^2 change, the model with the original variables only was retained based on considerations of simplicity. In order to compare the results of this study with previous research findings of caregivers who are support group members, findings from the bivariate as well as multiple regression analyses are presented.

FINDINGS

Characteristics of Clients

Sample characteristics for the predictor and dependent variables can be found in Table 7.2. Clients ranged in age from 19 to 81 years, with a mean age of 35.6 years. Almost two thirds of the clients are male, and just over one third are female. More than one third (39.4%) of the clients live in their own home whereas just over one quarter (27.3%) reside with the family caregiver. The remainder of clients live with friends or relatives or in a more restrictive environment such as a group home.

Clients had been ill for a considerable period of time, with the mean length of illness (ranging from 2 to 51 years) of 16.3 years. Almost all of the clients in the sample have been hospitalized for psychiatric illness, with a mean number of hospitalizations (ranging from 0 to 50) of 8.6. The mean length of most recent hospitalization, ranging from 3 to 270 days, is 46.9 days. The clients returned to the home of the caregiver following hospitalization an average of 5.4 times (range = 0-24 times). Caregivers reported that clients had moderate to low levels of behavioral problems, with a mean of 39.4 (ranging from 0 to 106) on the Client Behavioral Problems Scale.

TABLE 7.2 Sample Characteristics—Predictors and Dependent Variables (means, standard deviation [SD], and percentages; $N = 99$)

Variables I. Predictor Variables	Mean (or %)	SD
Client Characteristics		
A. Illness Severity		
1. Length of illness (years)	16.33	9.16
2. Number of hospitalizations	8.62	8.23
3. Number of days most recent hospitalization	46.86	57.18
4. Number of times returned home after hospitalization	5.37	4.67
5. Frequency of client behaviors (0 to 148, low to high frequency)	39.44	24.65
B. Client Demographic Characteristics		
1. Client age (years)	35.58	9.65
2. Client gender	63.3% M 36.7% F	
Caregiver Characteristics		
A. Caregiver Demographic and Socioeconomic Characteristics		
1. Caregiver age	61.45	9.71
2. Caregiver gender	21% M 79% F	
3. Caregiver marital status—married	66.3% Yes	
4. Caregiver social class (17 to 77, high to low class)	25.80	11.70
5. Family relationship to client—parent	84%	
B. Caregiver Health Status (1 to 5, excellent to poor)	2.59	1.02
C. Other Caregiving Responsibilities—Yes	19%	
D. Client Proximity and Contact With Caregiver		
1. Client living status—live with caregiver	27.3% Yes	
2. Frequency of contact between client and caregiver in past month (0 to 5, once a month to daily)	4.20	1.08
3. Frequency of contact between client and caregiver in past year (0 to 7, twice a year or less to daily)	6.00	1.29
E. Caregiver Social Support		
1. Overall social support (0 to 80, low to high support)	20.57	12.71
2. Sufficiency of family support (1 to 5, much less to much too much)	2.20	.87
3. Sufficiency of agency support (1 to 5, much less to much too much)	1.90	.91

TABLE 7.2 Continued

Variables II. Dependent Variables	Mean (or %)	SD
A. Perceived Overall Burden (0 to 108, low to high)	40.24	14.54
B. Burden Subscales		
1. Perceived disruption (0 to 44, low to high)	14.80	6.85
2. Perceived stigma (0 to 24, low to high)	7.25	4.57
3. Perceived strain (0 to 20, low to high)	8.95	3.52
4. Perceived dependency (0 to 16, low to high)	7.77	3.44

Caregivers' Characteristics

Caregivers range from 36 to 82 years of age (mean = 61.5 years). A majority (66.7%) of them are 60 years and above. The caregivers are predominantly female. A high proportion (66.3%) of them are married and a sizeable minority (26.5%) of them are widowed. Very few of them are separated, divorced, or never married. The annual family income of the caregivers is between $30,000 and $34,999. Using the Hollingshead and Redlich Two-Factor Index of Social Position, the scores range from 11 to 63, with a mean of 25.8 (S.D. = 11.7). This places them in social class II (upper middle), although the proportion of caregivers in social class III (middle) is fractionally higher than in social class II.

More than four fifths (84%) of caregivers are parents. A considerable number, about one fifth of them, also had additional caregiving responsibilities. Caregivers had frequent contact with their family member with chronic mental illness during the past month. The average amount of contact during the past month was in the category of several times per week. Almost all (90%) caregivers contacted their family members on a weekly basis or more frequently during the past month. The pattern of contact remained for the past year, with more than four fifths (86%) of them contacting their family member weekly or more frequently during the past 12 months. Caregivers' score on the overall social support scale was low (mean = 20.6), indicating a low to moderate level of overall social support. Concerning the adequacy of informal support in their caregiving roles, about one half of caregivers reported that they did not get enough help from their families, and two thirds of the

caregivers indicated not getting enough assistance from agency professionals. Finally, caregivers reported moderate to low levels of overall
burden. Among the four subscales of burden, caregivers reported higher
scores on disruption, strain, and dependency.

Predictors of Caregiver Burden

Bivariate Analyses

The correlations between the hypothesized predictors and caregiver's
overall burden were examined first. Only four variables had significantly strong zero-order correlations with overall burden ($\geq.25$ or $\leq-.25$)
(see Table 7.3). These were further used in the multiple regression
analysis for overall burden. These four variables are frequency of client
disruptive behaviors, caregiver health, sufficiency of informal support,
and sufficiency of formal support. The frequency of client behavioral
problems had the strongest association with burden ($r = .61$). The
greater the frequency of client behavior problems, the higher the burden.
None of the other illness variables was significantly associated with
caregiver burden. In addition, the poorer the caregiver's health ($r = .35$),
the higher the degree of burden. Two of the three caregiver social
network variables were related to the degree of overall burden. Thus,
caregivers who felt they were not getting enough support from family
members ($r = -.38$) or agency professionals ($r = -.27$) in caring for their
relative with mental illness reported higher levels of overall burden.

There were no statistically significant relationships between demographic and socioeconomic characteristics of either clients or caregivers
and the level of overall burden. Furthermore, neither client proximity and
degree of contact with the caregiver nor the respondents' other caregiving
responsibilities were related to level of overall burden.

After our examination of the bivariate predictors of overall burden, we
repeated the same sets of analyses for the predictors of each of the four
burden subscales: family disruption, stigma, strain, and dependency
(see Table 7.4). Findings reveal a number of differences between the
predictors of overall burden and the predictors of individual types of
burden. Only the frequency of client behavior problems and the sufficiency of family support were significantly associated with each type
of burden. In addition to these two variables, the correlates of each type
of burden were somewhat different. The higher the number of times the
client returned home after hospitalization ($r = .22$), the worse the

TABLE 7.3 Correlates of Caregiver Burden (*N* = 99)

Variable	Correlate
Conditions Conducive to Stress	
A. Illness Variables	
1. Length of illness	.08
2. Number of hospitalizations	.10
3. Number of days most recent hospitalization	−.11
4. Number of times returned home after hospitalization	.17
5. Frequency of client behaviors	.61**
B. Client Demographic Characteristics	
1. Client age	−.12
2. Client gender	.16
Conditioning Variables	
A. Client Proximity and Contact with Family	
1. Client living status (1 = live with caregiver)	.10
2. Frequency of contact between client and caregiver in past month	.004
3. Frequency of contact between client and caregiver in past year	.07
B. Characteristics of Caregivers	
1. Caregiver age	−.06
2. Caregiver gender (1 = male)	.07
3. Caregiver marital status (1 = married)	−.14
4. Caregiver social class	−.01
5. Relationship to client (1 = parent)	.18
C. Other Caregiving Responsibilities (1 = yes)	.17
D. Caregiver Health	.35**
E. Caregiver Social Network	
1. Overall social support	−.16
2. Sufficiency of family support	−.38*
3. Sufficiency of agency support	−.27*

*$p \le .01$
**$p \le .001$

caregiver health (*r* = .39), the less support from agency professionals that the caregivers had (*r* = −.28), and the higher the level of family disruption. Caregivers' perceived stigma was associated with worse caregiver health (*r* = .32) and less overall social support (*r* = −.25). Furthermore, male caregivers perceived more stigma than females (*r* = .21). Insufficiency of overall social support (*r* = −.28) and lack of support from agency professionals (*r* = −.36) were significantly correlated with

TABLE 7.4 Correlates of Caregiver Burden Subscales (N = 99)

Variable	Disrupt	Stigma	Strain	Depend
Conditions Conducive to Stress				
A. Illness Variables				
1. Length of illness	.05	.03	.002	.24[a]
2. Number of hospitalizations	.08	.04	.03	.13
3. Number of days most recent hospitalization	−.09	−.02	−.12	−.16
4. Number of times returned home after hospitalizations	.22[a]	−.08	.01	.20
5. Frequency of client behavior	.52[c]	.31[b]	.60[c]	.58[c]
B. Client Demographic Characteristics				
1. Client age	−.11	−.11	−.16	.05
2. Client gender (1 = male)	.11	.09	.21[a]	.03
Conditioning Variables				
A. Client Proximity and Contact With Family				
1. Client status (1 = live with caregiver)	.13	−.08	.04	.06
2. Frequency of contact between client and caregiver in past month	.07	−.17	−.08	.19
3. Frequency of contact between client and caregiver in past year	.10	−.10	.03	.18
B. Caregiver Demographic and Socioeconomic Characteristics				
1. Caregiver age	−.15	.02	.06	.11
2. Caregiver gender (1 = male)	−.01	.21[a]	.04	.06
3. Caregiver marital status (1 = married)	−.14	−.05	−.14	−.14
4. Caregiver social class	.02	−.07	.04	.12
5. Relationship to client (1 = parent)	.10	.16	.19	.11
C. Other Caregiving Responsibilities (1 = yes)	.18	.11	.11	.14
D. Caregiver Health	.39[c]	.32[c]	.13	.31[b]
E. Caregiver Social Network				
1. Overall social support	−.16	−.25[a]	−.28[a]	−.19
2. Sufficiency of family support	−.30[b]	−.28[b]	−.32[b]	−.40[c]
3. Sufficiency of agency support	−.28[b]	−.05	−.36[c]	−.26[a]

[a] $p \leq .05$
[b] $p \leq .01$
[c] $p \leq .001$

strain. Caregivers of male clients also had higher levels of strain (r = .21). The longer the client was ill (r = .24), the worse the caregiver health (r = .31), the less support from agency professionals that caregiver had

($r = -.26$), and the more the dependency that caregivers perceived from the family member with mental illness.

Our findings of the important role that client behavioral symptoms play in predicting caregiver burden are consistent with previous research. The finding of Thompson and Doll (1982) that caregiver burden did not disappear even when the client had few symptoms demonstrates that the level of client symptoms by itself is an insufficient explanation of caregiver burden. Indeed, other variables also were found in our analyses to be associated with caregiver burden and some of these variables, as is shown below in the discussion of our regression analyses, remain significant predictors even after controlling for the level of client behavioral problems.

The current study found no relationship between overall caregiver burden and other measures of the severity of illness, such as length of illness, number of hospitalizations, number of days of most recent hospitalization, and the number of times returned home after hospitalization. As can be seen in Table 7.1, previous research findings were inconsistent in this area. We found no relationship between client and caregiver characteristics and overall caregiver burden. Our findings concerning the lack of an association between the frequency of caregiver-client interactions and caregiver burden were not consistent with earlier studies by Grad and Sainsbury (1963) and Anderson and Lynch (1984). Finally, our findings concerning caregiver health and caregiver social networks break new ground, as other studies, except for our previous study of lower social class caregivers (Biegel, Milligan, et al., in press), have not addressed this area.

Bivariate findings of the current study, with some exceptions, were consistent with the findings of our previous study of lower social class caregivers. Both studies used the same predictor variables, though the scales used to measure overall social support were not the same in both studies. Some differences between the clients and caregivers in the two studies must be noted. Clients in the present study were slightly younger and had been hospitalized more times than clients in the lower social class sample. Caregivers in the present study were slightly older and more likely to be married and to be parents. By definition, caregivers in the present study were support group members (only 10% of the lower social class sample were support group members) and were of a higher social class. In addition, all of the caregivers in the present study were white, whereas about half the caregivers in the lower social class study were white with the other half being black. Caregivers in the present study had a higher level of self-reported health, lower levels of perceived support from agency professionals, and higher levels of burden.

Findings of bivariate analyses of the predictors of burden indicate that for both samples, frequency of client behavioral problems and lower perceived support from family members and agency professionals each were associated with higher levels of burden. In addition, for lower social class caregivers, lower levels of overall social support also were associated with higher levels of burden, whereas for higher social class caregivers, lower self-reported health was associated with higher levels of burden.

It should be noted that comparisons of the above bivariate correlates of caregiver burden with previous research are complicated by a number of factors. Most of the studies that have empirically examined variables associated with caregiver burden and that used standardized instruments to measure the study variables did not utilize samples of caregivers who were exclusively or predominantly members of support groups. Our comparisons are further complicated by the fact that sample characteristics, especially caregivers' SES data, are incomplete or not reported in a number of studies.

Multiple Regression Analysis

Utilizing our bivariate results to select predictor variables, four original predictor variables of burden (frequency of client behavioral problems, caregiver health, sufficiency of formal support, and sufficiency of informal support), as well as four interaction terms (client behavioral problems by family support, client behavioral problems by agency support, caregiver health by family support, and caregiver health by agency support), were entered into the model to predict the level of overall caregiver burden. The results indicated that the R^2 change (.06) induced by the interaction terms was not significant ($p >$ .05); therefore, the model with the four original variables was retained as the final model.

This regression model explained 46% of the total variance in caregiver burden ($F = 15.04$; $df = 4,63$; $p \leq .001$). However, only the frequency of client behavior and caregiver health were significant predictors of caregiver burden after controlling for the other independent variables (see Table 7.5). Thus caregivers who reported more client behavioral problems and had poorer health perceived a higher level of overall burden. Comparisons of these findings to our previous study of lower

TABLE 7.5 Results of Multiple Regression Analyses of Predictors of Caregiver Burden ($N = 68$)

Variable	Unstandardized Regression Coefficient (B)	Beta	T Value	p Value
Frequency of client behaviors	.33	.55	5.57	.000
Sufficiency of agency support	−.94	−.06	−.61	.546
Caregiver health	3.22	.23	2.49	.015
Sufficiency of family support	−2.67	−.17	−1.72	.090

Note: Adjusted R square = 46%, $F = 15.04$, $p \leq .001$, $df = 4,63$.

social class caregivers indicate that frequency of client behavioral problems is a common predictor for both populations. However, for lower-class caregivers lack of perceived family support is also a significant predictor, whereas caregiver health is not (Biegel, Milligan, et al., in press).

We repeated the same sets of analyses to identify the predictors for each burden subscale (see Tables 7.6 and 7.7). The interaction terms were not significant in increasing the variance explained in family disruption, stigma, and strain. As a result, only the original variables were retained in the models of regression analyses for these variables.

The variance explained for these three types of burden ranged from .27 to .45; the level of explain variance cannot be directly compared, however, because of the different composition of predictors for each model. As found in the analysis for the overall burden, frequency of client behavior was the strongest predictor of each type of burden after controlling for other predictors in the model. In addition, some different specific significant predictors were found for each type of burden. Caregiver health was a significant predictor of family disruption and stigma, respectively, as is the case in overall burden. Overall social support was associated with lower levels of caregiver strain.

Concerning the predictors of caregiver dependency, the four interaction terms explained 12% of the variance in dependency (see Table 7.7). Overall, the model with eight independent variables explained 49% of the variance. Dependency can be predicted by sufficiency of family support in addition to the frequency of client behavioral problems. As expected, caregivers with higher levels of perceived family support had

TABLE 7.6 Results of Multiple Regression Analyses of Predictors of
Caregiver Family Disruption, Stigma, and Strain

Variables	Unstandardized Regression (B)	Beta	T Value	p Value
Family Disruption (N = 69)[a]				
Frequency of client behaviors	.13	.44	4.20	.0001
Sufficiency of family support	−.84	−.11	−1.07	.29
Sufficiency of agency support	−2.00	−.13	−1.30	.20
Caregiver health	1.90	.29	2.97	.004
Stigma (N = 62)[b]				
Frequency of client behaviors	.06	.27	2.27	.03
Sufficiency of family support	−.49	−.10	−.80	.43
Caregiver health	1.43	.31	2.59	.01
Social support	−.06	−.17	−1.40	.17
Strain (N = 60)[c]				
Frequency of client behaviors	.08	.52	4.79	.000
Overall social support	−.08	−.30	−2.91	.005
Sufficiency of family support	.17	.05	.43	.67
Sufficiency of agency support	−.61	−.16	−1.53	.13

[a]Multiple R = .65; adjusted R^2 = .39; $F(4,64)$ = 11.82; $p < .001$
[b]Multiple R = .56; adjusted R^2 = .27; $F(4,57)$ = 6.57; $p < .001$
[c]Multiple R = .69; adjusted R^2 = 45; $F(4,55)$ = 12.83; $p < .001$

lower levels of caregiver dependency. In addition, t-tests for the individual interaction terms revealed that both sufficiency of family support and sufficiency of agency support had significant moderating effects on the relationship between the frequency of client behavioral problems and caregiver perceived dependency. Thus, for caregivers with higher levels of perceived family support, client behavioral problems had less of an effect on client dependency. However, the interaction effect was in the opposite direction for sufficiency of agency support. For those caregivers with higher levels of perceived agency support, client behavioral problems had a greater effect on client dependency.

In general, we found relatively little support for the hypothesis that social support moderates the effect of client symptoms upon caregiver burden. As indicated above, we did not find any moderating effects of

TABLE 7.7 Results of Multiple Regression Analyses of Predictors of Caregiver Dependency ($N = 69$)

Variables	Unstandardized Regression (B)	Beta	T Value	p Value
Original Variables[a]				
Frequency of client behaviors	.08	.58	5.58	.000
Caregiver health	.46	.14	1.56	.124
Sufficiency of family support	-.94	-.25	-2.60	.012
Sufficiency of agency support	.28	.08	.74	.461
Interaction Terms[b,c]				
Client behavior × family support	-.04	-.21	-2.30	.025
Client behavior × agency support	.06	.33	3.33	.002
Caregiver health × family support	.07	.02	.23	.820
Caregiver health × agency support	.54	.14	1.52	.134

[a]Multiple R = .66; adjusted R^2 = 39; $F(4,64)$ = 12.05; $p < .001$
[b]R^2 change = .12; F = 8.86; $p < .01$
[c]Multiple R = .74; adjusted R^2 = .49; $F(8,60)$ = 9.03; $p < .001$

social support in this regard for overall burden, family disruption, stigma, or strain. These findings are consistent with several previous studies, which also found that caregivers' social support did not moderate the effect of client symptoms on caregiver burden (Noh & Avison, 1988; Potasznik & Nelson, 1984).

The interpretation of the interaction effects of social support upon the relationship between client behavioral problems and caregiver dependency is limited due to our inability to specify causal direction, given the cross-sectional nature of the study design. We hypothesize, however, that family support reduces the relationship between client behavioral problems and caregiver dependency because other family members can share the caregiver's tasks and thus the caregiver who has family support does not feel that his or her ill family member is so dependent on him or her. Concerning agency professionals, we hypothesize that caregivers whose clients have more behavioral problems and who therefore feel that the client is overly dependent upon them have greater involvement with mental health professionals and thus feel more supported. However, unlike the support from family members, agency professionals cannot directly intervene to help make the client less dependent on the caregiver. This interpretation is supported by data from our study of lower social class caregivers, in which we asked caregivers who had ever sought help from anyone for a caregiving problem about their interactions with a wide range of formal helpers. Findings revealed that formal helpers understood their problems, took their problems seriously, were concerned about them, and treated them with respect. However, when the caregivers were asked how helpful these helpers were on a four-point scale from very helpful to not helpful at all, mean scores ranged between "somewhat" to "of little help" (Biegel, Milligan, et al., in press).

Findings from this study demonstrate that the frequency of client behavioral problems is the strongest predictor of both overall burden and each of the types of burden—family disruption, stigma, strain, and dependency—examined in this study. This finding is consistent with previous research with family caregivers of persons with mental illness indicating the important role that illness variables play in caregiver burden and is also consistent with the literature on caregiving with other chronic illnesses.

Caregiver health, which might be considered as a caregiver resource, was a significant predictor of the levels of overall burden and also of family disruption and stigma. As discussed above, the higher social class caregivers in this study reported their health as more positive than did the lower social class caregivers in our previous study, yet health was a significant predictor of burden only for the higher social class group. This difference might be explained by the fact that higher social class caregivers were older than the lower social class sample (mean of 62 years vs. a mean of 55 years), and the caregiving literature suggests that older caregivers worry about what will happen to their ill family member when they die. Therefore, older caregivers with lower self-reported health may feel more burdened because of their concern that their health problems may interfere with their continued caregiving role.

The lack of caregivers' perceived family support was found to be a significant predictor of overall caregiver burden on the bivariate level but was not a significant predictor of overall levels of burden when controlling for other variables, although it did predict higher levels of caregiver dependency. This finding needs to be interpreted in light of the fact that the sample for the study consisted of members of support groups. Such individuals are in a better position to obtain social support regarding the problems of caring for their relative with mental illness than are non-support group members. In fact, the emotional and informational support from members of their support group, which was not examined in this analysis, may have compensated, in part, for caregivers' perceived lack of support from family members.

It also should be noted, however, that caregivers in this sample had higher levels of burden than our previously studied lower social class caregiver group (only 10% of whom were in support groups) despite the fact that they had been support group members for an average of 48 months prior to the study. This suggests two things. First, individuals may self-select into support groups based on higher levels of burden. Second, support groups, though providing significant assistance to caregivers through informational and emotional support, may not have much of an effect in reducing the level of caregiver burden, especially because client behavioral problems are the strongest predictor of caregiver burden and support groups are not primarily focused on changing client behavior or helping caregivers in their interactions with their ill family member.

The variations in significant predictors (including interaction terms) other than client behavioral problems and to some extent caregiver health, for the types of burden, indicate the multidimensional nature of caregiver burden and the importance of segregating burden components. Significant predictors, such as sufficiency of informal support and overall social support, and the interaction effects between client behavioral problems and family support and between client behavioral problems and agency support on caregiver dependency may never be discovered if only the overall burden is assessed.

IMPLICATIONS FOR
PRACTICE, POLICY, AND RESEARCH

Results of this study have important implications for practice and policy in the mental health field. Findings show that the frequency of client behavioral problems is the strongest predictor of overall caregiver burden and each of the four components of burden: family disruption, stigma, strain, and dependency. In addition, lack of social support is an important predictor of caregiver strain and dependency.

Our findings concerning the importance of client behavioral symptoms in predicting caregiver burden suggest the need for specific interventions to help caregivers address behavioral problems and for interventions that assist caregivers in interactions with their ill relative. Family-based psychoeducational intervention models that combine education with behavioral change have proven to be effective in reducing client relapse rates and therefore would be expected to reduce caregiver burden (Hogarty, Goldberg, & Schooler, 1974; Hogarty, Schooler, & Ulrich, 1979; Schooler, Levine, Severe, et al., 1980). A recent statewide examination of multiple family psychoeducational groups found that this format leads to relapse rates of less than 10% (McFarlane, 1990). This approach is cost-effective as well, with McFarlane indicating the cost in New York was $240 per family per year (McFarlane, personal communication).

We believe, however, that the mental health system has to do more than develop and/or support specific programs and services for family caregivers of persons with mental illness. Rather, a change in orientation is needed. Despite the existence of ecological models of mental illness, such as the family systems model or the social rehabilitation model, mental health systems still are very much influenced by the traditional medical model. Thus mental health agencies treat patients, or clients, or consumers, as persons with mental illness are now called. Families of persons with mental illness are involved in the treatment process only in a tangential manner.

In our view families need to be seen as part of the treatment team, not left out of the process. Families shoulder significant amounts of caregiving responsibility for their relatives with mental illness and provide much support and assistance to their ill family member. Given the fact that many family members spend considerably more time with their ill family member than do mental health professionals, family members are in a unique position to help evaluate the effects of medication, especially medication changes, to help regulate medication use, and to help observe client behavior.

All too often clients' rights to confidentiality have been used as a rationale to prevent further involvement by family caregivers (Petrila & Sadoff, 1992). More comprehensive involvement of families by the mental health system does not mean infringement of clients' rights. Clients still have rights to confidentiality and case managers still would be required to obtain clients' permission to release confidential information about clients' illness and treatment to their family members. However, clients' refusal to involve their families in their care usually follows long periods of client and family conflict. By involving families at early stages of the treatment process and by providing general information and support to family members, perhaps such family conflicts can be avoided or minimized.

This study has addressed some limitations of previous research with caregivers of persons with mental illness by adapting a theoretical framework that has been used with caregivers of Alzheimer's patients. The study involved examination of the simultaneous effects of multiple independent variables on caregiver distress, the use of multiple measures of caregiver social support (overall social support as well as informal and formal support focused on the caregiving role), examining the role of both social support and caregiver health as predictors of caregiver distress, multidimensional conceptualizations of caregiver burden, and finally the use of standardized measures. The present study has its own limitations, however. The sample utilized—upper middleclass white caregivers who were members of the National Alliance for the Mentally Ill—is clearly not representative of all caregivers. In addition, the cross-sectional design does not allow an understanding of the effect of caregiving over time and how changes in the client's behavioral problems, hospitalization, or living status, or changes in caregiver health or social support, affect the level of caregiver burden. This is an important limitation as research has demonstrated that caregiver burden may continue over many years (Davis et al., 1974).

Future research with caregivers of persons with mental illness should use longitudinal designs with large, representative samples of caregivers. Building upon our finding from the bivariate analyses that sufficiency of agency support was a predictor of caregiver burden and upon our previous findings of the role of sufficiency of agency support in predicting caregiver burden with lower social class caregivers (Biegel, Milligan, et al., in press), future studies should examine, in more detail than was possible in the present study, the relationship between caregivers' interactions with mental health professionals and caregiver burden. In addition, building upon caregiver research with other chronic illnesses, future research should examine the long-term effects of caregiving upon caregivers' health and mental health status. Very few studies have examined the effects of burden on depression levels of family caregivers of persons with mental illness, despite the rich literature in this area with caregivers of Alzheimer's disease patients and stroke victims (Biegel et al., 1991; Cook, 1988).

NOTES

1. The latter variable would not be considered as caregiver burden, but rather as an objective stressor in the stress-coping model utilized in our research reported below.

2. The reader should be cautioned that not all of these studies used standardized instruments to measure caregiver burden.

3. Inconsistencies in the measurement of length of hospitalization make it difficult to compare these two studies.

4. Copies of the data collection instrument and scales used in this study are available from the first author.

REFERENCES

American Psychiatric Association. (1987). *Diagnostic and statistical manual of mental disorders,* 3rd ed., rev. Washington, DC: Author.

Anderson, E. A., & Lynch, M. M. (1984). A family impact analysis: The deinstitutionalization of the mentally ill. *Family Relations, 33,* 41-46.

Beels, C. (1978). Social networks, the family and the schizophrenic patient: Introduction to special issue. *Schizophrenia Bulletin, 4*(4), 512-521.

Biegel, D., Milligan, S., Putnam, P., & Song, L. (in press). Predictors of burden among lower socioeconomic status caregivers of persons with chronic mental illness. *Community Mental Health Journal.*

Biegel, D., Sales, E., & Schulz, R. (1991). *Family caregiving in chronic illness: Alzheimer's disease, cancer, heart disease, mental illness and stroke.* Newbury Park, CA: Sage.

Biegel, D., Tracy, E. M., & Corvo, K. (in press). Strengthening social networks: Intervention strategies for mental health case managers. *Health and Social Work.*

Biegel, D., & Yamatani, H. (1986). Self-help groups for families of the mentally ill: Research perspectives. In M. Z. Goldstein (Ed.), *Family involvement in the treatment of schizophrenia* (pp. 57-80). Washington, DC: American Psychiatric Press.

Brook, R. H., Ware, J. E., Davies-Avery, A., Stewart, A. L., Donald, C. A., Rogers, W. H., Williams, K. N., & Johnson, J. A. (1979). Overview of adult health status measures fielded in Rand's health insurance study. *Medical Care, 17,* 1-131.

Brown, G., Bone, M., Dalison, B., & Wing, J. (1966). *Schizophrenia and social care.* London: Oxford University Press.

Bruhn, J. G. (1977). Effects of chronic illness on the family. *The Journal of Family Practice, 4*(6), 1057-1060.

Bulger, M. W., Wandersman, A., & Goldman, C. R. (1993). Burdens and gratifications of caregiving: Appraisal of parental care of adults with schizophrenia. *American Journal of Orthopsychiatry, 63*(2), 255-265.

Carpenter, W. T. (1987). Approaches to knowledge and understanding of schizophrenia. In D. Shore (Guest Ed.), *Special Report: Schizophrenia 1987* [Reprinted from *Schizophrenia Bulletin, 13*(1)]. Rockville, MD: Department of Health and Human Services, Alcohol, Drug, and Mental Health Services Administration.

Cook, J. A. (1988). Who mothers the chronically mentally ill? *Family Relations, 37,* 42-49.

Cook, J. A., & Pickett, S. A. (1988). Feelings of burden and criticalness among parents residing with chronically ill offspring. *Journal of Applied Social Sciences, 12,* 79-107.

Crotty, P., & Kulys, R. (1985). Social support networks: The view of schizophrenic clients and their significant others. *Social Work, 30,* 301-309.

Crotty, P., & Kulys, R. (1986). Are schizophrenics a burden to their families? Significant others' views. *Health and Social Work, 11,* 173-188.

Davis, A., Dinitz, S., & Pasaminick, B. (1974). *Schizophrenics in the new custodial community.* Columbus: Ohio State University Press.

Doll, W. (1976). Family coping with the mentally ill: An unanticipated problem of deinstitutionalization. *Hospital and Community Psychiatry, 27*(3), 183-185.

Doll, W. S. (1975). Home is not sweet anymore. *Mental Hygiene, 59,* 2204-2206.

Francell, C. G., Conn, V. S., & Gray, D. P. (1988). Families' perceptions of burden for care for chronic mentally ill relatives. *Hospital & Community Psychiatry, 39,* 1296-1300.

George, L. (1980). *Role transitions in later life.* Monterey, CA: Brooks/Cole.

Gerhart, U. C. (1990). *Caring for the chronic mentally ill.* Itasca, IL: F. E. Peacock.

Goldman, H. H. (1984). Epidemiology. In J. A. Talbott (Ed.), *The chronic mental patient: Five years later.* Orlando, FL: Grune & Stratton.

Goldman, H. H., Gattozzi, A. A., & Taube, C. A. (1981). Defining and counting the chronically mentally ill. *Hospital and Community Psychiatry, 32,* 22-27.

Grad, J. P. D., & Sainsbury, P. M. D. (1963). Mental illness and the family. *Lancet, 1,* 544-547.

Gubman, G. D., Tessler, R. C., & Willis, G. (1987). Living with the mentally ill: Factors affecting household complaints. *Schizophrenia Bulletin, 13*(4), 727-736.

Hatfield, A. B. (1978). Psychological costs of schizophrenia to the family. *Social Work, 23,* 355-359.

Hatfield, A. B. (1979a). The family as a partner in the treatment of mental illness. *Hospital and Community Psychiatry, 30*(5), 338-340.

Hatfield, A. B. (1979b). Help-seeking behavior in families of schizophrenics. *American Journal of Community Psychology, 7,* 563-569.

Hatfield, A. B. (1987). Families as caregivers: A historical perspective. In A. B. Hatfield & H. P. Lefley (Eds.), *Families of the mentally ill: Coping and adaptation* (pp. 3-29). New York: Guilford.

Herz, M., Endicott, G., & Spitzer, R. (1976). Brief versus standard hospitalization: The families. *American Journal of Psychiatry, 133,* 795-801.

Hoenig, J., & Hamilton, M. (1966). The schizophrenic patient in the community and his effect on the household. *International Journal of Social Psychiatry, 12,* 165-176.

Hogarty, G. E., Goldberg, S. C., & Schooler, N. R. (1974). Drugs and social therapy in the aftercare of schizophrenic patients. *Archives of General Psychiatry, 28,* 54-63.

Hogarty, G. E., Schooler, N. R., & Ulrich, R. F. (1979). Fluphenazine and social therapy in the aftercare of schizophrenic patients. *Archives of General Psychiatry, 36,* 1283-1294.

Holden, D. F., & Lewine, R. R. J. (1982). How families evaluate mental health professionals, resources and effects of illness. *Schizophrenia Bulletin, 8,* 626-633.

Hollingshead, A. B., & Redlich, F. C. (1958). *Social class and mental illness.* New York: John Wiley.

House, J. (1974). Occupational stress and coronary heart disease: A review and theoretical integration. *Journal of Health and Social Behavior, 15,* 12-27.

Keith, S. J., & Matthews, S. M. (1984). Research overview. In J. A. Talbott (Ed.), *The chronic mental patient: Five years later.* Orlando, FL: Grune & Stratton.

Kint, M. G. (1978). Schizophrenia as a family affair: Problems of families in coping with schizophrenia. *Journal of Orthomolecular Psychiatry, 7,* 236-246.

Kreisman, D., & Joy, V. D. (1974). Family response to the mental illness of a relative: A review of the literature. *Schizophrenia Bulletin, 10,* 34-57.

Kreisman, D., Simmons, S., & Joy, V. (1979). Rejecting the patient: Preliminary validation of a self-report scale. *Schizophrenia Bulletin, 5,* 220-222.

Lamb, H. R. (1982). *Treating the long term mentally ill: Beyond deinstitutionalization.* San Francisco: Jossey-Bass.

Leff, J. P. (1983). The management of the family of the chronic psychiatric patient. In I. Barofsky & R. D. Budson (Eds.), *The chronic patient in the community: Principles of treatment.* New York: SP Medical and Scientific Books.

Leventhal, H., Leventhal, E. A., & Nguyen, T. V. (1985). Reactions of families to illness: Theoretical models and perspectives. In D. C. Turk & R. D. Kerns (Eds.), *Health, illness and families: A life-span perspective* (pp. 108-145). New York: John Wiley.

McFarlane, W. R. (1990). *Outcome results from the Family Psychoeducation in Schizophrenia Project* [Executive Summary]. New York: New York State Psychiatric Institute, Biosocial Treatment Research Division.

Noh, S., & Avison, W. R. (1988). Spouses of discharged psychiatric patients: Factors associated with their experience of burden. *Journal of Marriage and the Family, 50,* 377-389.

Pasaminick, B., Scarpetti, F., & Dinitz, S. (1967). *Schizophrenics in the community: An experimental study in the prevention of rehospitalization.* New York: Appleton-Century-Crofts.

Pearlin, L. I., Mullan, J. T., Semple, S. J., & Skaff, T. (1990). Caregiving and the stress process: An overview of concepts and their measures. *The Gerontologist, 30,* 583-591.

Pepper, B., & Ryglewicz, H. (1984). The young adult chronic patient: A new focus. In J. A. Talbott (Ed.), *The chronic mental patient: Five years later.* Orlando, FL: Grune & Stratton.

Petrila, J. P., & Sadoff, R. L. (1992). Confidentiality and the family as caregiver. *Hospital and Community Psychiatry, 43*(2), 136-139.

Potasznik, H., & Nelson, G. (1984). Stress and social support: The burden experienced by the family of a mentally ill person. *American Journal of Community Psychology, 12*(5), 589-607.

Robins, L. N., & Regier, D. A. (Eds.). (1991). *Psychiatric disorders in America: The epidemiologic catchment area study.* New York: Free Press.

Sainsbury, P., & Grad, J. C. (1962). Evaluation of treatment and services. In J. D. N. Hill, G. M. Carstairs, A. Cartwright, et al. (Eds.), *The burden on the community: The epidemiology of mental illness.* London: Oxford University Press.

Schooler, N. R., Levine, J., Severe, J. B., Brauzer, B., Di Mascio, A., Klerman, G. L., & Tuason, V. B. (1980). Prevention of relapse in schizophrenia: An evaluation of fluphenazine decanoate. *Archives of General Psychiatry, 37,* 16-24.

Schulz, R., Williamson, G. M., Morycz, R., & Biegel, D. E. (1992). A longitudinal study of the costs and benefits of providing care to Alzheimer's patients. In S. Spacapan & S. Oskamp (Eds.), *Helping and being helped in the real world: The Claremont symposium on applied social psychology* (pp. 153-181). Newbury Park, CA: Sage.

Spaniol, L., & Jung, H. (1983). *Families as a central resource in the rehabilitation of the severely psychiatrically disabled.* Boston: Boston University, Sargent College of Allied Health Professions, Center for Rehabilitation Research and Training in Mental Health.

Thompson, J. E. H., & Doll, W. (1982). The burden of families coping with the mentally ill: An invisible crisis. *Family Relations, 31,* 379-388.

Zarit, S. H., Reever, K. E., & Bach-Peterson, J. (1980). Relatives of impaired elderly: Correlates of feelings of burden. *The Gerontologist, 20,* 649-655.

8

Psychoeducational Programs

From Blaming to Caring

CATHERINE F. KANE

In recent years there has been a growing interest in developing psychoeducational programs for relatives of individuals with psychiatric diagnoses. These programs represent a shift in clinical models of psychopathology from psychodynamic frameworks that identify the family environment as the cause of psychiatric illness to biological models in which the family is perceived as a primary caregiver. Psychiatric illness can obstruct the normal course of family life (Lefley, 1987) with profound implications for the growth and development of family members. Family psychoeducational programs have the potential to assist family caregivers to cope with the impact of psychiatric illness. This chapter describes the evolution of psychoeducational programs, describes specific psychoeducational processes intended to support the caregiving abilities of family members, presents the existing models of family psychoeducational interventions, and evaluates the evidence regarding the effectiveness of such programs for caregivers and ill family members.

BLAMING FAMILY CAREGIVERS

Prior to the 1970s, the traditional individual cure motif dominated psychiatric treatment. During severe dysfunctional periods psychiatric patients were hospitalized for short periods in general hospital psychiatric units or, when the decompensation was lengthy and serious or repetitive, admitted to state psychiatric facilities. The recognition of the limitations of this type of treatment led to the evolution of the deinstitutionalization movement during the 1970s (Terkelsen, 1990). Thus, prior to the 1970s and given the limitations of the biological sciences regarding psychiatry at that time, the social/psychological sciences, influenced by Freudian or interactional theory and persuaded by the evidence of positive family history, focused on the *family* as the probable noxious agent precipitating psychiatric illness, particularly in the case of schizophrenia. This perspective dominated treatment and research.

However, as research findings conflicted, were not replicable, and proved inconclusive, the perspective that families caused mental illness was judged insupportable (Falloon, Boyd, & McGill, 1984; Goldstein & Doane, 1982; Liem, 1980). This is not to say that family research per se in major mental disorders was not productive. As Hahlweg and Goldstein (1987) aptly demonstrate, family interaction research particularly has contributed to our understanding of the impact of interpersonal processes on the course of major mental illness. However, with its emphasis on family dynamics and parent behavior to the exclusion of other factors, this literature also has contributed inadvertently to establishing and maintaining the perceptions that parents are to blame for psychiatric illness in their offspring.

Although empirical evidence of the effectiveness of family therapy was equivocal, family "therapy" was considered the appropriate route to take with families whose relatives were mentally ill, and certainly for those families who complained of having particular problems with the patient. The cure model took precedence based on the assumption that such a family's system was dysfunctional and in need of treatment.

Cause of Relapse

A confluence of factors led to a shift in emphasis from families as *cause* of the illness to families as influential in the course of major mental illness (Steinglass, 1987). This shift to evaluating the impact of the family on the course of mental illness was brought about, in part, by the effects of deinstitutionalization. Deinstitutionalization, in the early years, was expected to restore patients to their community environments. In the grand scheme, supportive services were considered essential, but they were not forthcoming early on and only recently are erratically available (Isaac & Armat, 1990). Thus patients were discharged to their families or single-occupancy residences. The issue of chronicity became salient as discharged patients relapsed, and patients who had never been institutionalized repeatedly relapsed in what is now commonly known as the "revolving door" phenomenon. The frequency of the relapse pattern emerged as a problem for which families once again were identified as the cause.

Working from a preliminary version of the stress-diathesis theory, British investigators (Brown, Birley, & Wing, 1972; Vaughn & Leff, 1976a) found stressful family environments associated with high relapse rates in schizophrenia and depression. These stressful environments were characterized by high levels of expressed emotion (EE), which is characterized by criticism directed at the patient and/or emotional overinvolvement with the patient, assessed through the Camberwell Family Interview (Rutter & Brown, 1966). Criticism is specifically a high number of critical comments expressed by a family member during the interview and is considered to represent a blaming disapproval of the patient. Emotional overinvolvement is a global rating of the evidence of enmeshment given during the interview. Patients who had high EE relatives relapsed more frequently than those patients with low EE relatives. In addition, patients who spent less time with high EE relatives had fewer relapses than those who spent more time with high EE relatives. This work was replicated in the United States (Vaughn, Snyder, Jones, Freeman, & Falloon, 1984). Though the effect of stressful family environments on the patient is clear, there remain many questions regarding the emergence of EE in families. Brown and colleagues (1972) emphasized that their early results suggested an interaction between the disturbed behavior of the patient and the emotional response of family members. It remains quite possible that the development of high EE occurs in response to characteristics of the illness symptomatology.

Families as Caregivers

During the 1970s, though the cure model continued in prominence, reports began to appear in the literature addressing the perspective of the family caring for a mentally ill relative (e.g., Creer & Wing, 1974; Doll, 1976; Hatfield, 1978; Leavitt, 1976). Concurrently, anecdotal reports of support groups for relatives of the mentally ill were being published (e.g., Atwood & Williams, 1978; Goldmeier, Hollander, & Sheehan, 1979; Schneideman, 1971). Goldstein was one of the first to publish the results of an experimental study evaluating the effect of family therapy and medications on the relapse rate for schizophrenics

(Goldstein, Rodnick, Evans, May, & Steinberg, 1978). This research team did not examine the EE phenomenon but made a telling change in their original structuring of the therapy. Though they had intended to apply relationally oriented family therapy, they recognized early on that this method was inappropriate for psychotically disorganized patients because the patients remained too disorganized *at discharge* to effectively participate in such an intervention. Thus a research team with the avowed purpose of implementing family therapy was unable to do so, due to the continued symptomatology of the patient following inpatient treatment. Essentially, the team developed a crisis-oriented strategy aimed at aiding the family to manage symptomatic patient behaviors during the crucial first weeks after discharge, including helping the family to learn about the illness, to recognize their vulnerability to various stressors, and to minimize or avoid future stressors.

Life-Cycle Issues

The occurrence of mental illness in a family member confronts the family with challenges that require reevaluation of family structures and roles, and adaptation of the family environment to respond to symptoms of the illness, exacerbations, and remissions. Rolland (1987) proposed a model of the interface between illness and the family life cycle. Two aspects of this framework are particularly relevant to families confronting psychiatric illness, these being the psychosocial typology of the illness and the life-cycle phase of the family. The typology of the psychiatric illness in terms of its onset, course, and prognosis profoundly impacts the family. For instance, an acute psychotic episode can take on crisis features that the family can recognize and respond to quickly. Given that it is a one-time occurrence, the family can return to its usual mode of functioning once the episode has subsided. The onset of chronic schizophrenia or depression can have a more insidious course, eventually becoming relapsing/episodic. The family life-cycle stage is integrally related to the effect of this illness on the family. For example, schizophrenia typically emerges during the later adolescent years and early adulthood. For the family of an individual with schizophrenia, the typical "launching" stage in the family life cycle is interrupted and the parents, who were expecting freedom from direct parenting responsibilities, find themselves coping with an individual whose cognitive abilities and capacity for good judgment are not dependable, requiring active parenting for protection and symptom management.

The family's desire to be helpful in such circumstances has been documented since 1961 when Evans, Bullard, and Solomon (1961) described the qualities of families that made them potential resources in the rehabilitation of the schizophrenic patient. Other studies supported this notion (Creer & Wing, 1974; Leavitt, 1976); however, families have been hindered in their effectiveness by treatment systems that have focused on patient treatment and rarely addressed family needs.

Hatfield (1983) investigated families' expectations of therapists and found that families wanted help to reduce anxieties about the patient, to learn what is appropriate to expect from the patient, to learn how to motivate the patient, and to understand mental illness, and also wanted therapist assistance in times of crisis. These educational needs are validated by other studies (Chavetz & Barnes, 1989; Francell, Conn, & Gray, 1988; Leavitt, 1976) and represent the family caregiver efforts to learn how to manage a complex illness.

Family Burden

Not surprisingly the consequences of family caregiving for psychiatric illness have been sparsely examined. However, over the years a meager but consistent group of studies has accumulated that attends to the reported distress of family caregivers. The resulting scenario is disturbingly bleak. Bernheim and Lehman (1985) summarize the findings of seven studies conducted between 1968 and 1984, including the early British studies by Grad and Sainsbury (1968) and Creer and Wing (1974). Overall these studies indicate that families experience many difficulties associated with the caregiver role, including financial strain, emotional stress, anxiety, worry, threats to employment, interference with social connections, and disruptions in family relationships. Each problem is attributable in some degree to patient illness. As noted earlier, patients are symptomatic even following inpatient treatment, and families are confronted with bizarre and abnormal behaviors, intrusive and disrupting behaviors, and symptoms of a more passive nature, such as social withdrawal, neglect of personal hygiene, and lack of motivation.

Early studies of family burden note a persistence over time, even with an improvement in patient functioning following the postdischarge adjustment period (Herz, Endicott, & Spitzer, 1976; Hoenig & Hamilton, 1966). More recent assessments of family burden have demonstrated that more than 25% of family members, on interview, report personal problems associated with personal health, emotional well-being, daily routine, finances, time off work, and tension in family relationships involving the patient (Falloon, Hardesty, & McGill, 1985; Jackson, Smith, & McGorry, 1990; Kane, 1990). Others have provided evidence that the strain of coping with a mentally ill relative is associated with higher levels of psychological distress (Chavetz & Barnes, 1989; Noh & Turner, 1987), that stressful life events contribute to the emotional distress of caregivers (Noh & Avison, 1988), and that decline in the physical health of caregivers may occur over time (Belcher, 1988).

Coping Frameworks

The growing literature on the family stress and burden associated with caring for a mentally ill relative has provided a basis for the development of coping and adaptation models for understanding the dynamics that occur in these families. These perspectives view the family as experiencing an insidious affliction in a loved one and interpret dysfunctional family behavior as predictable as the family struggles to recognize, understand, and contend with this misfortune (Hatfield & Lefley, 1987). Noh and Turner (1987) have demonstrated that applying a coping model to relatives living with psychiatric patients can elucidate the processes involved in the experience of family burden and patient relapse. Investigating the relationship between level of chronic strain and the extent of psychological distress among family members of discharged psychiatric patients, they examined how family members' perceptions of their own abilities to competently manage the challenge of their circumstances (mastery), social support, and chronic strain affected family members' mental health. Of all those variables, only mastery was associated with the mental health of family members living with schizophrenic/psychotic patients. This suggests that family members who do not have confidence in their ability to manage stressful circumstances experience more psychological distress than others who do feel confident.

Caring Versus Blaming

Blaming families for causing schizophrenia and relapse is no longer tenable. Blame has played a role in preventing families from receiving information and support for their caregiving role, and these deficits may lead families to blame the patient for behaviors that families do not attribute to illness. The view that families of the mentally ill are exhibiting normal responses to tragic circumstances allows a shift in viewpoint, which acknowledges that the family truly cares for the afflicted individual and lays the basis for active collaboration between clinicians and families to more effectively care for and about the patient by identifying and working toward meeting family needs.

Enabling Family Caregivers to Care

It is clear that the family's conceptualization of the reasons for the patient's behavior can influence how the family responds. Without adequate information, the family may not understand how to respond constructively to bizarre behavior. In 1980, Anderson, Hogarty, and Reiss published an article in *Schizophrenia Bulletin* using the terms "psychoeducational approach" to identify a family intervention model aimed at reducing the intensity of the patient's family environment. An important consideration concerning the author's description was the avoidance of the term "family therapy." There is no doubt that the intent was directed toward reducing relapse rates of schizophrenic patients. However, the process of the program was not described in the "cure" terms of "family treatment" or "family therapy." "Family intervention" was the descriptor chosen that had as its goal to increase the predictability and stability of the family environment by reducing family members' anxiety about the patient and improving their self-confidence, knowledge about the illness, and ability to react constructively to the patient. Teaching the family appropriate management techniques for coping with schizophrenic symptomatology was intended to decrease family pressure and overstimulation of the patient, particularly those affectively charged communications that were characterized by criticism and/or overinvolvement. This perspective marks the convergence of a number of concepts not previously associated in intervention models for families of the mentally ill: first, that families experience anxieties regarding this devastating illness; second, that families can learn facts and techniques that will enable them to cope more effectively with the patient; and third, that this change in the family's knowledge base would enable them to provide effective care to the patient. This intervention presented a model that could develop and maintain strategies for family caregiving in mental illness.

PSYCHOEDUCATION

Overview

This review of family psychoeducational programs covers published empirical reports beginning with Goldstein and colleagues (1978) to the present. There is a substantial body of research conducted on long-term interventions (more than a year; see Table 8.1) carried out with families, which can be distinguished from short-term interventions (less than 3 months; see Table 8.2). This review attempts to discriminate the purposes, programs, and outcomes of interventions that have been empirically tested.

Meeting the previously identified needs of families is the purpose of psychoeducational programs. These structured programs are designed primarily by clinicians to educate families about mental illness, its treatment, and skills to help the family cope more effectively. This perspective differs from that offered by Barter (1984), which describes psychoeducation as the use of educational techniques, methods, and approaches to aid in recovery from the disabling effects of mental illness. The former view emphasizes coping with the disruptive consequences of a disabling illness by developing interventions for the benefit of the family as advocated by Hatfield and Lefley (1987), Bernheim and Lehman (1985), and Anderson and colleagues (1980). The latter view emphasizes recovering from the illness by developing interventions for the benefit of the patient. This distinction regarding treatment focus is important to consider regarding psychoeducational programs for the family.

An emphasis on "recovery" drives a subtle expectation that the patient will be cured, rather than that the patient and the family will learn to cope more effectively with the short- or long-term disruptions caused by psychiatric illness. Certainly psychiatric illnesses can be time limited, but for the most part it is not known at the outset whether the illness will be a discrete episode or will take on a more chronic, intermittent course. Educating families and patients to cope rather than cure appears to be a more reasonable approach to designing interventions. Goldman (1988) contends that such programs for families should be labeled "education," and that the term "psychoeducation" should be reserved for psychosocial treatment programs for patients with psychiatric diagnoses.

TABLE 8.1 Long-Term Interventions

Study	Patient Type	Multifamily Group?	N	EE	Length	Family Program Description	Outcome
Leff et al. (1985)	Schiz.	Y (N)	FI 12, C 12	High and low	9 (avg.) multifamily groups, PTNi; 5 (avg.) in-home family sessions, PTI	Illness information-sharing problems and solutions; pragmatic approach to reducing EE and/or contact	9 mo.: FI less criticism, 9% relapse; C unchanged criticism, 50% relapse 2 yr., relapse: FI 40%, C 78%
Falloon et al. (1982); Falloon, Boyd, et al. (1985)	Schiz.	N (Y)	FI 20, C 19	High	25 weekly 1-hr. family sess.; 12 monthly 1-hr. family sessions	In home, illness information for 2 sessions; communication skills for subsequent sessions	9 mo., relapse: FI 6%, C 44% 2 yr., relapse: FI 17%, C 83%
Kotgen, et al. (1984); Dulz & Hand (1986)	Schiz.	Y (N)	FI 14, C 34	High and low	Weekly or monthly sessions for 2 years	Psychodynamic group psychotherapy	2 yr., relapse: FI 54%, C 36% (NS); both groups decreased EE 50%
Hogarty et al. (1986)	Schiz.	S = Y (N), FI = N (Y)	FI 22, SST 23, CB 23, DG 23	High	4-hr. session (S), then weekly, biweekly, and monthly family sessions for 1 year	S = illness info., medication, and management; family sessions to decrease EE and integrate S info.	1 yr., relapse: FI 23%, SST 30%, comb. 9%, drug 49% (no patients relapsed in the 33% of the families in which EE decreased)

Study	Diagnosis	Patient present?	N	EE level	Treatment	Description	Results
Tarrier et al. (1988, 1989)	Schiz.	FI, ED, C	FI 29, ED 23, C 25	High and low	9 months, 13 sessions	Illness info. for 2 sessions; FI = behavior tx to teach relatives to monitor sources of stress, reactions, and methods of coping; C = routine tx.	9 mo., relapse (high EE): FI 12%, ED/C 48%; EE: FI < ED/C. 2 yr., relapse (high EE): FI 33%, ED/C 59%
Leff et al. (1989, 1990)	Schiz.	FI = Y (Y), RG = Y (?)	FI 12, RG 11	High	FI = median of 17 sessions in 9 mo. and 12 sessions in final 15 mo.; RG = 45% nonattendance rate	2 in-home lectures followed by: FI = single-family in-home sessions; RG = multiple-family group sessions at facility (same program as Leff et al., 1982, 1985)	9 mo.: both groups less criticism, more warmth; relapse: FI 8%, RG 36% (NS). 2 yr.: both groups less overinvolvement; relapse: FI 33%, RG 36% (NS)
Cole et al. (1993)	Schiz.	N (Y)	FI 15, C 15	High and low	FI = structured communication skill training; C = family counseling	16 weekly sessions followed by 12 monthly sessions	16 mo.: both groups less emotional overinvolvement and improved communication

Notes: Y = yes; N = no; ( ) = patient present?; FI = family intervention; C = control; S = survival skills workshop; CB = combined; DG = drug; PTI = patient present?; FI = family intervention; C = control; S = survival skills workshop; CB = combined; DG = drug; PTI = patient included; PTNI = patient not included; RG = relatives' group; H = home; NS = not significant.

TABLE 8.2 Short-Term Interventions

Study	Patient Type	Multifamily Group?	N	EE	Length	Family Program Description	Outcome
Goldstein et al. (1978); Goldstein & Kopeikin (1981)	Schiz.	N (Y)	FI 52, DG 52	N/A	6 weekly meetings post-discharge	Family crisis intervention, shared problem solving	6 weeks and 6 months, relapse: high-dose drug and FI < low-dose drug tx. only 3 yrs.: no difference between groups
Berkowitz et al. (1984)	Schiz.	N (?)	FI 21, C 15	High and low	2 weekly in-home sessions	Illness information	6 weeks: FI less pessimism and more knowledge than C
Liberman et al. (1981); Wallace & Liberman (1985)	Schiz.	Y (Y)	FI 14, SP 14	High	9 weekly 2-hour sessions	FI: illness information and communication skills training; SP: mental health education, support, and insight-oriented intervention	1 yr., relapse: FI 21%, SP 51% (NS) 2 yr., relapse: FI 50%, SP 79% (NS)
Anderson et al. (1986)	Affect.	Y (Y)	PE 20, SP 20, C 17	N/A	Single 4-hour session	PE: illness information and coping strategies; SP: support and self-help	Immediate posttest: PE > SP satisfaction with the program, few other differences

Study	Diagnosis		N		Format	Content	Results
Hill & Balk (1987)	Schiz.	Y (N)	20	N/A	9 weekly 2-hour sessions	Illness information (5), treatment (2), and resources (2)	Stress decreased with attendance at more sessions
Smith & Birchwood (1987N)	Schiz.	Y (N)	PE 20, ML 20	N/A	PE: 4 weekly 1.5-hour sessions; ML: booklet only	Illness (3), resources and management (1)	Immediate posttest: knowledge improved for both groups 6 mo.: stress and burden decreased for both

NOTES: PE = psychoeducational; SP = support; ML = mail; NS = not significant.

Another issue regarding psychoeducation is whether or not it is family therapy. Though early reports on psychoeducation refer to the interventions as "family therapy," references to therapy gradually have dropped from the literature in favor of such terms as family "interventions" or "approaches." The long-term interventions are more likely to refer to family therapy than are the short-term interventions. Short-term interventions are more likely to be referred to as education groups.

Hogarty and colleagues' (1986) perspective is that psychoeducation should not be formally designated family therapy; they note that families become less anxious when they receive education about psychiatric disorders and therefore are able to become allies in the treatment process. Hogarty and colleagues specifically avoid traditional family therapy methods promoting disclosure, insight, or modification of family systems.

Family therapy is a treatment appropriate for families who perceive a problem in their family interaction that is unrelieved by acquisition of new information and directly learning new skills. An inherent assumption in this premise is that families should receive psychoeducation (information, support, and encouragement) early in their connections with the mental health service system. If information and solid collaboration between clinician and family do not relieve distress or enable families to feel more competent, then family therapy can be suggested as a possible pathway to change rigid family interaction patterns that may be preventing family members from making changes that would enable them to cope more effectively with the trauma of psychiatric illness in a loved one. Thus psychoeducation can be viewed as the foundation of the connection between family and service system. Once that connection is established the family can be open to the choices regarding their handling of the effects of mental illness within their family. Thus both family therapy and psychoeducation are family interventions with different goals. Family therapy explicitly intervenes to change family interaction patterns, whereas psychoeducation provides the family with information and training in skills to cope with the effects of the illness confronting the family.

Evaluations of various psychoeducational programs have used patient outcome rather than family caregiver outcome for assessing the effectiveness of family interventions (Falloon et al., 1982; Falloon, Boyd, et al., 1985; Goldstein et al., 1978; Hogarty et al., 1986; Liberman, Wallace, Falloon, & Vaughn, 1981; Wallace & Liberman, 1985). Family measures used in these studies were intended to inform patient outcome rather than family outcome. Emphasizing patient outcome over family outcome promotes the notion of family as cause of illness and relapse, whereas evaluating family outcomes for family interventions not only seems logical but also enables the determination of what, if any, positive changes have occurred in the family.

Models of Psychoeducation

A literature review was conducted to identify published reports of psychoeducational interventions to determine the dimensions that define such programs. Seven long-term programs and their outcomes were described in 12 published reports (see Table 8.1). Nine short-term programs and results were described in 13 published reports (see Table 8.2). The following discussion distinguishes long-term programs from short-term programs in terms of single-family versus multifamily interventions, patient participation in the family intervention, site of intervention, and content.

Long-Term Programs

Long-term interventions vary in the overall program design. Some are single-family focused (Falloon, Boyd, et al., 1985), in which specific information is given by clinicians to families in private sessions. Others are a mix of multifamily group activities and single-family sessions with clinicians (Hogarty et al., 1986; Leff, Kuipers, Berkowitz, Eberlein-Vries, & Sturgeon, 1982) where the multifamily activities are often lecture/discussion sessions in which information about the illness, course, and treatment is presented. Multifamily activities in the long-term interventions usually are designed to deliver information en masse, but also are described as opportunities for social connections to form between families coping with similar difficulties. Promoting social connections is often a goal of psychoeducational programs directed toward reducing the feelings of stigma and social isolation associated with caring for a mentally ill family member.

Leff and colleagues (1982, 1989, 1990; Leff, Kuipers, Berkowitz, & Sturgeon, 1985) have investigated and compared various models of long-term multifamily groups designed to enhance family caregiving practices. In the first study (Leff et al., 1982, 1985), families rated high in (EE) were purposely placed in groups with an equal number of low EE families, presumably so that through mutual helping, high

EE individuals would learn new behaviors from low EE individuals. This program was successful in reducing EE at 9-month follow-up and in significantly limiting patient relapse at 9 months. Relapses increased by 2-year follow-up but remained lower than in the control group in which patients and families received routine outpatient clinic care.

Patients often are included in the single-family sessions of the long-term interventions, whereas the multifamily activities of the informational sort are less likely to include the patient. It generally is presumed that families will learn to cope more effectively with patient symptoms if the patient is involved in the single-family sessions. When patients become too agitated to continue a family session, one strategy is to give the patient the opportunity to leave the session until he or she feels more under control. It likewise is presumed that symptomatic patients would be a detriment to the multifamily lecture/discussion information sessions. There is little empirical support for either presumption. Each of these long-term programs (Table 8.1) was carried out for families with patients suffering from schizophrenia. There have been no other reported studies that evaluate long-term programs for non-schizophrenic spectrum disorders.

The site for long-term interventions is usually a formal treatment setting, particularly for the multifamily activities. However, three programs have carried out single-family sessions in the home (Falloon et al., 1982; Leff et al., 1982; Leff et al., 1989). In comparing single-family sessions to multifamily groups, Leff and colleagues (1989, 1990) gave in-home presentations on illness information followed by single-family sessions or relatives' group. There was a large dropout rate in the relatives' group (45%), which may indicate that long-term interventions are best conducted with individual families.

The content of the long-term intervention varies considerably, but perhaps the clearest differentiation can be made along process lines. Falloon and colleagues (1982) and Tarrier and colleagues (1988, 1989) implemented a structured communications training program with families as the major portion of the intervention. Both models emphasize behavioral techniques. The Falloon model stresses communication and problem-solving training, whereas the Tarrier model trains relatives to monitor sources of and reactions to stress, and teaches them to learn more appropriate methods of coping, along with a problem-solving/goal-achievement program. Mueser and Glynn (1990) consider both Falloon and Tarrier to be examples of behavioral family therapy. However,

McGill and Lee (1986) have written of Falloon's model as psychoeducation. Hogarty's and Leff's programs, considered psychoeducational programs by Mueser and Glynn, provide more of an ongoing counseling intervention, advising families on emergent issues and problem solving with them concerning difficulties as such problems arise.

Thus these long-term programs are intensive efforts to educate families about psychiatric illness and to effect changes in family caregiving strategies and in the ways families cope with caregiver burden. Two major goals are reducing patient relapse by reducing the stress in the family environment and improving the family's ability to cope with stress. Two process modes are evident in these long-term programs. The primary process is either a behavioral approach to teaching families new skills to manage the illness and collateral stress or a counseling approach to advising families regarding emergent problems.

Short-Term Programs

Both schizophrenia and affective disorders have been addressed in studies of short-term interventions (Table 8.2). The programs reviewed here range in length from a single 4-hour session to 9 weekly 2-hour sessions. Most of the programs were conducted in multifamily groups. In the three programs that were single-family interventions (Berkowitz, Eberlein-Fries, Kuipers, & Leff, 1984; Goldstein et al., 1978; Spencer et al., 1988), the patient was included in the sessions; for the multifamily programs, the patient was not a participant. Only one of these programs (Berkowitz et al., 1984) was conducted in family homes.

Most of the programs are offered to families regardless of the patient's treatment situation; recruitment is primarily community-wide. Goldstein and colleagues (1978) conducted one of the first psychoeducational programs for families of schizophrenics immediately following patient discharge. Liberman and colleagues (1981), Spencer and colleagues (1988), and Kane, DiMartino, and Jimenez (1990) offered programs to families during the hospitalization period.

The content of these short-term interventions is fairly similar, although the proportion of time spent on each topic varies considerably. One program devoted seven sessions to helping families understand the patient's illness and treatment experience, with apparently no time dedicated to exploring family responses to the patient's behavior (Hill & Balk, 1987). Others appear to balance information about the illness and community resources with suggestions on managing problematic behavior and coping with the unpredictability of the illness. Two programs (Kane et al., 1990; Liberman et al., 1981) devote content specifically to communication and problem-solving skills. The two single-family interventions (Goldstein et al., 1978; Spencer et al., 1988) appear more similar in process to long-term interventions that implement a counseling intervention with families, giving advice and information as questions are asked and difficult situations arise.

Outcomes

Outcomes are reviewed in terms of patient outcomes, including symptoms and relapse, and family outcomes, including burden, knowledge, and emotional changes. It is beyond the scope of this chapter to describe and compare, in depth, the outcome measures used in these studies. Tables 8.1 and 8.2 summarize the main findings of each study.

Long-Term Programs

Expressed emotion, as rated from Camberwell Family Interviews (Vaughn & Leff, 1976b), is a variable of interest as a selection and/or an outcome criterion in each of these trials of long-term programs. Because EE has been associated with relapse rates, families rated as high EE are considered primary targets for family interventions to reduce EE. Most of the programs resulted in lower EE ratings for the treatment groups. Hogarty and colleagues (1986) found that no patients relapsed in families in which EE decreased. However, Dulz and Hand (1986) report, in a German population, that EE was equally reduced in both treatment and control groups with no significant difference in relapse rates. Structured communications training had effects similar to the more general counseling programs. The study by Cole, Kane, Zastowny, Grolnick, and Lehman (1993) produced findings similar to Dulz and Hand in terms of overall outcome. However, Cole and colleagues examined the interaction of patient and family variables and demonstrated that families coping with higher functioning, though persistently symptomatic patients were more critical of the patients. This suggests a complex relationship between caregiving and patient symptomatology that deserves further examination.

Presumably, different dynamics are inherent in criticism as opposed to emotional overinvolvement. The precise changes in family members' levels of criticism and emotional overinvolvement are not clearly delineated in the research, so it is not possible to say that communications training per se is more effective than a family counseling model, only that both seem to reduce patient relapse. Thus, whether family interventions effectively reduce EE, which in turn decreases patient relapse, is unclear. Long-term family interventions are associated with reduced relapse rates, but this may be due to families receiving ongoing information and support. These are interventions that enable family caregivers to continue to support the patient in warding off the effects of stress that induce relapse, and may enable families to maintain the patient at home during periods of family stress and transition.

These studies, on the whole, were well-executed, well-controlled experimental studies. Family outcome, however, is not reliably specified, nor is it clearly linked to patient outcome in these studies; therefore we remain uninformed as to what changed for families who received long-term family psychoeducational interventions that had such dramatic effects for patient function. Long-term evaluations of these programs suggest that patient relapse is delayed rather than completely prevented (Goldstein & Kopeikin, 1981).

Short-Term Programs

Of the short-term programs, one selected high EE families but did not evaluate change in EE (Liberman et al., 1981). In this study, difference in relapse rates was not significant when structured communication and problem solving were compared to supportive family counseling. The outcomes for these short-term programs generally were positive as a function of participation in the programs. However, the studies of short-term programs are not as a group as well controlled as the studies of long-term programs, and the maintenance of change over time was not examined, with the exception of Goldstein and Kopeikin (1981) and Wallace and Liberman (1985). Goldstein and Kopeikin specifically examined family interventions combined with high- or low-dose medication regimens. Patients who received the family intervention and high-dose drug treatments had fewer relapses at 6 weeks' and 6 months' postdischarge than patients who received a low-dose drug treatment. At follow-up, conducted more than 2 years later, no significant differences were found in outcomes by either Wallace and Liberman or Goldstein and Kopeikin.

An extensive series of evaluations were conducted by Glick, Clarkin, and colleagues (Glick et al., 1985; Haas et al., 1988; Spencer et al.,

1988) of their intervention for families of affective patients during hospitalization. On patient variables, they found a sex by treatment interaction, such that women patients had better outcomes in the family intervention, and male patients did better in the nonfamily intervention. Family measures demonstrated that those participating in the intervention were more positive about the patient's treatment and were more open to social interaction with friends and other relatives. A gender difference was found in the family measures as well: families were less rejecting of and felt less burdened by female patients.

Anderson and colleagues (1986) and Kane and colleagues (1990), conducting programs for families of affective-disordered and schizophrenic patients, respectively, compared a process/support group model of interventions to the psychoeducational model. In both programs families in the psychoeducational model reported more satisfaction with the program than those in the support group model. Kane and colleagues (1990) found that families in both groups gained knowledge and decreased burden. Families in the psychoeducational model also reported a decrease in depressive symptoms attributable to the intervention. These findings suggest that the more appropriate format for time-limited, short-term programs is a psychoeducational model. Such programs can be easily followed by an open-ended support group, or families can be referred to local self-help groups to build supportive social relationships.

In summary, the short-term programs appear to demonstrate positive outcomes for families. Two studies document reduced patient relapse, three document increased knowledge, five document reduced burden, one documents reduced depression, and one documents increased use of community resources. These programs have not been adequately evaluated for long-term outcomes.

Implications

These studies demonstrate that psychoeducational interventions with family caregivers have good potential for meeting the needs of families coping with psychiatric illness, and meeting these needs may have beneficial outcomes for the patient as well. Given that the patient is receiving optimum psychiatric management, long-term interventions may not be more effective than short-term programs for reducing patient relapse rate. Unfortunately, the long-term programs have been developed primarily in the context of research programs and generally do not exist outside this structure. Apparently, short-term interventions are being more widely provided.

These programs are provided primarily for families coping with schizophrenia. Because the onset of schizophrenia occurs during the launching phase of the family life cycle, the process of these programs is concerned with helping families to set limits and to renegotiate parenting responsibilities. Rolland (1987) illustrated the clash of illness and life-cycle stage when families in a centrifugal phase of the life cycle, such as launching, are faced with an illness that makes centripetal demands, such as the need for constant supervision. Families can become derailed from their natural momentum through the life course. Psychoeducational programs seemingly focus on the interface between illness and life-cycle stage, optimally enabling launching families to refocus inwardly to learn to manage new illness-related, task-oriented, and affective roles, but also enabling them to develop an effective balance between the centripetal demands of the illness and the centrifugal forces of the life stage. For a specific example, it would seem that caregivers high in emotional overinvolvement have become trapped by the centripetal demands of the illness and that psychoeducational programs can facilitate a realignment with the normal course of the life cycle to allow caregivers to attend to their own needs for growth and development. Given that these programs meet a crucial need for families by diminishing uncertainty and burden, it should be expected that any treatment program for the psychiatric patient should include, at the very least, a short-term psychoeducational program for the family.

SUMMARY

The evolution of the paradigm shift was reviewed from the blame/recovery emphasis of earlier years to a current coping/caring formulation with an appreciation for the lived experiences of families confronting these traumatic and often intractable mental illnesses. The advent of psychoeducational models heralds the lifting of blame from families by promoting collaboration between families and enabling clinicians to demonstrate their willingness to support families and help families enhance their caregiving abilities for the psychiatric patient. Though further evaluation is needed, psychoeducational programs in a variety of forms seem beneficial to caregivers and patients alike. Clearly, family developmental processes are disrupted by psychiatric illness. By providing information and supportive counseling to family caregivers, family psychoeducational programs promote collaborative relationships between family caregivers and clinicians, which in turn can maintain and foster healthy family development.

REFERENCES

Abramowitz, I. A., & Coursey, R. D. (1989). Impact of an educational support group on family participants who take care of their schizophrenic relatives. *Journal of Consulting and Clinical Psychology, 57*, 232-236.

Anderson, C. M., Griffin, S., Rossi, A., Pagonis, I., Holder, D. P., & Treiber, R. (1986). A comparative study of the impact of education vs. process groups for families of patients with affective disorders. *Family Process, 25*, 185-205.

Anderson, C. M., Hogarty, G., & Reiss, D. J. (1980). Family treatment of adult schizophrenic patients: A psychoeducational approach. *Schizophrenia Bulletin, 6*, 490-505.

Atwood, N., & Williams, M. (1978). Group support for families of the mentally ill. *Schizophrenia Bulletin, 4*, 415-425.

Barter, J. T. (1984). Psychoeducation. In J. A. Talbott (Ed.), *The chronic mental patient: Five years later* (pp. 183-191). Orlando, FL: Grune & Stratton.

Belcher, J. R. (1988). Mothers alone and supporting chronically mentally ill adult children: A greater vulnerability to illness. *Women & Health, 14*(2), 61-80.

Berkowitz, R., Eberlein-Fries, E., Kuipers, L., & Leff, J. (1984). Educating relatives about schizophrenia. *Schizophrenia Bulletin, 10*, 418-429.

Bernheim, K. F., & Lehman, A. F. (1985). *Working with families of the mentally ill.* New York: Norton.

Brown, G. W., Birley, J. L. T., & Wing, J. K. (1972). Influence of family life on the course of schizophrenic disorders: A replication. *British Journal of Psychiatry, 121*, 241-258.

Chavetz, L., & Barnes, L. (1989). Issues in psychiatric caregiving. *Archives of Psychiatric Nursing, 3*(4), 61-68.

Cole, R. E., Kane, C. F., Zastowny, T., Grolnick, W., & Lehman, A. (1993). Expressed emotion, communication and problem solving in the families of chronic schizophrenic young adults. In R. E. Cole & D. Reiss (Eds.), *How do families cope with chronic illness* (pp. 141-172). Hillsdale, NJ: Lawrence Erlbaum.

Creer, C., & Wing, J. K. (1974). *Schizophrenia at home.* London: Institute of Psychiatry.

Doll, W. (1976). Family coping with the mentally ill: An unanticipated problem of deinstitutionalization. *Hospital and Community Psychiatry, 27*, 183-185.

Dulz, B., & Hand, I. (1986). Short-term relapse in young schizophrenics: Can it be predicted and affected by family (CFI), patient, and treatment variables? An experimental study. In M. J. Goldstein, I. Hand, & K. Hahlweg (Eds.), *Treatment of schizophrenia: Family assessment and intervention* (pp. 59-75). Berlin: Springer Verlag.

Evans, A. S., Bullard, D. M., & Solomon, M. H. (1961). The family as a potential resource in the rehabilitation of the chronic schizophrenic patient: A study of 60 patients and their families. *American Journal of Psychiatry, 117*, 1075-1083.

Falloon, I. R. H., Boyd, R. L., & McGill, C. W. (1984). *Family care of schizophrenia: A problem-solving treatment for mental illness.* New York: Guilford.

Falloon, I. R. H., Boyd, R. L., McGill, C. W., Razani, J., Moss, H. B., & Gilderman, A. M. (1982). Family management in the prevention of exacerbations of schizophrenia: A controlled study. *New England Journal of Medicine, 306,* 1437-1440.

Falloon, I. R. H., Boyd, R. L., McGill, C. W., Williamson, M., Razani, J., Moss, H. B., Gilderman, A. M., & Simpson, G. M. (1985). Family management in the prevention of morbidity of schizophrenia: Clinical outcome of a two-year longitudinal study. *Archives of General Psychiatry, 42,* 887-896.

Falloon, I. R. H., Hardesty, J. P., & McGill, C. W. (1985). Adjustment of the family unit. In I. R. H. Falloon (Ed.), *Family management of schizophrenia: A study of clinical, social, family, and economic benefits* (pp. 102-114). Baltimore, MD: Johns Hopkins University Press.

Francell, C. G., Conn, V. S., & Gray, D. P. (1988). Families' perceptions of burden of care for chronic mentally ill relatives. *Hospital and Community Psychiatry, 39,* 1296-1300.

Glick, I. D., Clarkin, J. F., Spencer, J. H., Haas, G. L., Lewis, A. B., Peyser, J., DeMane, N., Good-Ellis, M., Farris, E., & Lestelle, V. (1985). A controlled evaluation of inpatient family intervention: Preliminary results of the six-month follow-up. *Archives of General Psychiatry, 42,* 882-886.

Goldman, C. R. (1988). Toward a definition of psychoeducation. *Hospital and Community Psychiatry, 39,* 666-668.

Goldmeier, D., Hollander, D., & Sheehan, M. J. (1979). Relatives and friends group in a psychiatric ward. *British Medical Journal, 1,* 932-934.

Goldstein, M. J., & Doane, J. A. (1982). Family factors in the onset, course and treatment of schizophrenic spectrum disorders. *Journal of Nervous and Mental Disease, 170,* 692-700.

Goldstein, M. J., & Kopeikin, H. S. (1981). Short- and long-term effects of combining drug and family therapy. In M. Goldstein (Ed.), *New dimensions for mental health services: New developments in interventions with families of schizophrenics* (pp. 5-26). San Francisco: Jossey-Bass.

Goldstein, M. J., Rodnick, E. H., Evans, J. R., May, P. R. A., & Steinberg, M. R. (1978). Drug and family therapy in the aftercare of acute schizophrenics. *Archives of General Psychiatry, 35,* 1169-1177.

Grad, J., & Sainsbury, P. (1968). The effects that patients have on their families in a community care and a control psychiatric service: A two year follow-up. *British Journal of Psychiatry, 114,* 265-278.

Haas, G. L., Glick, I. D., Clarkin, J. F., Spencer, J. H., Lewis, A. B., Peyser, J., Demane, N., Good-Ellis, M., Harris, E., & Lestelle, V. (1988). Inpatient family intervention: A randomized clinical trial: Results at hospital discharge. *Archives of General Psychiatry, 45,* 217-224.

Hahlweg, K., & Goldstein, M. J. (Eds.). (1987). *Understanding major mental disorder: The contribution of family interaction research.* New York: Family Process Press.

Hatfield, A. B. (1978). Psychological costs of schizophrenia to the family. *Social Work, 23,* 355-359.

Hatfield, A. B. (1983). What families want of family therapists. In W. R. McFarlane (Ed.), *Family therapy in schizophrenia* (pp. 41-65). New York: Guilford.

Hatfield, A. B., & Lefley, H. P. (Eds.). (1987). *Families of the mentally ill: Coping and adaptation.* New York: Guilford.

Herz, M. I., Endicott, J., & Spitzer, R. L. (1976). Brief versus standard hospitalization: The families. *American Journal of Psychiatry, 133,* 795-801.

Hill, D., & Balk, D. (1987). The effect of an education program for families of the chronically mentally ill on stress and anxiety. *Psychosocial Rehabilitation Journal, 10*(4), 25-40.

Hoenig, J., & Hamilton, M. E. (1966). The schizophrenic patient in the community and his effect on the household. *International Journal of Social Psychiatry, 12,* 165-176.

Hogarty, G. E., Anderson, C. M., Reiss, D. J., Kornblith, S. J., Greenwald, D. P., Javne, C. D., & Madonia, M. J. (1986). Family psychoeducation, social skills training, and maintenance chemotherapy in the aftercare treatment of schizophrenia. *Archives of General Psychiatry, 43,* 633-642.

Isaac, R. J., & Armat, V. C. (1990). *Madness in the streets: How psychiatry and the law abandoned the mentally ill.* New York: Free Press.

Jackson, H. J., Smith, N., & McGorry, P. (1990). Relationship between expressed emotion and family burden in psychotic disorders: An exploratory study. *Acta Psychiatrica Scandinavica, 82,* 243-249.

Kane, C. F. (1990). *Expressed emotion: An evaluation of the construct in relation to patient symptoms and family burden.* Unpublished manuscript, University of Rochester, School of Nursing.

Kane, C. F., DiMartino, E., & Jimenez, M. (1990). A comparison of short-term psychoeducation and support groups for relatives coping with chronic schizophrenia. *Archives of Psychiatric Nursing, 4,* 343-353.

Kottgen, C., Sonnichsen, I., Mollenhauer, K., & Jurth, R. (1984). Group therapy with families of schizophrenic patients: Results of the Hamburg Camberwell Family Interview Study III. *International Journal of Family Psychiatry, 5,* 83-94.

Leavitt, M. (1976). The discharge crisis: The experience of families of psychiatric patients. *Nursing Research, 2,* 566-574.

Leff, J., Berkowitz, R., Shavit, N., Strachan, A., Glass, I., & Vaughn, C. (1989). A trial of family therapy versus a relative's group for schizophrenia. *British Journal of Psychiatry, 154,* 58-66.

Leff, J., Berkowitz, R., Shavit, N., Strachan, A., Glass, I., & Vaughn, C. (1990). A trial of family therapy versus a relative's group for schizophrenia: Two year follow-up. *British Journal of Psychiatry, 157,* 571-577.

Leff, J., Kuipers, L., Berkowitz, R., Eberlein-Vries, R., & Sturgeon, D. (1982). A controlled trial of social interventions in the families of schizophrenic patients. *British Journal of Psychiatry, 141,* 121-134.

Leff, J., Kuipers, L., Berkowitz, R., & Sturgeon, D. (1985). A controlled trial of social intervention in the families of schizophrenic patients: Two year follow-up. *British Journal of Psychiatry, 146,* 594-600.

Lefley, H. P. (1987). Aging parents as caregivers of mentally ill adult children: An emerging social problem. *Hospital and Community Psychiatry, 38,* 1063-1070.

Liberman, R. P., Wallace, C. J., Falloon, I. R. H., & Vaughn, C. (1981). Inter-personal problem-solving therapy for schizophrenics and their families. *Comprehensive Psychiatry, 22,* 627-630.

Liem, J. H. (1980). Family studies in schizophrenia: An update and a commentary. *Schizophrenia Bulletin, 6,* 429-459.

McGill, C. W., & Lee, E. (1986). Family psychoeducational intervention in the treatment of schizophrenia. *Bulletin of the Menninger Clinic, 50,* 269-286.

Mueser, K. T., & Glynn, S. M. (1990). Behavioral psychotherapy for schizophrenia. *Progress in Behavior Modification, 26,* 122-149.

Noh, S., & Avison, W. R. (1988). Spouses of discharged psychiatric patients: Factors associated with their experience of burden. *Journal of Marriage and the Family, 50,* 377-389.

Noh, S., & Turner, R. J. (1987). Living with psychiatric patients: Implications for the mental health of family members. *Social Science and Medicine, 25,* 263-271.

Rolland, J. S. (1987). Chronic illness and the life cycle: A conceptual framework. *Family Process, 26,* 203-221.

Rutter, M., & Brown, G. W. (1966). The reliability and validity of measures of family life and relationships in families containing a psychiatric patient. *Social Psychiatry, 7,* 38-53.

Schneideman, J. (1971). Student nurses lead family groups. *Hospital and Community Psychiatry, 22,* 34-36.

Smith, J. V., & Birchwood, J. (1987). Specific and nonspecific effects of educational intervention with families living with a schizophrenic relative. *British Journal of Psychiatry, 150,* 645-652.

Spencer, J. H., Glick, I. D., Haas, G. L., Clarkin, J. F., Lewis, A. B., Peyser, J., DeMane, N., Good-Ellis, M., Farris, E., & Lestelle, V. (1988). Randomized clinical trial of inpatient family intervention: Effects at 6-month and 18-month followups. *American Journal of Psychiatry, 145,* 1115-1121.

Steinglass, P. (1987). Psychoeducational family therapy for schizophrenia: A review essay. *Psychiatry, 50,* 14-23.

Tarrier, N., Barrowclough, C., Vaughn, C., Bamrah, J. S., Porceddu, K., Watts, S., & Freeman, H. (1988). The community management of schizophrenia: A controlled trial of a behavioral intervention with families to reduce relapse. *British Journal of Psychiatry, 153,* 532-542.

Tarrier, N., Barrrowclough, C., Vaughn, C., Bamrah, J. S., Porceddu, K., Watts, S., & Freeman, H. (1989). Community management of schizophrenia: A two-year follow-up of a behavioral intervention with families. *British Journal of Psychiatry, 154,* 625-628.

Terkelsen, K. (1990). A historical perspective on family-provider relationships. In H. P. Lefley & D. L. Johnson (Eds.), *Families as allies in treatment of the mentally ill: New directions for mental health professionals* (pp. 3-30). Washington, DC: American Psychiatric Press.

Vaughn, C. E., & Leff, J. P. (1976a). The influence of family and social factors on the course of psychiatric illness: A comparison of schizophrenic and depressed neurotic patients. *British Journal of Psychiatry, 129,* 125-137.

Vaughn, C. E., & Leff, J. P. (1976b). The measurement of expressed emotion in the families of psychiatric patients. *British Journal of Social and Clinical Psychology, 15,* 137-165.

Vaughn, C. E., Snyder, K. S., Jones, S., Freeman, W. B., & Falloon, R. H. (1984). Family factors in schizophrenic relapse. *Archives of General Psychiatry, 41,* 1169-1177.

Wallace, C. J., & Liberman, R. P. (1985). Social skills training for patients with schizophrenia: A controlled clinical trial. *Psychiatry Research, 15,* 239-247.

9

The Home Care of a Patient With Cancer

The Midlife Crisis

CHARLES W. GIVEN
BARBARA A. GIVEN

CANCER, THE DISEASE AND DIAGNOSIS

Each year there are 1.1 million new patients and families who must deal with the diagnosis of cancer, plus another 7 million who are living with cancer—3 million of these were diagnosed 5 or more years ago. As treatments have become more complex and have moved to outpatient and home settings, families have become more actively involved in cancer care. Together, these developments place family caregivers in critical decision-making roles for the continuing care of their family members with cancer. Families now assume major roles in ensuring medication compliance, scheduling and transporting for treatments, pain and symptom management, and the emotional well-being of their relatives. These responsibilities ebb and flow with the site of cancer, its stage of progression, and the treatment modalities selected for the patient. For the family this means that they face periods in which they must assist, rearrange, and accommodate their own roles to provide care; assume some of the roles that the patient can no longer perform

AUTHORS' NOTE: This research was supported by grant #1 RO1 NR01915, "Family Home Care for Cancer—A Community-Based Model," funded by the National Center for Nursing Research, and by grant #PBR-32, "Family Homecare for Cancer," funded by the American Cancer Society.

during periods of active treatment; and, then, reallocate roles as patients improve.

As with other chronic diseases, the course of cancer is marked by periods of symptom exacerbation and disability followed by periods during which patients are relatively independent. Unlike other chronic diseases, treatment of cancer may actually bring about symptoms and periods of disability. For the middle-aged patient and his or her family, involvement in continuing care is highlighted by shifting role responsibilities couched in uncertainty about the prognosis and its impact upon the family members and the person for whom they are caring.

In this chapter we review and summarize families' involvement in caring for one of their members who has cancer and conclude with some proposals for future research. This chapter is divided into a number of sections. We begin with a brief discussion regarding how cancer, its stage at diagnosis, and the treatments employed are likely to affect patients and create needs for assistance. From this we move to describing how family composition, role responsibilities, relationships, and living arrangements may influence the availability and organization of caregiving. Next, family involvement is reviewed from two perspectives. First, reports of taxonomies of assistance that patients report are summarized. Second, we have reviewed family members' reports of care and how caring influences other aspects of their lives and relationships with other family members. In the course of these reviews we have given priority to those articles focused on patients and families in the middle years. Unfortunately, very few studies have revealed how site of cancer and stage at diagnosis influence variations in the amount of caregiver involvement or the types of tasks caregivers perform. Further, virtually no longitudinal studies have charted changes in caregiver involvement across the course of the disease and its treatment. Studies that do exist have examined the impact of only the terminal phase on caregiver's level of involvement (Grobe, Ilstrup, & Ahmann, 1981; McCorkle, 1987; Stetz, 1987).

Finally, outcomes are examined. There is a growing body of literature on how the caring processes influence caregiver outcomes. However, virtually no research details how patient needs in interaction with caregiver involvement are linked with patient outcomes. In many regards this is unfortunate, for if family care is to be given serious attention as a dimension of continuing therapy, its impact on patient outcomes must be identified and its role in the variation of those outcomes specified.

DURATION AND COURSE OF
CONTINUING CARE FOR
PERSONS WITH CANCER

Duration of the cancer illness and treatment episodes may vary from a few weeks to many years with periods of exacerbations and remission. The acute phase of care includes the diagnosis and initial treatment. During the diagnostic phase patients and families respond to the "diagnosis of cancer" and need emotional support and information about the disease and treatment. Following the diagnostic phase is the period of coping with the initial treatment, which often necessitates surgery, followed by adjuvant therapy, which is radiation or chemotherapy. In active treatment, reactions to the aggressiveness of therapy and subsequent side effects impact both the patient and family members. It is during this period that patients may experience severe disability and dependency on family members for transportation and assuming tasks that the patient cannot perform or with which assistance is needed.

If the disease is responsive to the initial treatment, adjuvant therapy patients may recover, sometimes with some loss of function. At this time families go through a period of uncertainty and fear as they await the "cure" or "recurrence" message that comes during the maintenance and follow-up, which may span 5 to 10 years. If the cancer recurs or spreads, the patient and family may experience a crisis followed by periods of uncertainty as they wait for future reports. In the progressive and advanced stages of the disease there may be increased demands upon the family for complex medical treatments, technology, and care activities as the patient becomes increasingly dependent.

Unfortunately, in the cancer literature there are relatively few descriptions of family activity and involvement in cancer care. Most examinations focus on hospitalized patients, on patient needs, or, if home care is mentioned, on those with advanced disease where the focus is only on palliative or terminal care. The palliative and terminal care literature focuses on family and patient support, comfort, and pain management. Only recent work, primarily by nurse researchers, has focused on family members caring for patients with cancer in the home, primarily husbands caring for their wives with breast cancer (Lewis & Woods, 1991; Northouse, 1988, 1989; Northouse & Swain, 1987).

In the cancer literature most work links family care to caregiver stress, coping, and adjustment (Lewis & Woods, 1991; Northouse, 1989; Northouse & Swain, 1987; Oberst, Thomas, Gass, & Ward, 1989).

The literature is filled with discussions about caregiver burden, or caregiver stress and distress, which has been associated with levels of patient's dependency and the nature of the family relationships. Researchers have spent much time trying to explain the causes and relationships between a variety of factors and caregiver burden and stress. For example, in their review article in *Family Caregiver in Chronic Illness,* Biegel, Sales, and Schulz (1991) discuss caregiving in cancer patients. These reviewers did examine initial diagnosis, treatment, post-treatment, relapse, and terminal stages to the psychosocial reactions of cancer patients. They briefly describe family reactions to cancer in which they describe interpersonal crisis; disruption of family equilibrium; and role disruption leading to such reactions as denial, anger, depression, fear, and anticipatory grieving. These stress studies rarely examine actual tasks (assistance) performed by caregivers. As a result, we know little about whether the assumption of new roles within the family or the caregiving tasks are related to caregiver distress, or how much of this stress is due to family or changes in long-standing relationships or to the general threat of loss of a loved one. For the adult middle-aged cancer patient and family, little description is available on how the family carer incorporates cancer care into his or her everyday life. Not only are the patient and family coping with the disease and treatment, but also they are providing most of the needed cancer care. As families assume greater responsibility for care, we need to understand how the course of the disease and its treatment impact patients' needs and the care demands upon family members. That is the focus of this chapter. In the next section we examine the availability and family organizational arrangements that arise during care for the middle-aged adult with cancer.

CANCER AND FAMILY DISRUPTION IN MIDLIFE

Families are the primary source of support and assistance to patients with cancer (Lewis, 1986). Lewis, Ellison, and Woods (1985) describe families as having two lives: the life related to illness and treatment and the life of a family with the need to deal with each of the members.

The role changes experienced in providing assistance have been described in the elderly but not among middle-aged cancer patients. Many of the cancers, such as breast, colorectal, uterus, ovary, brain, and lymphoma, occur commonly in the mid-adult years. For the middle-aged family, the impact of cancer care upon work and social role activities of both the patient and the caregiver is profound at this stage in the life cycle. The organization of family roles, patterns of communication, self-esteem, member independence, social support, and family cohesion all are impacted by the care requirements (Cassileth et al., 1985; Lewis, 1989; Lewis, Woods, Hough, & Bensley, 1989; Northouse & Northouse, 1987; Oberst & Scott, 1988).

To provide care for the middle-aged cancer patient, family caregivers often make changes in their own employment situation and add patient care to their other family responsibilities. Women, more than men, appear likely to give up work roles. Among middle-aged caregivers, 16% quit jobs, 17% took leaves, 36% decreased hours worked, 39% missed days worked, and 7% took early retirement. More than 40% of the working caregivers had an alteration in work schedule necessitated by cancer care (Given & Given, 1991). Although this is less of an issue for many elderly spouse caregivers who are retired, it remains an important issue for adult children who are caring for elderly parents (Brody, 1985).

Caregiving arrangements vary according to the patient-caregiver relationship. In most cases, spouses care for middle-aged adult cancer patients (Lewis et al., 1989; Northouse, 1989). This differs for older cancer patients, for whom adult children provide care (Given & Given, 1991). In these situations living arrangements may be altered either temporarily or permanently. The patient may move into the home of a relative in order to facilitate care. Many times family members will move into the home of the patient to care for him or her. The conditions that dictate the direction of these moves have not been carefully documented. However, when a patient is widowed, single, or divorced, more caregivers are involved. In a study of 315 patients with cancer, Wellisch and colleagues (1989) and Olson (1989) found that home care was provided by one caregiver in 66% of cases when the patient was married, that among widowed patients one caregiver was involved in only 24% of the situations, and that among single or divorced patients one caregiver was involved in only 29% and 30%, respectively, of these situations. Clearly, 60-70% of patients with no spouse caregivers have more than one individual involved in their care. Thus others, generally female, assist with care when a spouse is not available (Olson, 1989). During the middle years spouses may carry an excessively heavy burden of responsibility in caring for a husband or wife with cancer. They may have few others to assist them and they may be forced to lead, at least temporarily, multiple other roles or to assume the added care responsibilities of caregiving while also carrying out multiple other roles (Stommel & Kingry, 1991).

Family stage in the life cycle dictates which roles have to be reallocated when caring for a spouse or parent with the diagnosis of cancer. Stages of life cycle reflect the developmental tasks facing the family and the resources available to them to carry out cancer care. Families have to mobilize new ways of functioning as a family and as a household, according to Woods, Lewis, and Ellison (1989), to provide care. For families in childbearing or child-rearing stages, there are additional complexities as they physically care for and socialize children in addition to caring for a family member with cancer. Those who are older may be retired, so that care does not interfere with other roles (Krause, 1990; Townsend, Noelker, Deimling, & Bass, 1989). A supportive and functional family care environment should enhance the capacity of the patient with cancer to adapt to cancer and cancer treatment (Cassileth et al., 1985; Stommel & Kingry, 1991).

Perhaps the impact that cancer has upon the family was summarized most succinctly by Corbin and Strauss (1988), who describe how cancer superimposes "illness-related work" upon "everyday life work." Illness-related work contains within it the emotional burdens of caring and the reorganizing of long-established role relationships. Although always difficult, this work may be particularly demanding for families with small children. The caregiver must assume the illness-related work and parental roles, as well as customary work and household roles. Spouses appear to assume responsibilities for caregiving alone. This may be more problematic for the middle-aged couple who tries to maintain all their normatively defined roles than for the elderly, who may have fewer pressing daily demands (Given & Given, 1991; Krause, 1990). As we examine the needs that families must address when caring for patients at home, it is essential to consider the impact that care has upon each member of the family, how those impacts might vary depending upon who provides the care, the other demands that caregivers face upon their time, the information they have, the amount of assistance from others available to caregivers, and the family stage. In the next section we summarize the literature describing needs for assistance.

RESEARCH ON CANCER PATIENTS'
NEEDS AND CAREGIVER INVOLVEMENT

Approaches to Classifying Cancer Patients' Needs

Mor, Guadagnoli, and Wool (1987) summarized the work of several major studies and classified the concrete needs of cancer patients into three major categories: physical needs, instrumental needs, and administrative needs. Mor and colleagues (1987) suggest that despite the heterogeneity of the samples and cross-study comparison, the needs of cancer patients vary as a function of disease progression and increase with the severity or duration of the disease. Patients diagnosed at earlier stages had fewer needs than did patients with metastasis. Unfortunately, Mor, Guadagnoli, and Wool (1988) do not provide any indication of the order in which these responsibilities might occur. For example, do these categories form a Guttman-type scale, with increasing needs progressing from assistance with administrative tasks to instrumental and physical tasks? Or is there any evidence to link these categories according to treatment or to disease progression? Other research seems to indicate that administrative needs may occur across the disease trajectory. Families must interact and negotiate with the health-care system to obtain information, services, and equipment and with family and friends to mobilize support for assistance with care. In addition, families make financial decisions regarding the purchasing of supplies, medicines, and equipment (Lewandowski & Jones, 1988; Lewis & Woods, 1991; Mor et al., 1987, 1988; Tringali, 1986; Wellisch, Fawzy, Landsverk, Pasmau, & Wolcott, 1983; Wright & Dyck, 1984).

In the categorization, Mor and colleagues (1988) do suggest that needs arise from domains in life functioning, such that patients who are more active and involved may require more assistance to compensate for the additional roles they must relinquish. If this is correct, then middle-aged patients may have more needs than older individuals. However, even though middle-aged patients may have far more role responsibilities than do elderly patients, the question remains as to just how many of these roles actually are assumed by others when they cannot be performed by the patient. Certainly, care of children residing at home must, to some extent, be assumed by others (Stommel & Kingry, 1991). Work roles, outside the home, remain unfilled, as do many family tasks that simply go unattended. The point is that for the middle-aged patient and family, future research needs to inventory patient roles and then assess which ones are assumed by other family members and which remain unattended. This would provide important information regarding just which needs are met and which remain unmet and the implications of the unmet needs for care of the patient and his or her family. We need to examine what assistance middle-aged cancer patients require and how families have to be involved. We need to seek an alternative way to categorize and describe assistance to these middle-aged families as compared to the usual focus on activities of daily living (ADL) and instrumental activities of daily living (IADL) dependency so often described in the geriatric literature. For the middle-aged family, assistance is more than a focus on maintaining independent functioning, which is the prime focus of families caring for the elderly. The focus is on care tasks, symptom management, and dealing with the emotional responses to disease and treatment.

Although Mor and colleagues (1988) do not include uncontrolled symptoms in their classifications, they note that symptoms can lead to impaired function as well as requiring intervention and assistance. In their 1988 article Mor and colleagues indicate that fatigue, dry mouth, pain, and nausea frequently occur and are unrelieved in 20% of the cancer patients. With adjuvant therapy, symptom management is important. In addition, Mor and colleagues do not have a specific category for the treatments in the home but did report that 10-15% of the patients had treatments such as dressings and infusions.

Other researchers have constructed more loosely organized classifications of patients' needs. Googe and Varrachio (1981) assessed 15 families providing home care to cancer patients. They classified family activities into household help, assisting with expenses and transportation, pain management, and information. In another classificatory schema, Welch (1981) sampled 41 family members of adult cancer patients and found physical care, care of children, special meal preparation, providing emotional needs, and balancing work and family roles were activities performed by family members to their patient with cancer. Following interviews with 28 families, Grobe and colleagues (1981) investigated families' needs for education with respect to care for terminally ill patients with cancer. Their classification was based on the skill needs that family members required for care and included ambulation, bowel management, comfort care, dietary control, pain management, skin care, and wound care. Finally, even though each used different methods, Hinds (1985), Stetz (1987), and Wellisch, DiMatteo, and colleagues (1989) arrived at similar conclusions regarding the needs of cancer patients with advanced to terminal disease. All investigators reported that patients needed assistance with managing symptoms, personal care, complying with treatment regimens, financial management, and assisting patients with their anxiety and depression. Needs such as these appear to be consistent across age groups.

Approaches to classifying the needs of middle-aged cancer patients were formulated from varying perspectives: self-reports from patients, reports from caregivers, and, in some cases, observations made by researchers. Unfortunately, it is not always clear which perspective was employed to develop the classification. Moreover, the prevalence of patients' needs for assistance often was obtained using predefined categories. Thus the extent to which these classification schema encompass the possible range of needs remains open to question, and no classification specifically dealt with needs based on family life cycles. In the next section we review and summarize research from the perspective of caregivers, focusing on the tasks and activities they perform while caring for their patients at home.

Approaches to Describing Caregiver Involvement

Definitions of involvement in providing care generally include direct care and those indirect activities of caregivers that allow the patient to remain in the home. Direct care includes the supervision of, arrangement for, assistance with, or performance of those self-care and other tasks related to physical comfort and emotional support that maintain the comfort of patients and their involvement in physical and mental health. Direct care may include personal care; pain and other symptom management; and assisting with such medical care activities as taking medications, care for tracheostomies, assisting with infusion pumps, and emotional care for the patient.

Family caregiver involvement in indirect tasks includes all those activities that allow the patient to remain at home and to receive care there, including cooking, cleaning, shopping, money management, and scheduling and transporting patients to their cancer treatments. There is very little evidence indicating how the number, amount, or ratio of direct to indirect tasks may be related to cancer site. For example, in head and neck cancer, families become involved with oral hygiene; nutrition concerns; nasogastric feedings; total parenteral nutrition; and assistance with lifting, pushing, and carrying (Jacobs, Goffinet, & Goffinet, 1987). Cancer of the breast—compared to lung cancer, bone cancer, head and neck cancer, or pancreatic cancer, for example—poses different demands on the family carer and results in different levels of intensity and periods of time over which the cancer care will be needed. Finally, cancer involves family members in such responsibilities as making judgments and decisions regarding when and how to obtain care; giving medications, including pain management; and counseling and comforting patients. Most of these activities require a more sophisticated and complex level of decision making than that with which family members are familiar.

For example, Oberst and colleagues (1989), using the Appraisal of Caregiving Scale, assessed the demands placed on 47 caregivers of patients receiving radiotherapy. Family caregivers reported spending most of their time providing transportation, giving emotional support, and performing extra household tasks. Patients received the most assistance from family and friends and made minimal use of health-care professionals. Patient dependency and length of time in treatment were correlated positively with the caregiver assistance. Other caregiver activities included managing illness-related finances, monitoring symptoms, managing behavior, and assisting with treatments, and were considered more demanding than assistance with mobility and personal care.

Stommel, Given, and Given (1991) calculated the average hours of family labor over a 3-month period devoted to caring for 191 middle-aged cancer patients with solid tumors. The average daily involvement for cancer care was about 5 hours. In Stommel and colleagues' work, patient dependency and not duration of disease or site of cancer influenced the amount of family assistance required.

McCorkle and Wilkerson (1991), using the concept of enforced social dependency, which they define as needing help or assistance from others to perform activities or roles that an adult should be able to do, found that caregivers assist with self-care (eating, dressing, and toileting). In addition, they found that caregivers were involved in supervision of care, arranging for care by others, and providing assistance to the patient during the night. Finally, McCorkle and Wilkerson found that across 6 months, even though patient symptoms and functional abilities improved, caregivers continued to report that they were providing assistance to patients. Caregivers still had to modify schedules to assist patients to deal with cancer and cancer treatments, provide care during the night, and be available for care 24 hours a day at the 3-month follow-up. At intake, caregiver involvement was related to patients' physical care needs; however, 3 months later associations were found between caregivers' involvement and the physical problems of patients as well as their psychological status.

In other longitudinal studies of caregiver involvement, Oberst and colleagues (1989) and Given and colleagues (1991) found that the level of middle-aged family members' involvement in caring was related to their treatment trajectory and patient level of dependency. Given and colleagues (1991), reporting on data from 303 middle-aged caregivers of patients with solid tumors undergoing adjuvant therapy, found that symptom management, providing support and encouragement, and dealing with the patient's emotional status and psychological distress required the most caregiver assistance. These activities, along with managing symptoms and structuring care activities, consumed more caregiver time than assistance with self-care. Using structural equation models, Given and colleagues (1991) found that the severity, number, and frequency of such symptoms as fatigue, decreased appetite, nausea, and vomiting influenced patients' mobility, which in turn was related to the impact upon caregivers' daily schedules.

Estimates of family involvement in cancer care have been based largely on indicators of direct assistance for self-care and such instrumental activities as shopping, transportation, money management, and arranging for treatments and other services. However, symptom management and control become a major focus for both the patient and the family as they struggle to manage the disease and treatment (Dodd, 1984; Given et al., 1991; McCorkle & Quint-Benoliel, 1983; McCorkle & Wilkerson, 1991; Nail, Greene, Jones, & Flannery, 1989). Symptom distress influences social and physical function, curtails caregiver-patient interaction, and affects role interactions with others. Patients' symptom distress also may lead to such emotional responses as anger, frustration, or depression. The severity, number, and frequency of symptoms may dictate the level and type of involvement or care required from the family caregiver. Although symptomatology is discussed in the cancer literature, the involvement of family members in symptom management is rather limited.

Pain is a major symptom that prompts family members to seek ways to provide comfort to the person with cancer (Blank, Clark, Longman, & Atwood, 1989; Hull, 1989). Ferrell, Rhiner, Cohen, Grant, and Rozek (1991); Ferrell, Wenzl, and Wisdom (1988); and Ferrell, Wisdom, and Schneider (1989) have studied pain management performed by families of cancer patients at home. They reported on family assistance to patients related to pain medications and what activities other than giving pain medications were done to help relieve the pain. Caregivers assisted in both nonpharmacological and pharmacological approaches to pain management. With regard to pharmacological management, families were involved in deciding what medication to use for pain relief and when to give the pain medication; administering pain medications at night; reminding and encouraging the patient to take the medication; and keeping records about decisions, dosages, and pain assessment both for themselves and for health-care professionals. Families described how they communicated with health-care professionals, obtained prescriptions, and, for those patients on continuous infusion pain medications, became involved in the technical details of pain relief.

With respect to nonpharmacological pain management, family members assisted patients to position themselves by using pillows, with ambulation, or applying lotions and ointments or heat and cold to painful areas of the body. Further, families reported that simply being present, touching, distracting, or talking to patients may help to manage pain. It is interesting to note that caregivers reported that nonpharmacological pain interventions usually were acquired through trial-and-error approaches and were seldom the result of instruction from the health-care professionals (Ferrell et al., 1991). Thus families' involvement (assistance) in symptom management ranges from direct care, to complex monitoring and decision making, to emotional comforting. Each form of involvement demands different skills, organizational capacities, role demands, and psychological strengths that family members have not had to draw upon before.

THE OUTCOMES OF CARING
FOR PATIENTS AND THEIR FAMILIES

Patient Outcomes

Research describing the impact of family care upon patients' outcomes is virtually nonexistent. This is surprising in view of its potential importance for such clinical parameters as adherence to treatment cycles, symptom management, and limiting the impact of and promoting recovery from therapy. Further, family care may have important implications for such system costs as readmission to the hospital and loss of time from work. Future research needs to develop strategies for examining how the care that families provide in the home contributes to medical and to possible cost savings for the care of middle-aged patients with cancer. To do so models will have to be developed and tested that link the care provided in the home to specific patient health states.

The Impact of Caregiving Upon Family Members

The impact of caring upon middle-aged family members depends upon the level of dependency of the patient, the patient's stage in the course of treatment, the progression of the disease, and the number of other roles the caregiver occupies. For example, Vess, Moreland, and Schwebel (1985) focused on the impact of cancer on the family's reallocation of roles and the psychosocial environment. They found that spouse communication patterns strongly influenced how well roles were enacted and the strain and role conflict that resulted from cancer care. Intragenerational caregivers may suffer from role entrenchment if they isolate themselves in order to meet care for their spouse. Caregiving may impose considerable demands and offer little variation in daily routines, leading spouses to focus all their energies on the cancer care experience.

Role changes include restrictions and alterations in homemaking, parenting, and companionship. Blank and Gotay (1984) and Welch (1981) found that caregivers experienced changes in household roles, restricted role activities, and altered responsibilities. White, Zahlis, and Shands (1991) reported that in the early phase, after newly diagnosed breast cancer, 61% of the caregivers had to alter their roles. Patients could no longer do their share of tasks so caregivers performed their own tasks and those of their patient. Spouses who work must provide care, shop, interact with health-care agencies, cook, and provide transportation and child care. In addition, the spouse may be involved in bathing, dressing, and cleaning—very personal tasks that may be distressing for both parties, especially in the middle-aged group. Older couples with functional dependencies are more likely to be expected to be involved in care tasks.

Oberst and James (1985) found that lifestyle disruptions, such as changes in work, household schedules, and child-care arrangements, caused concern in 50% of spouses of newly diagnosed cancer patients with bowel or genitourinary cancer. Some care tasks were flexible, whereas others required immediate attention and high levels of judgment, making them more difficult to fit into a daily schedule. Each time changes occurred in the illness or treatment, these necessitated an adjustment in the activities of family members; sometimes this meant taking on new tasks, whereas at other times it involved giving up care activities. Such changes are disruptive to those with multiple role demands, such as the middle-aged caregiver (Stoller & Pugliesi, 1989; Townsend et al., 1989).

In a later study Oberst and Scott (1988), in one of a few longitudinal studies, documented the types of problems reported by 40 spouses of cancer patients at 10, 30, and 60 days after hospital discharge. Problems were patient symptoms, emotional concerns, dealing with uncertainty, and impact of disease on lifestyle. Alteration in household roles exists for families with cancer, especially with patients 46-64 years of age, as roles were relinquished, partly filled, or inadequately performed.

Changes in role performances among family caregivers were reported in a 1979 American Cancer Society study in which 35% of families reported roles had changed due to caring for a patient with cancer. Lewis and Woods (1991) also reported role alteration. Perry and Roades de Meneses (1989) found that fully half of their caregivers were having difficulty maintaining their work roles while assisting with a family member who had cancer. Given and Given (1991) estimated the lost work hours due to caregiving for patients with cancer. However, the impacts of caring for cancer patients upon employment, promotion, and job shifts have not been discussed in the literature on home care for cancer patients. Employment confirms both economic as well as personal benefits to the caregiver and his or her family. As family members take leaves of absence, miss work, or leave early to provide care, they may be sacrificing economic rewards and benefits as well as diversion from caring and the loss of self-esteem and personal rewards confirmed by their work. Finally, little mention is made in the literature regarding how cancer care may compromise child-rearing for the middle-aged care-giver except for the work by Lewis and Woods (1991). The literature suggests that caregivers may make considerable personal sacrifices, but at this time there is little documentation of exactly how families integrate caregiving into their lives, which roles they compromise, which they simply forgo, and which ones they strive to protect and maintain and what impact this has on other family members.

CONSIDERATIONS FOR FURTHER RESEARCH

Although never stated explicitly, a major goal of the research reviewed in this chapter seems to be directed toward the development and testing of interventions that will assist cancer patients and their families at home to manage more effectively the course of their disease and the sequelae of its treatment. However, with the exception of Mor and colleagues (1988), Oberst and Scott (1988), McCorkle and Wilkerson (1991), and Given and Given (1989), research designs have not been fit to the onset of the cancer nor have they been sensitive to important clinical milestones in the course of treatment. It is difficult to generalize patients' needs and caregivers' skills or possible role changes from cross-sectional studies using data collected from patients having different types of cancer, who are at different stages of their disease, and who are undergoing different modalities of treatment. To design and test interventions to assist cancer patients and their families, it is essential that descriptive, and preferably longitudinal, designs be fit to the course of the disease. Research that employs more carefully selected inception cohorts will be in a far better position to describe how the course of the disease and associated treatment influence patients' needs and caregivers' responses. Beginning with initial treatment and proceeding through adjuvant and palliative therapy, researchers must appreciate the variation that patients experience in the severity, types, or duration of their needs. Without this information it is difficult to understand the needs of patients and their families and the extent to which these care needs drive the dynamics of family accommodation to caregiving. Such designs will enable researchers to identify correctly the proportion of patients who need assistance, or the variations in the types and duration of the assistance as patients proceed from initial diagnosis through different modalities for continuing treatment. Research such as that of Oberst and Scott (1988) indicates that needs do change over the course of illness and that patients and the family caregivers may differ as to when and what types of assistance they are more likely to require (Mor, Masterson-Allen, Houts, & Siegel, 1992). By accruing patients who are at different points along the course of the disease and its treatment, and where no attempts are made to assess how different treatments may variously impact upon continuing care needs and caregiver demands, it is virtually impossible to appreciate which families entangle those aspects of cancer care for which patients and which families may need assistance, the types of assistance that are needed, and the likely duration of this need.

In Figure 9.1 we attempt to depict schematically our argument regarding the importance of understanding the interplay between the formal and informal systems for the ongoing care of persons with cancer. The formal system has been separated into the acute and continuing care domains for several reasons. First, system decisions will be influenced by the age or the comorbid status of the patient. The role of patient characteristics in the stage at diagnosis and type and aggressiveness of the treatment have been discussed by Yancik and Yates (1989) and by Swanson, Satariano, Satariano, and Osuch (1990). Age and comorbidity may influence decision making in the acute care system, which in turn will determine the amount and type of contact patients have with formal continuing care. Although one could argue that these decisions would have important implications for families and the care they provide, there is very little research to suggest how variations in contact with the formal continuing care system are related to the amount and types of responsibilities faced by families.

Second, the site and stage of the disease and the initial treatment decisions will be related to the types of continuing therapy, and these in turn will be related to the needs of the patient for symptom relief and assistance with self-care as well as the patient's ability to perform other customary activities. For example, more aggressive treatments are likely to produce greater disability and to demand more from family caregivers. The stage of disease and the aggressiveness of the therapy may prove to be important variables signaling the intervals between measurement observations. To date, all longitudinal research has become accomplished on uniform intervals between observations. Such intervals may remain uniform; however, they may differ depending upon the stages of disease or the treatment. Mor and colleagues (1992) did compare patients undergoing similar types of therapy at 3 and 6 months and found no differences in their reports of needs for self-care or symptom management. By fitting designs to the site, stage, and treatment modalities, researchers can specify more precisely the optimum observation intervals in order to better specify when patients and their families are more likely to need assistance.

Third, the capacity of family caregivers to adequately implement complex therapeutic regimens, to manage home care technology, to meet patients' needs for symptom management, to help patients follow good dietary regimens, and to maintain patients' emotional health is likely to influence patients' capacities to remain in treatment and may well lead to fewer readmissions to the hospital for pain or symptom

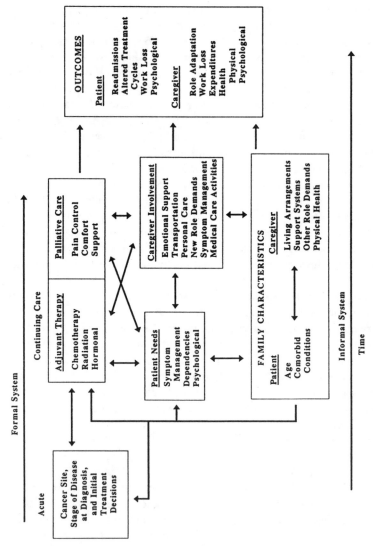

Figure 9.1. An Integrative Model Linking Continuing Care Across the Formal and Family Care Systems

management and to more favorable treatment outcomes. Again, more research is needed to understand the roles that continuing care, especially care provided by families, plays in effecting favorable outcomes. Fourth, as Figure 9.1 depicts, the optimal interaction between the formal and informal systems of care depends upon the living arrangements, other role demands, and the capacity of the family caregivers to incorporate these added demands into their daily schedules. These relationships are summarized by the double-headed arrows linking caregiver assistance with patients' needs and to the formal continuing care systems. These issues are especially important to patients and/or to family caregivers who are in their middle years. Treatment sequelae may be particularly problematic to patients who are attempting to maintain their employment and other responsibilities. In some cases this may even extend to basing the choice of treatment upon its impact on patients' abilities to maintain their other social roles. Caregivers who face conflicts related to caring for children, spouse, or parent and to maintaining their work roles are particularly threatened by the demands for continuing care that treatment options may impose upon them.

Finally, it is most unfortunate that virtually all research on continuing care, whether for patients with cancer, the elderly, or those with dementias, has focused exclusively on the impact of caring upon the families who are involved. If there are preferable ways to provide home care, then the more efficacious approaches should be reflected in improved patient and caregiver outcomes. Although past research has focused on interventions to improve the mental health of caregivers, none appears to have linked family caregiving to patients' outcomes. This was mentioned above, and its importance is highlighted by the diagram in Figure 9.1 that indicates that more appropriate home care may lead to fewer readmissions, fewer interruptions in treatment cycles, shorter periods of work loss, and better patient mental health. These dimensions need to be addressed in future studies. Particularly interventions that can demonstrate improved patient outcomes are essential to building a high-quality system of continuing care.

In future studies, then, patients should be accrued at the time of their initial diagnosis of cancer or at known and uniform times following diagnosis and stratified according to site, stage, and treatment regimen. Patients and their families should be followed over time to determine their needs and the ability of their family caregivers to respond. Some important research questions that may be addressed through this approach include:

1. Does the site of cancer pose any special problems for families who care for the cancer patient at home?

2. Do families caring for patients with cancer at the more advanced stages have to provide more and/or different care from that provided by those who have been diagnosed at earlier stages?

3. Is there some logical progression in the tasks of caregiving that corresponds to the progression of the disease or the aggressiveness of the therapy?

4. Are there patients' needs and caregivers' assistance cycles that correspond to the age comorbidity status of the patient and the prescribed treatment regimen?

5. Is there an interaction between the site of cancer and the stage at diagnosis and the demands for home care?

6. How do these demands affect caregivers' outcomes at various points along the life cycle, and are patients' outcomes related to caregivers' abilities to meet patients' needs effectively?

In this chapter we have used the course of cancer and its treatment to frame discussions about the continuing care needs of patients and the demands that are placed upon their families during the middle years. We have argued that future research should consider carefully how to fit research designs that seek to describe the continuing care needs of cancer patients and their families to clinical parameters in order to identify how cancer and its treatment influences the functional, behavioral, and psychological states of the patients and how these states change over the course of care. By pairing the observed range and duration of responses to cancer and its treatment against the stage of disease and the initial and continuing treatments, it will be possible to time the introduction and the extent of interventions so as to better meet the needs of patients and their caregivers. Further, by following the course of care and the demands made upon family caregivers such as deficiencies in their knowledge, inappropriate decisions and their approaches to care can be addressed and improved. Proceeding in this way, future research can identify and test patient and family-directed interventions and chart their impact upon the quality and outcomes for patients and their family caregivers. The outcomes of these interventions should preserve normal functioning for patients and families in the middle years, reduce unnecessary days lost from work and customary activities, and shorten the impact of cancer upon the family.

REFERENCES

Biegel, D. E., Sales, E., & Schulz, R. (1991). Overview of family caregiving. In D. E. Biegel, E. Sales, & R. Schulz (Eds.), *Family caregiving in chronic illness* (pp. 1-19). Newbury Park, CA: Sage.

Blank, J., Clark, L., Longman, A., & Atwood, J. (1989). Perceived home care needs of cancer patients and their caregivers. *Cancer Nursing, 12*(2), 78-84.

Blank, J., & Gotay, C. (1984). The experience of cancer during early and advanced stages: The views of patients and their mates. *Social Science & Medicine, 18*(7), 605-613.

Brody, J. (1985). Parent care as a normative family stress. *The Gerontologist, 25,* 19-29.

Cassileth, B., Lusk, E., Stouse, T., Miller, D., Brown, L., & Cross, P. (1985). A psychological analysis of cancer patients and their next-of-kin. *Cancer, 55*(1), 72-76.

Corbin, J., & Strauss, A. (1988). *Unending work and care: Managing chronic illness at home.* London: Jossey-Bass.

Dodd, M. (1984). Patterns of self care in cancer patients receiving radiation therapy. *Oncology Nursing Forum, 11*(3), 23-27.

Ferrell, B., Rhiner, M., Cohen, M., Grant, M., & Rozek, A. (1991). Pain as a metaphor for illness. *Oncology Nursing Forum, 18*(8), 1315-1321.

Ferrell, B., Wenzl, C., & Wisdom, C. (1988). The pain management team: Five years' experience. *Oncology Nursing Forum, 15,* 285-289.

Ferrell, B., Wisdom, C., & Schneider, C. (1989). Quality of life as an outcome variable in the management of cancer pain. *Cancer, 63,* 2321-2327.

Given, B., & Given, C. (1989). *Family homecare for cancer—A community-based model* (Grant No. RO1 NR01915). Bethesda, MD: Michigan State University and National Center for Nursing Research.

Given, B., & Given, C. (1991, April). *Cancer survivorship: Long term effects on family caregivers.* Address given at the Oncology Symposium, University of North Carolina at Chapel Hill.

Given, C. W., Stommel, M., Given, B., Dwyer, T., Osuch, J., Kurtz, M. E., & Kurtz, J. C. (1991). *The influence of cancer patient symptoms, functional states on patient depression and family caregiver reaction and depression.* Manuscript submitted for publication.

Googe, M., & Varrachio, C. (1981). A pilot investigation of home health care needs of cancer patients and their families. *Oncology Nursing Forum, 8,* 24-28.

Grobe, M., Ilstrup, D., & Ahmann, D. (1981). Skills needed by family members to maintain the care of an advanced cancer patient. *Cancer Nursing, 4*(5), 371-375.

Hinds, C. (1985). The needs of families who care for patients at home: Are we meeting them? *Journal of Advanced Nursing, 10,* 575-581.

Hull, M. (1989). Family needs and supportive nursing behaviors during terminal cancer: A review. *Oncology Nursing Forum, 16*(6), 787-792.

Jacobs, C., Goffinet, D., & Goffinet, L. (1987). Chemotherapy as a substitute for surgery in the treatment of advanced resectable head and neck cancer. *Cancer, 60,* 1178-1183.

Krause, N. (1990). Stress, support, and well-being in later life: Focusing on salient social roles. In M. A. P. Stephens, J. H. Crowther, S. E. Hobfoll, & D. L. Tennenbaum (Eds.), *Stress and coping in later life families.* Washington, DC: Hemisphere.

Lewandowski, W., & Jones, F. (1988). The family with cancer: Nursing interventions throughout the course of living with cancer. *Cancer Nursing, 11*(6), 313-321.

Lewis, F. (1986). The impact of cancer on the family: A critical analysis of the research literature. *Patient Education & Counseling, 8,* 269-289.

Lewis, F. (1989). Attributions of control, experienced meaning, and psychosocial well-being in advanced cancer patients. *Journal of Psychosocial Oncology, 7,* 105-119.

Lewis, F., Ellison, E., & Woods, N. (1985). The impact of breast cancer on the family. *Seminars in Oncology Nursing, 1*(3), 206-213.

Lewis, F., & Woods, N. (1991). *Family functioning in chronic illness* (Final Report Vols. 1-2, No. RO1 NR01000). Bethesda, MD: National Center for Nursing Research/University of Washington.

Lewis, F., Woods, N., Hough, E., & Bensley, L. (1989). The family's functioning with chronic illness in the mother: The spouse's perspective. *Social Science & Medicine, 29*(11), 1261-1269.

McCorkle, R. (1987). The measurement of symptom distress. *Seminars in Oncology Nursing, 3*(4), 248-256.

McCorkle, R., & Quint-Benoliel, J. (1983). Symptom distress: Current concerns and mood disturbance after diagnosis of life-threatening disease. *Social Science & Medicine, 17,* 431-438.

McCorkle, R., & Wilkerson, K. (1991). *Home care needs of cancer patients and their caregivers* (Final Report No. NR01914). Bethesda, MD: National Center for Nursing Research/University of Pennsylvania.

Mor, V., Guadagnoli, E., & Wool, M. (1987). An examination of the concrete service needs of advanced cancer patients. *Journal of Psychosocial Oncology, 5*(1), 1-17.

Mor, V., Guadagnoli, E., & Wool, M. (1988). The role of concrete services in cancer care. *Advanced Psychosomatic Medicine, 18,* 102-118.

Mor, V., Masterson-Allen, S., Houts, P., & Siegel, K. (1992). The changing needs of patients with cancer at home. *Cancer, 69*(2), 829-838.

Nail, L., Greene, D., Jones, L., & Flannery, M. (1989). Nursing care by telephone: Describing practice in an ambulatory oncology center. *Oncology Nursing Forum, 16*(3), 387-395.

Northouse, L. (1988). Social support in patients' and husbands' adjustment to breast cancer. *Nursing Research, 37*(2), 91-95.

Northouse, L. (1989). A longitudinal study of the adjustment of patients and husbands to breast cancer. *Oncology Nursing Forum, 16*(4), 511-516.

Northouse, P., & Northouse, L. (1987). Communication and cancer: Issues confronting patients, health professionals, and family members. *Journal of Psychosocial Oncology, 5,* 15-41.

Northouse, P., & Swain, M. (1987). Adjustment of patients and husbands to the initial impact of breast cancer. *Nursing Research, 36,* 221-225.

Oberst, M., & James, R. (1985). Going home: Patient and spouse adjustment following cancer surgery. *Topics in Clinical Nursing, 7*(1), 46-57.

Oberst, M., & Scott, D. (1988). Postdischarge distress in surgically treated cancer patients and their spouses. *Research in Nursing and Health, 11,* 223-233.

Oberst, M., Thomas, S., Gass, K., & Ward, S. (1989). Caregiving demands and appraisal of stress among family caregivers. *Cancer Nursing, 12*(4), 209-215.

Olson, M. (1989). Family participation in post hospital care: Women's work. *Journal of Psychosocial Oncology, 7*(1-2), 77-93.

Perry, G., & Roades de Meneses, M. (1989). Cancer patients at home: Needs and coping styles of primary caregivers. *Home Healthcare Nurse, 7*(6), 27-30.

Stetz, K. (1987). Caregiving demands during advanced cancer: The spouse's needs. *Cancer Nursing, 10*(5), 260-268.

Stoller, E. P., & Pugliesi, K. L. (1989). Other roles of caregivers: Competing responsibilities or supportive resources. *Journal of Gerontology: Social Sciences, 44,* S231-S238.

Stommel, M., Given, C. W., & Given, B. (1991). *The cost of cancer care to families.* Manuscript submitted for publication.

Stommel, M., & Kingry, M. (1991). Support patterns for spouse-caregivers of cancer patients: The effect of the presence of minor children. *Cancer Nursing, 14*(4), 200-205.

Swanson, G. M., Satariano, E. R., Satariano, W. A., & Osuch, J. R. (1990). Trends in breast-conserving treatment of female breast cancer in the Detroit metropolitan area, 1980-1987: The effects of tumor size, age, and race. *Surgery, Gynecology & Obstetrics, 171,* 465-471.

Townsend, A., Noelker, L., Deimling, G., & Bass, D. (1989). Longitudinal impact of interhousehold caregiving on adult children's mental health. *Psychology and Aging, 4,* 393-401.

Tringali, C. (1986). The needs of family members of cancer patients. *Oncology Nursing Forum, 13,* 65-69.

Vess, J., Moreland, J., & Schwebel, A. (1985). A follow-up study of role functioning and the psychological environment of families of cancer patients. *Journal of Psychosocial Oncology, 3*(2), 1-14.

Welch, D. (1981). Planning nursing interventions for family members of adult cancer patients. *Cancer Nursing, 4*(5), 365-370.

Wellisch, D., DiMatteo, R., Silverstein, M., Landsverk, J., Hoffman, R., Waisman, J., Handel, N., Waisman-Smith, E., & Schain, W. (1989). Psychosocial outcomes of breast cancer therapies: Lumpectomy versus mastectomy. *Psychomatics, 30*(4), 365-373.

Wellisch, D., Fawzy, F., Landsverk, J., Pasmau, R., & Wolcott, D. (1983). Evaluation of psychosocial problems of the home-bound cancer patient: The relationship of disease and the sociodemographic variables of patients to family problems. *Journal of Psychosocial Oncology, 1*(3), 1-15.

White, E., Zahlis, E., & Shands, M. (1991). Breast cancer: Demands of the illness on the patient's partner. *Journal of Psychosocial Oncology, 9*(1), 75-93.

Woods, N. F., Lewis, F. M., & Ellison, E. S. (1989). Living with cancer: Family experiences. *Cancer Nursing, 12*(1), 28-33.

Wright, K., & Dyck, S. (1984). Expressed concerns of adult cancer patients' family members. *Cancer Nursing, 7*(5), 371-374.

Yancik, R., & Yates, J. W. (Eds.). (1989). *Cancer in the elderly.* New York: Springer.

10

Caregiving Issues
After a Heart Attack

Perspectives on Elderly Patients
and Their Families

ROSALIE F. YOUNG
EVA KAHANA

Illness is not singularly experienced. As family sociologists have long asserted (Litman, 1974; Parsons & Fox, 1952; Pratt, 1976), illness invariably involves the family unit. This is particularly evident to family members of older people. The health problems of later life are generally chronic, so they continue and may cause deterioration of organs and bodily systems that result in reduced functional ability (National Center for Health Statistics, 1985). The family is intricately involved in the management of illness because it is the main source of aid for ailing elders (Shanas, 1979). Although families, and caregivers in particular, can be adversely affected by illness situations (Litman, 1971), the range of family responses is not well documented. Therefore, this chapter addresses the family-illness intermesh among older persons and their families facing a common chronic health problem of later life. It presents perspectives on caregiving and care receiving after a heart attack, and the major focus is on dyadic effects.

The risk of myocardial infarction (MI), the medical term for a heart attack, increases significantly with each decade of life (National Center for Health Statistics, 1985). MI is a very serious condition that poses a basic threat to life and well-being. Rather than cancer or Alzheimer's disease, heart conditions are responsible for more deaths, hospitalizations, and physician visits than any other condition of later life (U.S. Department of Health and Human Services, 1986). Limitations in activities of daily living are reported among 13% of heart patients (Manton, 1990). MI also is associated with severe emotional stress, decline in social functioning, and reduction in the patient's quality of life (Krantz & Deckel, 1983).

The family of the heart patient is very involved in care, and the nature of this involvement has been examined previously (Croog & Levine, 1982; Finlayson & McEwen, 1977). Two areas have received extensive attention: services provided by family caregivers and the aftereffects of caregiving, especially for wives. As in most illness situations (Stone, Cafferata, & Sangl, 1987), the heart patient has diverse needs and family members are called upon to assume many duties. Their activities may be in the category of "ordinary" or "extraordinary" care. The latter refers to care provided over an extended period of time; thus it is characteristic of many chronic physical and mental illness situations (Hirshorn, 1991). Most families respond to this need by providing continuous assistance for as long as they can (Kingston, Hirshorn, & Connor, 1986). In cases in which a heart attack has caused hospitalization, family members provide hands-on care and services when the patient returns home and is confined to bed. Because this may involve only the immediate aftermath of a heart attack, the family subsequently moves to a different level of care and continues to provide diverse types of assistance with instrumental activities of daily living such as shopping, meal preparation, and laundry (Speedling, 1982). Other family responsibilities besides care provision and household management include interaction with medical providers and provision of social and emotional support (New, Ruscio, Priest, Petritsi, & George, 1973).

This characterization of the family role in illness is suggestive of unidirectional activity. Families respond to MI by offering their time, muscles, and minds to help the patient with his or her needs. Yet it has been shown that the family role can be much broader. The role can be that of a proactive unit. Indeed, "energized" families not only respond to the demands of an illness situation but also can effectively promote health and recovery (Pratt, 1976).

Declining health of a family member is the beginning of a multifaceted caregiver-care recipient interaction (Miller, McFall, & Montgomery, 1991). Caregiving, which represents one of the most prevalent dyadic relationships of later life (Kahana & Young, 1990), has been studied extensively. In the field of gerontology, caregiving has become an important area of inquiry because growing numbers of functionally impaired elders require a great deal of assistance from both families and formal organizations. Because needs for care and challenges of dependency characterize the old-old (Kahana, Kahana, & Kinney, 1989), one might logically expect that the effectiveness of care providers or responses to care by elderly care recipients would represent the focus of inquiry in this field. Curiously, however, the thrust of such research in caregiving has dealt with the burden of caregivers (Biegel, Sales, & Schulz, 1991). Many useful findings have emerged from these investigations, but it is clear that some essential issues have eluded us. Perhaps foremost is that investigators seldom consider the patient and his or her caregiver as a dyad (Montgomery, Stull, & Borgatta, 1985). The units of analysis for studies of caregiving have been the care provider and, to a lesser extent, the recipient of care. However, they are not considered jointly.

In attempting to broaden our investigations beyond the focus on caregiver responses to care provision, it becomes apparent that, depending on the type of caregiver being considered, very different research traditions and theoretical contexts might apply. To the extent the caregiver is an older person such interest represents a special case of stress research in which (a) caregiving is a chronic stressor and (b) burden or diminished psychological well-being is an adverse consequence of stress. Another theoretical context pertains to intergenerational relationships. In cases in which younger family members (typically adult children) serve as caregivers, caregiving may be meaningfully studied as a special case of intergenerational exchange (Kingston et al., 1986). Hence the multiple family roles of adult-daughter caregivers (e.g., wife, parent) may need to be considered in the context of elder care provision (Young & Kahana, 1992).

Undoubtedly, other theoretical perspectives also can be applied to a dyadic focus. However, regardless of the particular conceptual focus, dyadic approaches to caregiving permit both a clear and a more comprehensive understanding of the parameters of this field. Use of dyadic perspectives compels investigators to explicate their assumptions about the domains related to independent and dependent variables in their research. It also ensures that researchers avoid drawing unidirectional and unidimensional conclusions that may distort holistic understanding of the caregiving phenomenon. It may be argued that caregivers with certain attributes, such as avoidant coping strategies, experience little burden, and therefore that such attributes are desirable. However, simultaneous consideration of outcomes of elders cared for by the same group of caregivers might reveal that those same attributes may be associated with perceived neglect by care recipients.

The field of gerontology is moving beyond this limited view of caregiving. Noelker (1991) has presented a strong argument for addressing the care recipient's view of caregiving. Furthermore, Malone-Beach and Zarit (1991) critiqued the caregiving literature and indicated that many of the deficiencies could be overcome both by using a systems approach and by focusing on dyads. They argued that addressing the caregiver-care recipient dyad would enable better understanding of caregiving situations. In this work, it is proposed that the caregiving paradigm, family reactions to illness, and recovery (or nonrecovery from later life illness) can be better appreciated if the conceptual and empirical foci are on the caregiver-care recipient dyad.

CONCEPTUAL AND EMPIRICAL APPROACHES TO CAREGIVER-CARE RECIPIENT INTERACTIONS

It was noted that there have been few conceptual or empirical explorations of the caregiver-care recipient dyad. However, theoretical approaches that include the family unit have been present in the literature for some decades. Although Parsons and Fox (1952) depicted illness as dysfunctional to the family system because it disrupted other roles, other theories from family sociology have presented a more diverse view of the family-illness interface. Hansen and Hill (1964) addressed family crises, emphasizing the management of stressful situations by families. Their theory formed the basis of a resource approach to family adjustment to illness situations, the ABCX model of illness adaptation (McCubbin & Patterson, 1983). The ABCX model posits that an event such as illness (A) elicits the family's resources (B) and, depending on how the family defines the event (C), a crisis (noncrisis) results (X). The model has been applied to studies of childhood illness (McCubbin & Patterson, 1983), and although such tests fall short of proposing caregiving activity as a resource that can help to avert crises, the work suggests the important contribution of family-based care. A similar approach is represented by Engel's biopsychosocial model (1981). This work proposed a series of factors that influence positive outcomes of heart disease. Among these were family functioning variables. This conceptualization indicated the therapeutic value of family involvement in illness management.

Other family theories have posed a systems approach to the management of illness. These family-oriented approaches to understanding social and psychological sequelae of illness generally focus on a group of individuals with primary ties to the patients. Family members may play significant roles in contributing to the etiology of illness, may provide a context for fulfillment of the sick role, or may be involved in the treatment of the patient, either contributing to success or posing impediments to recovery. It is recognized that the family constitutes a dynamic system wherein the illness of one member may have a ripple effect impacting significantly on interactions among individual family members and the well-being of the entire unit (Kazak, this volume). Family therapy is built upon such an approach that treats the family unit for conditions that one member experiences (Satir, 1976). The focus of this approach is on treatment, but in designing appropriate treatment strategies the shared etiology of mental health problems by patient and family is addressed. Interestingly, in this tradition families are viewed less in terms of their caregiving roles and more in the capacity as copatients.

Still other family theories propose diversity of family responses; these include both positive and negative outcomes for the family unit (Leventhal, Leventhal, & Nguyen, 1985). Given the threat of illness to lifestyle, life quality, and family finances, to name a few, families may unify rather than divide. They often close ranks, attempting to maximize the quality of their lives, and closeness and cohesion can result from an illness experience (Boss, 1986). Family caregiving can be an emotionally satisfying activity that benefits both caregiver and care recipient (Masciocchi, Thomas, & Moeller, 1984). Theories introduced to explain positive aspects of caregiving are based on this premise, even though they do not explicitly propose mutuality in patient-caregiver outcomes (Kahana & Young, 1990).

Thus theoretical work of the past decades has paved the way for a conceptualization of caregiver-care recipient interactions at later life that is based upon diversity rather than uniformity. Further, such work has enabled us to characterize caregiver-care recipient illness responses as dyadic in nature, not just as circumstances faced by two individuals. It is thus suggested that, to fully capture a dyadic approach, a model should be posed that depicts a range of dyadic outcomes. Such a model should be anchored in the prior caregiving literature and should reflect the limits of much of the caregiving work, with its singular focus on caregivers (Zarit, 1990). Caregiving generally has been considered as a stressor that impinges on the primary caregiver resulting in burden and adverse effects on psychological well-being. Conversely, the caregiver is viewed as a significant source of social support to the care recipient (Kahana & Young, 1990). The dyadic perspective advocated here represents an intermediate step between conventions of caregiving research and the far more complex approaches of family studies. It reflects the recognition that a system orientation that considers complex interactions of all family members does not readily lend itself to empirical investigations using traditional survey research orientations. A system view is more consistent with qualitative and clinical approaches to understanding the social context of illness. Although a dyadic model of caregiving is more simplified than a systems approach, it has appeal for advancing research and conceptual understanding of caregiving. Because the dyadic model allows for simultaneous consideration of the impact on both of the major actors in the caregiving encounter, as well as the capacity for both to affect the illness and, of course, to influence outcomes for each other, it can enable us to conceptualize family illness situations in a broader and perhaps more accurate way.

A CONCEPTUAL APPROACH
TO LATE-LIFE CAREGIVING AND
CARE RECEIVING FOR HEART PATIENTS

A caregiver-care recipient dyadic outcomes model applicable to later life chronic illness is introduced next. The model is directly related to two assumptions that were presented previously. First is that there are diverse rather than uniform outcomes of an illness situation. Second, the dyad can be simultaneously considered as it affects and is affected by illness at later life.

Figure 10.1 presents the dyadic outcomes model. It depicts, in cells A-D, four possible outcomes that range from positive to intermediate to negative. Inspection of the model shows that both caregiver and care recipient may prosper (cell A); that the caregiver may prosper while the care recipient declines (cell B); that the care recipient may prosper and the caregiver declines (cell C); or that both members of the dyad may decline (cell D). Clearly, cells A and D are symmetrical dyadic outcomes

	Care Recipient Positive Outcomes	Care Recipient Negative Outcomes
Caregiver Positive Outcomes	A Dyad prospers	B Caregiver prospers Care recipient declines
Caregiver Negative Outcomes	C Care recipient prospers Caregiver declines	D Dyad declines

Figure 10.1. Dyadic Outcomes Among Elderly Care Recipients and Care Providers

because the unit responds uniformly. In contrast, cells B and C show mixed outcomes—one segment of the dyad thrives while the other fails to thrive. In discussing the model, appropriate literature is presented that supports the outcome indicated by each cell. Much of this literature was derived from studies of Alzheimer's disease, as this has been the foremost area of investigation for caregiving researchers. However, wherever literature about heart patients exists it is included, because the focus of this chapter is on family caregiving issues after a heart attack.

Cell A presents a dyadic outcome that is positive for both the caregiver and the care recipient, and hence is symmetrical. This depiction of favorable outcomes for caregiver and care recipient alike generally has been overlooked in research efforts. However, there is some conceptual work about positive aspects of caregiving. On the theoretical level, altruism has been proposed as an explanation of why persons perform acts that are difficult, distasteful, or even dangerous. In the case of caregivers to the elderly, this can account for their willingness to engage in many care provision tasks (Kahana, Midlarsky, & Kahana, 1987). Theories that emphasize social exchange (Blau, 1964) also may help to explain caregiving activities as well as others that focus on mutuality, reciprocity, and sense of duty in families (Adams, 1968). The service role has been found to be gratifying to many people (Masciocchi et al., 1984; Schulz, 1990). Caring for an ailing person helps caregivers feel useful (Stone et al., 1987). The belief that they are helping the patient recover is uplifting to many care providers (Kahana & Kinney, 1991; Kinney, Stephens, & Brockman, 1987). It is suggested that caring for a loved one contributes to a mutually satisfying patient-caregiver relationship (Sangl, 1985). The psychological bonding that occurs can be important to caregiver and care recipient alike (Hirshorn, 1991). Although this recent work has not directly tested the assertions of cell A, that dyadic progress will occur, it lends support to the family cohesion approach represented by the work of Boss (1986).

Cell B delineates a mixed response by the dyad that rarely has been conceptualized or tested. The assertions are that there will be asymmetrical outcomes whereby the caregiver may prosper while the care recipient declines. This represents an odious view of caregiver-care recipient interactions.

Research that can verify this outcome is exceedingly scant. There are many studies of death and/or decline among care recipients. Yet not only is investigation linked to patient outcomes, without including the caregiver in the analysis, but also little information is included in postmortem inquiries about familial activities prior to death. An exception may be in cases in which *elder abuse* is suspected. Interestingly, research on elder abuse does not provide extensive evidence of abuse perpetrated by caregivers (Pillemer & Wolf, 1986).

There is some literature about dependency states that may be helpful in surmising whether patients decline while caregivers have positive outcomes. Patients that are the object of dependency-inducing behaviors by their care providers may acquire a state of learned helplessness (Kahana & Kinney, 1991). The caregiver, on the other hand, may feel fulfilled. If the illness situation has increased the power a woman caregiver has over her spouse, she may have some sense of fulfillment (Troll, Miller, & Atchley, 1979). Although the caregiver may have rewards that are associated with keeping the care recipient physically or psychologically dependent, it is likely that the patient does not perceive this situation as beneficial. As noted, this pattern has the fewest empirical tests.

Cell C is another example of mixed dyadic response in which the care recipient prospers as the caregiver declines. This represents a care recipient-centered one-directional model (Kahana & Young, 1990) and is consistent with the overwhelming research focus on poor caregiver outcomes (Zarit, 1990). An overwhelming number of investigations are based on the assumption of patient progress (recovery, stabilization, or delay in institutionalization) at the expense of caregivers (burden). This work investigates the price of caregiving and, clearly, burden is the predominant topic. Although work of the future may affirm the usefulness of burden studies (George, 1990), the concept has received a great deal of scrutiny because of its methodological and conceptual deficiencies (Schulz, 1990; Zarit, 1990).

Caregiver strain has been the subject of many studies, and these investigations provide ample evidence that caregivers experience adverse effects such as emotional exhaustion and physical, mental, and/or social morbidity (George & Gwyther, 1986; Miller et al., 1991; Poulshock & Deimling, 1984). Yet it is not at all clear how these adverse caregiver outcomes relate to the welfare of the care recipient. There is some limited support for a caregiver strain-patient recovery model from the heart disease literature. Heart patients are predominantly cared for by their spouses (Finlayson & McEwen, 1977), and wives of patients who have suffered MI experience severe emotional distress (Croog & Levine, 1982). Yet, although care of persons with heart disease is associated with strain, fatigue, and other adverse consequences, most older patients recover (Tofler et al., 1988), even while the family experiences strain (Speedling, 1982).

Assertions of dyadic decline, as depicted in cell D, also are supported by the literature. However, this is generally from studies of Alzheimer's disease (AD), which results in inevitable physical and intellectual decline. Theories from the early family literature were based on this premise (e.g., Parsons & Fox, 1952). They proposed that family strain, family dysfunction, and other adverse effects (e.g., dyadic decline) would result from prolonged or even short-term illness. Although this poorest dyadic outcome may occur among AD families, this situation may not characterize other illnesses and even may be typical of only a relatively small proportion of AD families.

Reviewing the research finding of poor patient and caregiver outcomes, it has been shown that poor mental and physical health of elders is associated with similarly poor states among their caregivers (George & Gwyther, 1986; Miller et al., 1991; Poulshock & Deimling, 1984; Pruchno & Resch, 1989; Zarit, Todd, & Zarit, 1986). The most consistent findings have been that caregivers experience symptoms of anxiety or depression and their subjective well-being is poor if they care for elders with psychological problems. These caregivers experience considerable emotional distress if they aid an elder who behaves in a disruptive or embarrassing way (Schulz, 1990). Some limited evidence suggests that caregivers deal with the stress of caring for an emotionally impaired person by "letting it out" on the elder (Bernatavicz, 1982; Kosberg, 1983; Pillemer & Wolf, 1986; Shelby-Lane, 1991). The impaired person may become the victim of his or her caregiver's rage or even abuse.

Time also may be a factor in poor caregiver-care recipient outcomes. A spiral of decline can be found among many patient-caregiver dyads as caregiving is prolonged. Clearly, as the patient's health declines, the caregiver is found to have increasing levels of stress (Schulz, 1990). Emotional response on the part of the caregiver can then affect his or her ability to provide the patient with the care that is needed. Should the caregiver suffer physical or mental health consequences or "burnout," there can be a very serious impact on the care recipient. Although predictors of institutional placement are not well understood (Kosloski, Montgomery, & Borgatta, 1988), Zarit and colleagues (1986) showed that the removal of elders from the home often follows reports of burden among caregivers. Breakdown in the ability of the caregiver to provide the type and level of assistance that is needed is thought to be a probable cause of patient institutionalization, even though studies of nursing home admissions link demographic and functional characteristics with most placements (Liu & Manton, 1984).

Research conducted among heart patient families has not focused on dyadic decline. However, there is abundant evidence that if a patient dies, the caregiver exhibits poor mental and physical aftereffects (Finlayson & McEwen, 1977). Some caregivers even hold themselves responsible for the death or failure to recover and subsequently suffer severe guilt.

In summary, conceptual approaches to caregiver-care recipient interactions that derive from a dyadic perspective on family response to illness can be modeled. This chapter introduced such a model with four types of dyadic responses as its components. These responses represented a continuum of positive to negative outcomes. Two dyadic patterns were symmetrical and the other two were asymmetrical. Having proposed the model, we believe it can be widely used to consider several types of caregiving issues. Furthermore, it can be used as the basis of empirical tests of the range of responses that characterize the family-illness interface at later life.

EMPIRICAL TESTS
OF A DYADIC OUTCOMES MODEL

A goal of this chapter is to present a dyadic conceptualization of late-life illness that proposes diverse patient-family outcomes. Yet the ultimate value of a theoretical formulation is whether it is applicable to the real world. To seek verification of the model, a test was designed that might demonstrate differential predictors of the four typologies of dyadic outcomes. Families facing heart disease of an older member were the subjects for this empirical test.

The sample for this study was based upon elderly patients with confirmed myocardial infarction (MI) and their family caregivers. These elderly patients, who represented 534 consecutive admissions, were referred by the cardiac and intensive care units of 7 hospitals in a major metropolitan area and approached for participation in the first 3 days after the MI. Patients who died, were admitted to nursing homes, had no family caregivers, were cared for in a distant geographic area, or could not be interviewed at the 6-week post-MI period for various reasons were excluded ($n = 204$), as were 84 patients who subsequently refused to participate. These factors reduced the sample to 246 patients. Of this number, data were collected from 63 patients only, and from 183 patient-caregiver dyads. The 183 patient-caregiver dyads thus comprise the sample for this study.

Patients were recruited for the study during their hospital stay and identified the person who would serve as their primary caregiver upon their return home. Upon discharge, both patient and caregiver were contacted. Only those dyads in which both patients and caregivers agreed to participate were included.

The first of two postdischarge interviews occurred six weeks after hospitalization (Time 1). The second interview, which determined the longer term effects of caregiving on the family, took place one year later (Time 2). Comparable survey instruments were used for both patients and their caregivers. Parallel questions pertaining to health, family caregiving, and psychosocial factors were included on the patient and caregiver versions of the instruments.

Psychological distress was evaluated as the dyadic outcome measure. The focus upon mental health was due to the previously presented evidence showing the severe emotional impact of MI among patients and caregivers alike (Croog & Levine, 1982; Finlayson, 1974; Krantz & Deckel, 1983). Based on the proposed model, dyads were expected to experience a range of outcomes from positive to negative. Accordingly, it was anticipated that some patient-caregiver units might have a great deal of distress, others would have very little, and still others would exemplify an intermediate type of response with one member being found to have a great deal of distress while his or her partner had little.

Measurement of psychological distress was by the 58-item Symptom Checklist (SCL-58) by Derogatis, Lipman, and Covi (1973). This scale lists complaints indicative of psychiatric symptomatology. Subjects rate discomfort on a scale of 1 to 4. There is a possible scale range of 58-236, indicating low to high global distress. The measure also has five factors validated in previous research, of which two (anxiety and depression) were separately analyzed in this work. Intercorrelations of the anxiety and depression scales were low.

During the first interview patients averaged 67 years of age and were predominantly male (66%). Most were married (67%) and white (69%). Their health status ranged from fair to poor. Patients averaged 2.1 post-MI cardiac symptoms (of a possible 6) and most required extensive help from their caregivers with activities and instrumental activities of daily living. The assistance averaged more than 30 hours weekly during the first 2 weeks after hospital discharge. The caregiver sample averaged 60 years of age and most (80%) were female. Spouses predominated as caregivers (63%), although daughters were the second most typical type of caregivers (16%). This sample was also 69% white.

To determine dyadic outcomes, scores on the mental health measures first were determined for caregiver and patient samples. Analysis of global SCL scores showed similar levels of distress for patient and caregiver samples ($M = 81.7$ for patients and 76.7 for caregivers). These scores indicated greater levels of distress for the caregivers and care recipients than has been shown for general community living samples (Derogatis et al., 1973). Similar results were obtained when anxiety and depression were considered. Average patient and caregiver scores on the anxiety measure were 7.96 and 7.85, respectively. Depression scores averaged 15.02 for patients and 14.67 for caregivers.

The extent to which mental distress symptomatology was congruent among caregivers and care recipients was a major research focus. Data showed that there was only a small degree of similarity. Pearson's product-moment correlations of caregiver-patient scores ranged from −0.04 to 0.16 on global SCL, anxiety, and depression measures. These data provided tentative support for two assertions. First, the range of responses to the illness included positive and negative reactions by both patients and caregivers. Second, these responses were often incongruent for the two samples.

Because the previous analyses were made using statistical tests of aggregate scores for the patient and caregiver groups, additional tests were performed to compare the responses of each member of a patient-caregiver dyad. This enabled the test of the four outcomes proposed in cells A-D of the model. Data representing each patient-caregiver unit first were analyzed by determining whether each member's score on the SCL measure was elevated or non-elevated. Elevated referred to scores that were greater than one standard deviation of the mean for that sample (patients or caregivers). Next, this score was compared with that of the other member of the dyad to determine the status of the unit. The dyad then was categorized as prospering (neither elevated, indicative of cell A), distressed (both elevated, representing cell D), or showing mixed response whereby one person was elevated and one was not (cells B & C). Finally, the proportion of dyads that were prospering, declining, and had mixed response types was calculated.

As shown in Table 10.1, cell A represented the modal pattern for the sample. Indeed, in 45% of the cases both members of the dyad had non-elevated scores on the global SCL measure. In contrast, 13% of the dyads had the outcome represented by cell D, elevated scores for both members. Figures for the mixed response that was indicated by cells B and C were 26% (B) and 16% (C). Examination of types of mental distress—depression and/or anxiety—elicited similar response patterns to those shown for the global measure. Half of the dyads had the positive outcome represented by cell A (51% on the depression scale and 53% on the anxiety scale). Few had the poor dyadic outcomes of cell D (11% and 8% for the depression and anxiety subscales, respectively). Mixed response was found among 38% of dyads on both the depression and the anxiety subscales.

The preceding analysis demonstrated that although few dyads had universally poor mental health outcomes and many had good outcomes, a substantial group of dyads failed to respond uniformly. Clearly, there were four patterns of dyadic response, as had been predicted. A logical extension of these conclusions is that if divergent outcomes result from the same type of health problem, there may be specific factors that account for them. Indeed, identifying variables that are associated with divergent family responses to illness is a key research question (Leventhal et al., 1985).

TABLE 10.1 Distribution of Dyadic Outcomes and Psychological Distress (in percentages)

Variable	Cell A (dyad prospers)	Cell B (CG prospers, CR declines)	Cell C (CR prospers, CG declines)	Cell D (dyad declines)
SCL	45 ($N = 83$)	26 ($N = 47$)	16 ($N = 29$)	13 ($N = 24$)
Depression	51 ($N = 94$)	23 ($N = 42$)	15 ($N = 27$)	11 ($N = 19$)
Anxiety	53 ($N = 97$)	19 ($N = 35$)	19 ($N = 35$)	8 ($N = 15$)

Note: CG = caregiver, CR = care receiver

To determine whether certain distinguishing factors might be identified that contributed to each dyadic mental health pattern, several variables were considered. These pertained to caregiver and care recipient health status, characteristics of the caregivers, and characteristics of the caregiving situation. Health is a basic consideration in influencing caregiving outcomes. Seriously impaired patients are generally more difficult to care for than their healthier counterparts and often are institutionalized (Montgomery & Kosloski, 1991). The caregiver's health is also a consideration because it can limit the amount or quality of help the caregiver is able to provide (George & Gwyther, 1986). Prior research suggests that health of the caregiver mediates the association of task provision and caregiver burden (Miller et al., 1991). Characteristics of the caregiver are also potential predictors of outcomes. Some studies show that they offer better prediction than care recipient characteristics (Colerick & George, 1986; Montgomery, 1989). Sex and age of the caregiver frequently have been analyzed as predictors of caregiving outcomes (Schulz, 1990; Stone et al., 1987). Although women predominate as caregivers to elders, they also seem to suffer more adverse effects (Horowitz, 1985; Stoller, 1983). Age, interestingly, is not highly correlated with caregiving strain and older spouse caregivers actually may suffer fewer adverse effects than child caregivers (Young & Kahana, 1989). Characteristics of the caregiving situation, which sometimes are referred to as the objective stressors of a caregiving situation (Schulz, 1990), are also of importance (Kahana & Young, 1990). The amount of care required by the patient and corresponding caregiving effort have been shown to be associated with caregiver burden (Morycz, 1985; Zarit, 1991). However, a recent study of caregiving stress gives us reason to question these findings because neither anxiety, depression, nor affect balance were associated with the patient's receipt of ADL and IADL assistance (Chiriboga, Weiler, & Nielsen, 1990).

The above-noted patient, caregiver, and caregiving situational variables were analyzed for their potential effect on dyadic mental health outcomes. In this analysis of predictors of dyadic outcomes the focus was on depressive symptomatology, which was the most frequent type of distress reported by respondents using the elevated/non-elevated distinction that was previously presented. Four dyadic groups were distinguished corresponding to cells A-D of the model: (a) low symptomatology among both patients and caregivers; (b) high symptomatology for patients, low for caregivers; (c) low symptomatology for patients, high for caregivers; and (d) high symptomatology for both. Discriminant function analysis was used and the predictor variables were age and health of the caregiver; age, sex, and health of the patient; and the task assistance and emotional support offered by the care provider. Findings showed that age and health of the caregiver, the extent of the caregiving support, health of the patient with regard to cardiac distress level, and his or her sex were significant factors that distinguished the groups with regard to depression. They correctly classified 57% of the dyads. With regard to each pattern, the variables predicted 81% of the dyads in cell A, 42% in cell B, 11% in cell C, and 39% in cell D. Clearly, the predictive power varied and was poor only for the caregiver prospers/care recipient declines dyad.

The significant predictors differed for each of the four groups. Dyads representing positive outcomes for the dyad (cell A) were characterized by male patients with little cardiac distress. Little caregiving support and care provided by a younger family member was associated with the mixed dyadic outcome in which patients prospered but caregivers suffered, presented in cell B. Good health status of caregivers was associated with cell C outcomes (high symptomatology for patients, low for caregivers). The dyads experiencing shared negative outcomes (cell D) were comprised of patients who were cared for by older caregivers and who had more cardiac distress and required a great deal of caregiving assistance. Overall, this method of data analysis provided evidence that health of the patient and the amount of caregiving assistance are important predictors of good, poor, and mixed dyadic outcomes. These findings are both logical and consistent with much of the heart disease and gerontology literature.

DISCUSSION

The preliminary data obtained in our research to consider the nature and predictors of dyadic outcomes for caregivers and care recipients provide a useful glimpse into the complexities as well as the promise of viewing family caregiving in a more holistic and relational manner. Having recognized that caregiving involves an important dyadic interaction we attempted to operationalize one consequence of this interchange (i.e., mental health outcomes) in a manner that incorporates both of the key actors in the relationship: the caregiver and the care recipient. Results of our analyses reveal that diverse patterns of dyadic mental health outcomes exist in heart-disease caregiving. Alternative typologies are associated with demographic characteristics of caregivers, care recipients, illness characteristics, and demands of the caregiving situation. The fact that age of caregivers comprised one of the significant predictors of poor dyadic caregiver outcomes points to the potential importance of the life stage of members of the caregiving dyad in shaping well-being outcomes. Because our study focused on elderly heart patients variability was primarily present in age and life stage of caregivers. It is plausible, however, that age and life stage of care receivers may be equally potent influences on well-being outcomes for both members of the dyad. Thus it is possible that younger heart patients, whose heart attack is an "off time" life-stage event, would be particularly prone to high levels of psychological distress because of both the disruptiveness of their illness and the need to accept care from others during a life stage in which independence or even generativity toward others comprises salient developmental tasks. It is also possible that situations with a woman providing care to a middle-aged husband in good health up to a sudden heart attack would result in greater stress and more adverse mental health outcomes for both the patients and the caregivers. Consequently, more adverse dyadic outcomes may be anticipated.

Alternatively, psychological well-being outcomes may be enhanced during life stages in which the caregiving relationship is "on time." Thus, for example, an older husband who had always been protective of his somewhat younger wife and concerned for her well-being, should he die first, may derive uplifts from his ability to provide care or be of assistance to her in the aftermath of the heart attack. She, too, may derive solace from being cared for by her husband, resulting in relatively positive dyadic outcomes for caregiver and care recipient.

Introducing a conceptual model for analysis of the effects of heart disease on psychological well-being of the caregiving dyad was a goal of this chapter. The premise was that illness is a family rather than an individual matter that may strain the patient-caregiver dyad. Alternatively, it can be a life experience with potentially good outcomes for the unit or for one of its members. Thus, to understand how illness affects older patients and their families, it is important to concentrate on the caregiver-care recipient dyad.

To present this in a manner that might be helpful to researchers and practitioners alike, a model of the family illness response was introduced. Because there is considerable heterogeneity in caregiver and care recipient populations related to sociodemographic characteristics, and also expectations (Stone et al., 1987; Whitehouse, 1990), this model proposed several ways that the caregiver-care recipient units might respond to serious illness at later life. A range of dyadic outcomes was proposed that would represent both uniform and discrepant aftereffects among the dyads.

Data from a study of older patient-family caregiver dyads were analyzed as an empirical test of the model. This was based on longitudinal research conducted among elderly heart patients and their primary caregivers. Several findings emerged that provided support for the contention that families respond to demands and challenges of caregiving in diverse ways. The outcomes were not necessarily poor and the range of responses were from dyadic progress to mixed response to dyadic decline. Although it was shown that half of the dyads were adversely affected by the illness situation to the extent that both were quite symptomatic on mental health measurement tools, the other half were not. Indeed, among the considerable variation shown in the family's response to the illness situation, good dyadic outcomes occurred more often than other singular reactions.

The proposed dyadic outcome model can help clarify how older families react to serious illness. The model used also may be used to explore diversity in outcomes for dyads confronting different caregiving challenges or operating in different personal or situational contexts. Thus, for example, it is quite likely that the care recipient's health status has an impact on the outcome that the dyad experiences. Some of the data from this study confirm that this may be the case. The mental distress of both caregivers and care recipients was higher if the patient either suffered continuation of cardiac distress or experienced decline in cardiac status over a 1-year period (Young & Kahana, 1990). However, based on the present study it is difficult to determine the extent to which differing dyadic caregiving outcomes are a function of characteristics of the caregiver, the care receiver, or the illness. Determining the relative influences of illness, caregiver, and care receiver characteristics and situational factors represents a useful and challenging research area for future caregiving research concerned with dyadic outcomes.

Another promising area for further inquiry relates to understanding normative family expectations as they influence dyadic outcomes. It is quite possible that the family's normative expectations for care of ailing persons might influence the extent to which favorable or unfavorable outcomes ensue. Family members are socialized to accept norms of family solidarity, elder care, and intergenerational continuity of values (Adams, 1968; Brody, 1985; Nydegger, 1983). This extends to both spouses and children who assist older people. There are also fairly universal marital expectations that include aiding one's spouse during illness (Troll et al., 1979). Parent care is also an expectation in many cultures and can even be governed by religious dictates (e.g., filial responsibility) (Markides, 1989). Children of frail parents often are motivated internally to care for their elders (Hirshorn, 1991). This can be due to a belief in reciprocity, sense of duty, and moral obligation, or, for many persons, an unquestionable desire to aid a person they love. This suggests that variation in dyadic outcomes might be directly related to norms of family responsibility and elder care held by both members of the dyad. However, because child-parent care units differ extensively from dyads comprised of marital partners (Stone et al., 1987; Young & Kahana, 1989), to effectively consider this issue would require that norms and values of adult child caregivers be distinguished from those held by spouses.

Using the proposed four-cell model of caregiving outcomes, researchers can design a variety of studies that would test the dyadic patterns that were observed for a variety of caregiver-care recipient situations. Examples include how specifically constituted dyads (e.g., adult child caregivers of older parents with cognitive and behavioral problems associated with dementia) may fit into the patterns that were found in this study of heart patient-family caregiver dyads. It is possible that the proportion of dyads that have poor outcomes may vary significantly from the results shown in this study if either the care recipient or the caregiver has different characteristics. Ethnic and racially distinct caregiver-care recipient dyads also should be investigated.

Although different types of illness and caregivers or care receivers with different characteristics may experience different dyadic outcomes, the four-cell typology of outcomes proposed here has general applicability as it is exhaustive of potential outcomes in any illness situation. It would be difficult to envision all dyads responding well just as it is hard to conceive of all having poor or mixed outcomes. Therefore, it can be useful to conceptualize the family illness paradigm in terms of dyadic response to illness with a range of positive and negative outcomes. As this study of older heart patients and their families showed, the caregiver-care recipient dyads had diverse, rather than uniform, outcomes; not all were desirable, but only a small proportion had universally bad aftereffects of the illness situation.

The model also has implications and applications for health and human service professionals. Practitioners who encounter persons suffering from chronic diseases can have a more thorough understanding of the family involvement in illness as the result of reviewing this model. By considering a model of dyadic caregiver outcomes they can recognize that there are mutual aspects of the family-illness intermesh. Practitioners need to approach the family as a unit and consider the effects on each key member of the caregiver-care receiver unit, if they are to benefit their patients or clients. Because the aftereffects of an illness situation may not be uniform for all family dyads, as indicated by the data from the heart patient-caregiver dyads, practitioners should try to determine whether the family is experiencing symmetrical or asymmetrical outcomes in developing treatment. Not only will this be illuminating, but also it can enable practitioners to consider benefits and desirability of alternative interventions. Treatment or aid by members of the health-care team thus may be targeted where its benefits are greatest (Leventhal et al., 1985). Assistance may be provided to either or both members of the caregiver-care receiver dyad or to the entire family to ensure maximum recovery or at least minimal adverse effects for those involved in caregiving.

REFERENCES

Adams, B. A. (1968). *Kinship in an urban setting*. Chicago: Markham.
Bernatavicz, F. (1982). Family, neighbors, and friends. In *Improving protective services for older Americans*. Portland, ME: University of Southern Maine, Human Services Development Institute.

Biegel, D. E., Sales, E., & Schulz, R. (1991). *Family caregiving in chronic illness.* Newbury Park, CA: Sage.

Blau, P. (1964). *Exchanges and power in social life.* New York: John Wiley.

Boss, P. (1986). Family stress: Perception and context. In B. Sussman & S. Steinmetz (Eds.), *Handbook on marriage and the family.* New York: Plenum.

Brody, E. M. (1985). Parent care as a normative family stress. *The Gerontologist, 25,* 19-25.

Chiriboga, D. A., Weiler, P. G., & Nielsen, K. (1990). The stress of caregivers. In D. E. Biegel & A. Blum (Eds.), *Aging and caregiving* (pp. 121-138). Newbury Park, CA: Sage.

Colerick, E., & George, L. (1986). Predictors of institutionalization among caregivers of patients with Alzheimer's disease. *Journal of the American Geriatric Society, 34,* 493-498.

Croog, S., & Levine, S. (1982). *Life after a heart attack: Social and psychological factors eight years later.* New York: Human Sciences Press.

Derogatis, L. R., Lipman, R. S., & Covi, L. (1973). SCL-90: An out-patient psychotic rating scale—preliminary report. *Psychopharmacology Bulletin, 1,* 13-28.

Engel, G. L. (1981). The clinical application of the biopsychosocial model. In M. R. Haug (Ed.), *Elderly patients and their doctors* (pp. 3-21). New York: Springer.

Finlayson, A. (1974). Social networks as coping resources: Lay help and consultation patterns used by women in post-infarction cancer. *Social Science and Medicine, 10,* 97-103.

Finlayson, A., & McEwen, J. (1977). *Coronary heart disease and patterns of living.* New York: Prodist.

George, L. K. (1990). Caregiver stress studies: There really is more to learn. *The Gerontologist, 30*(5), 580, 581.

George, L. K., & Gwyther, L. P. (1986). Caregiver well-being: A multi-dimensional examination of family caregivers of demented adults. *The Gerontologist, 26,* 253-259.

Hansen, D. A., & Hill, R. (1964). Families under stress. In H. T. Christensen (Ed.), *Handbook of marriage and the family* (pp. 782-819). Chicago: Rand-McNally.

Hirshorn, B. (1991). Family caregiving is an intergenerational transfer. In R. F. Young & E. A. Olson (Eds.), *Health, illness, and disability in later life* (pp. 101-112). Newbury Park, CA: Sage.

Horowitz, A. (1985). Family caregiving to the frail elderly. *Annual Review of Gerontology and Geriatrics, 5,* 194-246.

Kahana, E., Kahana, B., & Kinney, J. M. (1989). Coping among vulnerable elders. In Z. Harel, P. Erlich, & R. Hubbard (Eds.), *Understanding and serving the vulnerable aged* (pp. 64-85). New York: Springer.

Kahana, E., & Kinney, J. (1991). Understanding caregiving interventions in the context of the stress model. In R. Young & E. Olson (Eds.), *Health, illness, and disability in later life: Practice issues and interventions* (pp. 122-142). Newbury Park, CA: Sage.

Kahana, E., Midlarsky, E., & Kahana, B. (1987). Beyond dependency, autonomy, and exchange. *Social Justice Review, 1*(4), 439-459.

Kahana, E., & Young, R. (1990). Clarifying the caregiving paradigm. In D. E. Biegel & A. Blum (Eds.), *Aging and caregiving* (pp. 76-97). Newbury Park, CA: Sage.

Kingston, E. R., Hirshorn, B. A., & Connor, J. M. (1986). *Ties that bind: The interdependence of generations.* Cabin John, MD: Seven Looks.

Kinney, J. M., Stephens, M. P., & Brockman, A. M. (1987). Personal and environmental correlates of territoriality and use of space: An illustration in congregate housing for older adults. *Environment and Behavior, 19,* 722-737.

Kosberg, J. L. (1983). The special vulnerability of elderly parents. In J. L. Kosberg (Ed.), *Abuse and maltreatment of the elderly: Cause and intervention* (pp. 263-275). Boston: John Wright.

Kosloski, K., Montgomery, R., & Borgatta, E. (1988, November). *Factors influencing the nursing home placement of the elderly.* Paper presented at the 41st annual meetings of the Gerontological Society of America, San Francisco.

Krantz, D. S., & Deckel, A. W. (1983). *Coping with chronic disease: Research and applications.* New York: Academic Press.

Leventhal, H., Leventhal, E. A., & Nguyen, T. V. (1985). Reactions of families to illness: Theoretical models and perspectives. In D. C. Turk & R. D. Kerns (Eds.), *Health, illness, and families: A life span perspective* (pp. 108-145). New York: John Wiley.

Litman, T. (1971). Health care and the family: A three generational analysis. *Medical Care, 9,* 67-81.

Litman, T. (1974). The family as a basic unit in health and medical care: A social behavioral overview. *Social Science and Medicine, 8,* 495-519.

Liu, K., & Manton, K. (1984). The characteristics and utilization pattern of an admission cohort of nursing home patients. *The Gerontologist, 24,* 70-76.

Malone-Beach, E. E., & Zarit, S. H. (1991). Current research issues in caregiving to the elderly. *International Journal of Aging and Human Development, 32,* 103-114.

Manton, K. G. (1990). Mortality and morbidity. In R. H. Binstock & L. K. George (Eds.), *Handbook of aging and the social sciences* (3rd ed., pp. 64-87). San Diego, CA: Academic Press.

Markides, K. S. (1989). Aging, gender, race/ethnicity, class, and health: A conceptual overview. In K. S. Markides (Ed.), *Aging and health: Perspectives on gender, race, ethnicity, and class* (pp. 9-22). Newbury Park, CA: Sage.

Masciocchi, C., Thomas, A., & Moeller, T. (1984). Support for the impaired elderly: A challenge for family caregivers. In W. Quinn & G. A. Hughston (Eds.), *Independent aging: Family and social systems perspectives* (pp. 115-131). Rockville, MD: Aspen Systems.

McCubbin, H., & Patterson, J. (1983). The family stress process: The doubled ABCX model of adjustment and adaptation. In H. McCubbin, M. Sussman, & J. Patterson (Eds.), *Social stress and the family: Advances and developments in family stress theory and research.* New York: Haworth.

Miller, B., McFall, S., & Montgomery, A. (1991). The impact of elder health, caregiver involvement, and global stress on two dimensions of caregiver burden. *Journal of Gerontology, 46,* S9-S19.

Montgomery, R., & Kosloski, K. (1991). *Secondary analysis of effects of intervention on family caregivers: Correlates of nursing home placement* (Final Report to the Health Care Financing Administration, Contract #HCFA-90-0435). Unpublished report.

Montgomery, R. J. V. (1989). Investigating caregiver burden. In K. S. Markides & C. L. Cooper (Eds.), *Aging, stress, and health* (pp. 201-218). New York: John Wiley.

Montgomery, R. J. V., Stull, D. E., & Borgatta, E. F. (1985). Measurement and analysis of burden. *Research on Aging, 7,* 137-152.

Morycz, R. K. (1985). Caregiving strain and the desire to institutionalize family members with Alzheimer's disease. *Research on Aging, 7,* 329-361.

National Center for Health Statistics. (1985). *Health, U.S.* (DHHS Publication No. PHS 86-1232). Washington, DC: Government Printing Office.

New, P. K., Ruscio, A. T., Priest, R. P., Petritsi, D., & George, L. A. (1973). The support structure of heart and stroke patients: A study of the role of significant others in patient rehabilitation. *Social Science and Medicine, 2,* 185-199.

Noelker, L. S. (1991). Older persons as care receivers: The Benjamin Rose Institute. *Gerontological Society of America,* pp. 1-4.

Nydegger, C. N. (1983). Family ties of the aged in cross-cultural perspective. *The Gerontologist, 23,* 26-32.

Parsons, T., & Fox, R. (1952). Illness, therapy, and the modern family. *Journal of Social Issues, 8,* 31-44.

Pillemer, K. A., & Wolf, R. S. (1986). *Elder abuse: Conflict in the family.* Dover, MA: Auburn.

Poulshock, S. W., & Deimling, G. T. (1984). Families caring for elders in residence: Issues in the measurement of burden. *Journal of Gerontology, 39,* 230-239.

Pratt, L. (1976). *Family structure and effective health behavior: The energized family.* Boston: Houghton Mifflin.

Pruchno, R. A., & Resch, N. L. (1989). Husbands and wives as caregivers: Antecedents of depression and burden. *The Gerontologist, 29,* 159-165.

Sangl, J. (1985). The family support system of the elderly. In R. Vogel & H. Palmer (Eds.), *Long-term care: Perspectives from research and demonstration* (pp. 307-336). Rockville, MD: Aspen Systems.

Satir, V. (1976). *Conjoint family therapy* (rev. ed.). Palo Alto, CA: Science and Behavior Books.

Schulz, R. (1990). Theoretical perspectives on caregiving. In D. E. Biegel & A. Blum (Eds.), *Aging and caregiving* (pp. 27-52). Newbury Park, CA: Sage.

Shanas, E. (1979). The family as a social support system in old age. *The Gerontologist, 9,* 169-174.

Shelby-Lane, C. (1991). Elder abuse: A case analysis for health care providers. In R. Young & E. Olson (Eds.), *Health, illness, and disability in later life: Practice issues and interventions* (pp. 73-82). Newbury Park, CA: Sage.

Speedling, E. J. (1982). *Heart attack: The family response at home and in the hospital.* New York: Tavistock.

Stoller, E. P. (1983). Parental caregiving by adult children. *Journal of Marriage and the Family, 45,* 851-858.

Stone, R., Cafferata, G. L., & Sangl, J. (1987). Caregivers of the frail elderly: A national profile. *The Gerontologist, 27,* 616-626.

Tofler, G. H., Muller, J. E., Stone, P. H., Willich, S. N., Davis, V. G., Poole, K., Braunwald, E., & MILIS Study Group. (1988). Factors leading to shorter survival after acute myocardial infarction in patients ages 65 to 75 years compared with younger patients. *American Journal of Cardiology, 62,* 860-867.

Troll, L., Miller, S., & Atchley, R. (1979). *Families in later life.* Belmont, CA: Wadsworth.

U.S. Department of Health and Human Services. (1986). *Current estimates from the National Health Interview Survey, United States* (Series 10, No. 156) (DHHS Publication No. PHS86-1584). Washington, DC: Government Printing Office.

Whitehouse, P. J. (1990, August). *Special challenges in research on the mental health/physical health interface in caregivers: Future directions.* Paper presented at the National Institute of Mental Health Workshops on the Mental Health of Family Caregivers in Alzheimer's Disease and Related Dementias, Washington, DC.

Young, R., & Kahana, E. (1989). Specifying caregiver outcomes: Gender and relationship aspects of caregiving strain. *The Gerontologist, 29,* 660-666.

Young, R., & Kahana, E. (1990). *Mental health adaptation and caretaking to ailing aged* (Final Report to National Institute on Aging). Unpublished report.

Young, R., & Kahana, E. (1992). Adult daughters and parent care: Roles and role strain. *Sociological Abstracts, 40,* 6.

Zarit, S. H. (1990). Interventions with frail elders and their families: Are they effective and why? In M. A. P. Stephens, J. H. Crowther, S. E. Hobfall, & D. L. Tennenbaum (Eds.), *Stress and coping in later-life families* (pp. 241-265). New York: Hemisphere.

Zarit, S. H., Todd, P. A., & Zarit, J. M. (1986). Subjective burden of husbands and wives as caregivers: Longitudinal study. *The Gerontologist, 26,* 260-266.

PART III

The Interface Between Formal Care Providers and Caregiving Families

11

Care at Home

Family Caregivers and Home Care Workers

LUCY ROSE FISCHER
NANCY N. EUSTIS

This chapter examines the interrelationship of two important components of long-term care systems: family caregiving and paid home care. What are the linkages between these "informal" and "formal" systems of care? How different is home care by family members versus paid workers? What conditions lead to cooperation or conflict between family caregivers and paid home care workers? How are services coordinated?

BACKGROUND

A number of gerontologists and specialists on long-term health care have noted that more understanding is needed of the intermeshing of formal and informal care. Cantor and Little (1985), for example, commented: "With informal care such a crucial part of the social care

AUTHORS' NOTE: This research received funding from the Blandin Foundation, the Graduate School of the University of Minnesota, the All-University Council on Aging/Center for Urban and Regional Affairs at the University of Minnesota, and St. Olaf College. The authors express special thanks to Terri Karis, Royanna Lindtvedt, Carol Felton, and Nathan Almquist, who were interviewers for the project; to Jill Olivieri, Scott Parks, and Sally Losness, who served as research assistants; and to the home care agencies, clients, workers, and family caregivers who participated in the study.

system, the question of the proper interface between informal and formal subsystems becomes critical. We need to know more about the appropriate balance between individual, family and societal responsibility for the care of dependent elderly" (p. 773). Similarly, McAuley and Arling (1984) have argued that an important policy issue is how to foster a more reasonable mix of formal and informal care in home and institutional settings. There has not been much research, however, on the intersection of formal and informal care systems. Most research on long-term care is about *either* "informal" caregiving or "formal" care.

One factor that has been well established is the dominance of the informal system of care. Most long-term care is provided by families. Horowitz (1985), in her review of caregiving literature, concludes: "Families provide 80% of all home health care for older people . . . ; conversely, 80% of all older people with home health care needs depend primarily on their family" (p. 198). Various estimates have suggested that for every elderly patient in a nursing home, there are between 1 and 2.5 patients with equivalent impairments who are being cared for at home by their families. The cost borne by families is considerable. Montgomery (1982) wrote that although more than a fourth of the federal budget is spent on the aged and disabled, far more is spent by families.

Families continue to provide care even when formal services are used (Horowitz, 1985; Newhouse & McAuley, 1987). Conversely, however, most elderly who receive family care do *not* use formal services. Stone, Cafferata, and Sangl (1987), in their analysis of data from a national sample of caregivers, found that less than 10% used paid services, and formal care was viewed as a last resort. Horowitz (1985) reports that "When family caregivers do approach formal service providers, they tend to be very selective and modest in their service requests, often requesting far less than professionals would have recommended" (p. 224).

Much research on formal/informal care has focused on finding ways to reduce costly institutional care. A number of experimental programs have attempted to substitute limited home care for more costly institutional care, particularly by supporting caregivers. The idea is that respite care and supplemental home care should alleviate the burden of family care and encourage families to continue to provide care in their homes. To a large degree, however, attempts to reduce governmental costs through such programs have been unsuccessful from a cost-saving perspective (Callahan, 1989). A recent study (Newman, Stuyk, Wright, & Rice, 1990), in fact, found that formal, community-based support may *increase* the likelihood of institutionalization. Elderly who received both paid and unpaid care were institutionalized more often than those who had only unpaid caregivers (see also Christianson, 1988; Kemper, 1988).

The dominance of the informal care system reflects, in large part, the lack of access to paid home care (Heumann, 1991). When asked what kind of care they would want if they had long-term care needs, elderly have about equal preference for receiving paid care or family care—in their own homes (McAuley & Blieszner, 1985). Elderly are twice as likely to prefer paid home care to any form of institutional care and more than four times more likely to someone else's (a relative's) home to be cared for. Being cared for in one's own home might be, in fact, a universal value. And yet, there are few resources for paid home care, especially in this country. Cantor and Little (1985) point out that in the United States, out of every dollar for the elderly spent by government, only 1.5 cents are for community-based social services. Virtually the only public funding for long-term care is through Medicaid, eligibility for which is determined by financial need. The consequence is that paid long-term care is available only to the very rich or the very poor. People in the middle class gain access to care only by spending down most of their assets and becoming impoverished in order to qualify for Medicaid.

One linkage between informal and formal care is through the case management role of family caregivers. In a recent paper (Fischer & Eustis, 1988a) on family caregiving and the impact of DRGs (Medicare's Prospective Payment System), we described the "managerial family," in which family caregivers mediate between the patient and the health-care bureaucracy, arrange for post-hospital care, and supervise paid caregivers both in the hospital and at home. One critical component of the managerial role is arranging for and supervising home care. We noted that "the post-DRG health care environment exacerbates managerial responsibilities for family caregivers" because patients tend to leave the hospital "quicker and sicker" (Fischer & Eustis, 1988a, p. 388; see also Archbold, 1990; Daatland, 1983; Fischer & Eustis, 1990; Horowitz, 1985; Sussman, 1985).

A theoretical perspective on systems of formal and informal care is Litwak's theory of complementary roles (see Chapter 4 in this volume; Litwak, 1985; Litwak & Szelenyi, 1969; Sussman, 1985). Litwak and his associates argue that support systems differ in structure and function. They note that large, formal bureaucracies (such as long-term care institutions) have a number of distinct characteristics: They concentrate on technical knowledge, allow a division of labor, and offer standardized services at low costs because of economies of size. Conversely, informal primary groups (such as families) have opposite structures: They are small in size, they specialize in "everyday" rather than technical knowledge, they are characterized by long-term commitments, and they offer idiosyncratic rather than standardized services. Litwak and his coauthors argue that the elderly, in order to have their needs met for long-term health care, need both formal and informal support systems. Formal providers are best at handling areas requiring expert knowledge and large-scale resources. The informal system is necessary for providing nonuniform aspects of care, which are both technically simple and unpredictable. Although these support systems have opposite "structures," the roles they provide are complementary rather than mutually contradictory. Thus, for example, a patient in a nursing home might receive routine care from the institution, whereas visiting relatives might provide "watchdog" supervision and special "treats"—based on commitment to and knowledge of the individual. Litwak (1985) reports that nursing home patients who have no close family ties tend to lose those types of idiosyncratic services that families are best able to provide.

When we apply the Litwak model to home care rather than institutional care, however, the distinctions between formal and informal care may not be entirely appropriate. What are the economies of scale in home care? How is family work distinct from tasks provided by paid home care workers? One characteristic of both paid home care and family caregiving is that the care essentially is unsupervised because it is provided in private settings, behind closed doors. Litwak (1985) therefore contends that, for home care agencies, standardization of care is critical: "When the organization does not standardize the task, supervising help is very difficult—given the lack of internal commitments such as altruism or duty—and the task has a low probability of being done effectively" (p. 413). Ostensibly, there is more risk from home care workers in an unsupervised setting than from family caregivers who have "internal commitments" to the care recipient. It is not clear, however, that standardizing a home care task would have much impact on the effectiveness or efficiency of paid home care, because there still would be no supervision. Moreover, family "commitments" are not always reliable, as we know from research on family violence and elder abuse.

THE HOME CARE RELATIONSHIPS STUDY

This chapter is part of a qualitative study on relationships between home care workers and their clients (see Eustis & Fischer, 1991; Fischer & Eustis, 1988b). A central purpose of this research was to explore how worker-client relationships affect the quality of care. Family caregiving was included in this study both because family caregivers are a critical component of the health-care system and because we suspected that the client-worker-caregiver triangle could have a significant impact on home care quality. We tried to interview as many family members as possible who were directly involved in providing care at home and/or arranging for paid home care.

The data in this study are largely qualitative. We conducted in-depth interviews with home care clients, their paraprofessional workers (home health aides or personal care attendants), and, in some cases, their family caregivers. The interview data were dictated, transcribed, and analyzed contextually. There were 54 cases, with each case comprised of a home care client, a worker, and, when appropriate, a family member. We interviewed 54 clients, 39 workers (some workers had several clients in the sample), and 15 family members. In addition, there were some precoded questions as well as written questionnaires that were mailed to clients 6 months following the interview (about four fifths of the sample responded to the follow-up).

The study focused on long-term (rather than short-term) home care clients—operationally defined as clients who have received or are projected to receive at least 6 months of home care and have at least two visits per week. All of the clients in our sample had chronic disabilities, such as heart disease, neurological disorders, multiple sclerosis (MS), cerebral palsy, or spinal cord injuries.

A stratified, nonrandom sampling design was used so the home care cases included both urban and rural settings; elderly and working-age clients; and agency and direct-hire workers. These characteristics—location, age, and hiring arrangement—served as "independent variables" in some of our analyses. Conclusions about the effects of these variables, however, need to be drawn with caution because the variables are confounded. The young (working-age) clients tend to have more extensive needs for home care and are more likely to hire workers directly rather than through agencies, which is considerably more expensive. There is, furthermore, a much larger percentage of young clients in the urban than in the rural sample (48% versus 25%). It is likely that young clients with heavy home care needs may opt to live in urban areas where there are more resources and opportunities for disabled adults. Eight home care agencies were contacted and the names of clients and workers were obtained from them. To obtain clients who hire workers directly, newspaper classified ads were scanned, and persons who advertised for home health workers during the previous year were recruited for the study. Some direct-hire clients came to us by word of mouth and one volunteered for the study after reading about it in a small town newspaper. The sampling technique introduces some biases. Of particular concern is the likelihood that selections made by the agencies omitted problematic clients and workers.

The sample is roughly half from the Minneapolis metropolitan area (28 cases) and half from southeastern Minnesota (26 cases). There were 30 elderly clients ranging in age from 65 to 99, with an average age of 79. The 24 working-age clients ranged in age from 27 to 64, with an average age of 42. Thirty-four of our clients had workers provided by agencies, and 20 had workers hired directly. The 15 family caregivers who were interviewed included 8 spouses, 2 daughters, 1 daughter-in-law, 2 mothers, and 2 sisters; they ranged in age from 35 to 88. A third of the family caregivers had health problems themselves. The large majority of respondents in the sample—the clients, workers, and family caregivers—were female.

The elderly clients, compared to the working-age clients, were more likely to be housebound and to be in pain. They also were more likely to live with and receive help from family members. Younger clients were much more likely to be unable to walk and were more than twice as likely to hire home care workers directly, rather than through an agency. Not surprisingly, younger clients pay less per hour ($7.67 versus $8.60) but hire workers for substantially more hours per week. Workers for younger clients are more likely to be part-time in home care, to be students, and to be single. Workers for the elderly clients are more likely to be Certified Nurse Assistants and to think of home care as their career.

CARE AT HOME

Home care clients tend to require individually tailored packages of home care services, and each type of disability has a range in severity, both across individuals and over time for a particular person. The clients in our sample varied in their disabilities and in their needs for service. A few cases will illustrate the variability in both needs and services.

> An 81-year-old married man requires a hoyer lift to move from his bed to a wheelchair or from his chair to the toilet. He receives both personal care and homemaking for a few hours every day. His wife helps with his care but is herself too frail to either lift her husband or do extensive homemaking.

> A 70-year-old never-married, minimally retarded woman needs help getting drops in her eyes for her cataracts. Each of her several daily visits lasts only a few minutes.

> A 41-year-old never-married woman with severe arthritis needs a live-in caregiver since she moved out of her parents' home.

> A 74-year-old widowed woman is both physically and mentally incapacitated from a recent stroke. Her children live at a distance and her paid caregiver was legally appointed as her guardian *ad litem* to manage her affairs.

> A 35-year-old married woman gave birth to her fourth child *after* a car accident that left her paralyzed. With the help of health-care insurance, she has hired a full-time personal care attendant who comes every weekday and does a variety of chores—including homemaking, personal care, and child care.

How much paid home care is received by a particular client is determined by a number of factors, including the nature and severity of the disability or illness, access to unpaid helpers, and financial resources. Clients who live with relatives, such as spouses or children, often have access to a considerable amount of unpaid help. In contrast, disabled persons who live alone, even if they have paid help, may have problems managing tasks at night or early in the morning. Moreover, clients who either have high incomes or qualify for public or private insurance are likely to have much more extensive home care than low-income clients with no home care funds—regardless of need. In fact, "needs" are determined in large part by resources. One divorced woman with MS, for example, earns less than $15,000 a year and spends nearly $3,000 each year to hire unskilled helpers to stay overnight (at $8 a night) because she cannot lift her legs onto her bed; she needs help at 11:00 p.m. and again at 2:00 a.m. (when she gets up to use the bathroom). In addition, she must pay for a limited amount of other care—homemaking and personal care during the day. Clearly, she has little money to pay for extensive home care.

Our data suggest that clients tend to "make do"—that is, to find ways to manage on their own while lacking a variety of ostensibly necessary services. For example, one man who lives alone has trained himself to restrict his use of the toilet to once a day when his home care worker is there. A few women said that they do not take regular baths or showers—just sponge baths. (The interviews were conducted during a hot summer!) Many of the clients rarely or never go outside because they cannot manage to do so without help.

The term "making do," however, is ours—and not a concept explicitly suggested by the interviewees. About one third of the home care clients said they had had experiences when they lacked needed help. Although there can be problems between workers and clients, most of the clients in our study appeared to be grateful for the care they received and felt that their "needs" for care were being met. Most of the clients interviewed for this study maintain their independence in their own homes or apartments and avoid institutional living—through a combination of limited home care, paid and/or unpaid, and "making do."

FAMILY CAREGIVERS VERSUS HOME CARE WORKERS

Help from "informal" caregivers—family caregivers (or friends and neighbors)—ostensibly is based on affection and/or obligation. In contrast, relationships with paid home care workers are contractual and are based on an exchange of services for monetary compensation. From Litwak's framework, we can infer that these divergences in structure are associated with differences in functions. Specifically, we might anticipate that paid home care would differ from family caregiving in the following functional parameters: *longevity, motivation, scope,* and *responsibility.* Our data on home care workers, in some ways, conform neatly to the Litwak formulation. In other ways, however, we find that the distinctions are not so clear-cut, largely because there is much "informality" in the "formal" role of home care worker.

According to Litwak, because kinship relationships are permanent, a central feature of family support is long-term commitment.[1] Conversely, we would expect to find problems in long-term availability for paid home care workers—the "revolving-door" phenomenon. To some degree, our findings illustrate the lack of longevity for paid home care arrangements. We observed, in fact, that impermanence was taken for granted by both clients and workers in our sample. Very few of the home care clients assumed that their workers would remain available as long as they needed help, and most of the workers in our sample simply did not know how long they either would continue in home care or would work for their particular clients. Virtually all of the workers implied that the choice to continue or not was theirs. Family caregivers, whose role tends to subsume a strong sense of obligation, rarely convey the same freedom of choice. Even so, our sample of home care workers may be atypically stable. About 80% of the home care workers had worked in their current home care position (for the same agency or the same direct-hire client) for more than a year, and more than a quarter had worked in their position for more than five years. Potentially, the age of the workers in this sample helps to account for the stability in their jobs. Nearly two thirds of the workers were women in their middle years—35 to 55; only six workers were under age 30.[2]

In terms of motivation, it is clear that home care workers do not express the same degree of obligation or affection that we might expect from family caregivers. Nonetheless, because of the nature and setting of home care, relationships between workers and clients often become more informal than formal. Almost two thirds of home care clients and about half of workers used noncontractual terms in defining their relationships; that is, they depicted one another as "a friend" or "like family." Rural clients and older clients were particularly likely to see their workers in friend/family terms. Given the low salaries and the minimal benefits (most workers in our sample were part-time and did not receive health insurance), there may need to be other motivations besides the economic contract. Most of the home care workers we interviewed indicated altruistic motivations for doing this type of work: "I love people and I feel very needed"; "I feel I am helping [my clients] to stay out of the nursing home"; "I love to wait on people"; "I think it is a mission" (see Chichin, 1991).

Paid home care and family care are most similar in the scope and nature of the work. Care at home, whether by paid workers[3] or family caregivers, entails a diffuse set of services that are designed uniquely for the patient. For paid home care, this means the parameters of the work role have to be defined idiosyncratically rather than by a clear set of job responsibilities. Ostensibly, home care workers—unlike family caregivers—are paid by the hour. But about a quarter of the clients said their workers at times spent more time with them than the hours they were paid. In fact, workers were far more likely to spend "extra" time than they were to come late or leave early. Furthermore, about two thirds of the workers in our sample provided "extra" services beyond their scheduled time and duties. Our respondents reported that their workers, on their own time, ran errands for clients, baked cookies, took clients to special events, and so forth. Because clients' needs are diffuse, it may not always be easy to define what is "extra"—especially for some of the younger, disabled clients with live-in personal care attendants. Even so, it is apparent that many workers develop personal ties with their clients and the boundaries around their responsibilities tend to expand.

Family caregivers tend to have a diffuse sense of responsibility for the spouse, parent, or other relative whom they are caring for. This means they care about the whole person—for his or her emotional as well as physical well-being—and they are accountable for the care. The "managerial" role emerges from this caregiver responsibility, in the sense that the caregiver makes sure care is provided by someone—by herself or himself or by another caregiver, paid or not (see Fischer, 1986; Fischer & Eustis, 1988a; Fischer, Rogne, & Eustis, 1990). Interestingly, in this research we observed that some home care workers approximate such managerial functions. We found examples of workers arranging for and training other workers. We also noted instances of workers taking responsibilities for matters that clearly went beyond in-home care. For example, one worker arranged for an electric door to be installed in her client's building so he could enter and leave the building. Such examples were found particularly in the rural sample. The fact that most workers provide "extra" services for their clients also indicates that home care workers tend to have a sense of accountability and, especially in small towns, may function as quasi-family members who take responsibility for providing whatever is needed.

It appears, in effect, that family caregivers and home care workers are not completely "opposite" in terms of their functions or the structure of their relationships with care recipients. Although the commitment of workers to clients may not be as "permanent" as family relationships, sometimes care arrangements are long term and may be based on affection and caring—not simply monetary reward. Moreover, the services are essentially the same whether the caregiver is a relative or a stranger, and the work is diffuse and idiosyncratically defined.

Of course, we should not exaggerate the similarities. Relationships with paid home care workers lack the emotional complexity and legitimacy of family relationships, as we have noted in other reports on caregiving relationships (see Fischer, 1986; Fischer et al., 1990). Even when paid workers serve as surrogate family caregivers, the boundaries around their responsibilities are much more defined. This point can be illustrated by a counter-example—a case in which a paid worker functioned essentially as a family caregiver. The client, a 74-year-old woman, was disabled from a stroke, her two sons lived far away and rarely visited, and her paid caregiver had been appointed as her guardian *ad litem.* The sons had agreed to the legal procedure. Not only did the sons rarely contact their mother, but also the guardian noted that it usually was not possible to contact them (she had tried once in an emergency, without success, because, she said, the sons tend to move around a lot). The client appeared to have a strong emotional attachment to and dependence on her guardian, who described her role in home care as a "mission." This worker was not available during the summer months, when she went with her husband, a high school teacher, to their summer home in northern Minnesota, and she had arranged for a substitute worker. The client, during her interview (which took place in August), talked, with tears in her eyes, about her loneliness for her usual worker. Nonetheless, neither the worker nor her client seemed to have any expectation that she might forgo any of her own summer plans. Moreover, we can note in this case that a legal procedure was required to set up this relationship, and that under the terms of the guardianship the caregiver is accountable to the courts!

Interestingly, it seems that many younger disabled persons lack family caregivers and/or prefer paid home care to family care. The younger clients in our sample, in fact, were more likely than the elderly clients to talk about the importance of maintaining a job-oriented relationship. One young urban client stated: "Rhonda is basically a worker and it's important to me to keep it that way." She added, however, that, given the setting and nature of the relationship, it is impossible to remain just "businesslike." Young adults with disabilities, especially those who are associated with the Independent Living Movement, view access to paid care as a critical resource in maintaining independent lives. As an employer or consumer, the person who requires personal assistance is relatively in control of his or her own care—symbolically and emotionally, as well as in practical terms. Conversely, reliance on family members to provide care invites dependence—in several ways. A family constitutes a limited pool and, to the extent that the disabled person has no or few other alternative resources, he or she is literally dependent on the persons who provide care. There is the potential for emotional blackmail; if the care recipient refuses to comply with demands from the caregiver, there is the risk that care will be refused. Alternatively, even without such negative implications there is the inherent emotional complexity of family relationships. The care recipient, for example, may be reluctant to "burden" a loving spouse, parent, sibling, or other relative—thus restricting the care that is available. There is also the risk of loss: Family caregivers can move away or die. Spouses also can choose to divorce their disabled partners (this is, apparently, quite common for younger persons who are disabled after being married). For all these reasons, younger disabled persons, especially, are aware that paid home care provides more of a potential for autonomy than family care (see Heumann, 1991; Simon-Rusinowitz & Hofland, 1989).

FAMILY CAREGIVERS
AND HOME CARE WORKERS:
COOPERATION OR CONFLICT?

For some home care clients, the home becomes a meeting place between family members and home health-care workers. Under what circumstances is there cooperation or conflict between family caregivers and paid home care workers? To what extent do family-worker interactions affect the quality of home care—either positively or negatively?

The Caregiving Alliance

In our sample there were three examples of family caregivers and home care workers who created a caregiving alliance. In all of these cases the clients were uncooperative male patients, and the workers and the clients' wives worked together to manage the care and support each other under adverse conditions. In one case, a home care worker said that he and the wife of his client, a man who had been brain damaged in a work-related injury, "teamed up to get George [the client] out of bed in the morning." George, because of his disability, had difficulty communicating, frequently refused to get out of bed until the afternoon, had a tendency to become angry and violent, and was in many ways difficult to handle. When the worker arrived in the morning, the worker and the client's wife (before she left for work) would discuss how George seemed to be feeling, what activities might be appropriate for that day, and whether George was likely to be particularly "stubborn" that morning about getting up. The worker also generally reported to the wife at the end of the day, letting her know about George's activities and whether there were any problems. This worker and his client's wife did *not* develop a close friendship out of their brief interactions. Nonetheless, their caregiving alliance helped both of them to help George, particularly because each of them individually had difficulty in managing George's behavior.

The caregiving alliance is a benign conspiracy. The goal of George's wife and his home care worker is to manage George—that is, not to do what George wants, but to have George do what they believe is good for George. From the client's point of view, in fact, this alliance may be a challenge to his or her authority and may not seem so benign. In this case, as in the others with similar situations, the caregiving alliance may be less important in its practical effects than in the mutual support. For both family caregivers and home care workers who are faced with problematic caregiving conditions, support from someone who shares in and therefore understands the situation may help them to continue providing care despite the difficulties. In this sense, a family-worker caregiving alliance facilitates care.

Conflict Over Care

At the other extreme, family-worker interactions sometimes complicate caregiving. In our sample there were several examples of difficulties in family-worker relationships.[4]

From the perspective of family caregivers, the tasks completed by paid home care workers may directly or indirectly affect them. Work by paid workers can relieve them of some care duties; especially for family members in the same household, cooking and cleaning by home care workers may be as much for their benefit as for the client. In several cases there was some conflict between the workers and the wives or live-in daughters of clients over the quantity and/or quality of housework done by the home care workers (see Chichin, 1991). One elderly client, who lives with her daughter, taught her worker how to play certain card games; they also watch soap operas together during the worker's scheduled visit. In this case, the daughter wishes that the worker would help out more with housecleaning (i.e., in the daughter's home). This case illustrates the ambiguity of home care workers' responsibilities. What are the parameters of this job? Is socializing an "extra"—or can it be a central purpose for the paid visit? Who is the "client"—the person who needs care, the family caregiver, or both? The social versus medical parameters are not always clear in actuality, even when the care is provided under restrictive Medicare guidelines (see Mundinger, 1983).

Family caregivers also have an emotional stake in the well-being of the client and, therefore, a concern about how well the client is being treated. In one case a sister called the home care agency to complain about workers. In another case the mother of the client, who was a 36-year-old woman with multiple sclerosis, disliked her daughter's personal care attendant, whom she described as a "manipulator," but she also was concerned that personal care attendants are hard to find and she did not want to "rock the boat."

From the perspective of home care workers, there are a number of risks in interacting with family members. It was common in our sample for home care workers to complain that the family members of their clients were negligent in one way or another. They did not help enough ("It wouldn't hurt if they would come over and relieve me so I could have a day off"). Or they did not offer much social or emotional support ("They aren't there as much as I thought they would be to take her out"; "It would be nice to have them around for the holidays"). Some of the workers commented that families interfere with care or challenge their authority. One worker quipped: "Families are the hard thing to work with. One usually takes care of the whole thing and the others tell you what to do." In a few cases workers resented the fact that children in the household created extra work for them and suggested that the children ought to do more chores for the household. Another worker noted that she does not know the family well, but:

> her granddaughter will walk around me when I am sitting on the floor taking care of Judith's feet. It is much nicer when they are gone. Sometimes they argue with her when I am there. I don't like that. There is no reason why they couldn't do the personal care for her, although I enjoy doing it. When I am there, it seems like they are sitting watching over me, hovering. They could be doing something else.

This case illustrates the interweaving issues of responsibility and authority. This worker simultaneously complains that the family is inadequate in their role (they argue with her client, and they do not fulfill all their family duties, such as personal care) and that the family members are diminishing her authority ("watching over me, hovering") and, therefore, implicitly impugning her competence (see also Chichin, 1991; Surpin & Grumm, 1990).

SEPARATE WORLDS

In assessing patterns of interactions between family caregivers and home care workers, we find that neither caregiving alliances nor conflicts are common in our sample. Rather, *the most frequent type of relationship entails no interaction* at all. In more than half of our sample, home care workers have virtually no contact with their clients' relatives. In the rest of the sample, even when workers and family members have contact, the relationship often is perfunctory—that is, the relative and worker occasionally say "hello" or sometimes have a brief conversation if they happen to be in the household at the same time. Sometimes even family members who live in the same households are at work when the home health aides come and therefore have little or no contact with the aides. In effect, family caregivers and paid home care workers often operate in separate worlds or parallel domains. Even when both provide care, they do not necessarily operate as a "team," and, in most situations, they neither coordinate nor clash over their respective services.

Given our previous work on managerial roles for family caregivers, we were surprised to find so little direct involvement between family and workers. We had anticipated that many, perhaps most, home care clients would have family members whose managerial responsibilities would include arranging for home care. In fact, only about a quarter of the home care clients in our sample had family members who played a major role in deciding on and arranging for home care. It should be noted, however, that we are viewing these clients and their families at only one point in time. It is possible that family members may have been involved in home care decisions or supervision at other times—and with other paid home care workers. Moreover, only a few of the clients in our sample had any mental impairments. It is likely that family involvement is much more necessary in care at home for cognitively impaired persons.

Several factors appear to account for the separation between family and paid home care workers in our study. One factor is the absence of close relatives because of geographical and/or emotional distance. Those clients who lack family caregivers also do not have relatives who can serve as supervisors of their paid caregivers. Many relatives of the home care clients in our sample are not available as caregivers because they live far away. When relatives who live in other towns or cities serve as caregivers, the distance is *the* major hurdle. One daughter-in-law, for example, lives in the Twin Cities but helps her frail 82-year-old mother-in-law in a small town in southern Minnesota. She says: "We put 200 miles on our car every week just from going to ____ [town], and in an emergency, we're helpless." It is not very surprising that this daughter-in-law does not know her mother-in-law's home health aide.

A second factor is the involvement of various "formal" social service organizations and home health agencies in case management. For some clients, their home care arrangements were made, or at least initiated, by hospital social workers. The social workers contacted the home care agencies directly, and arrangements were made, with the agreement of the client, with little need for family intervention.

Finally, many clients, especially working-age disabled adults, manage their own care. When clients serve as their own case managers, the implication is that paid workers, family caregivers, and other helpers are all parallel components of a care network, which is overseen and managed by the clients themselves. Thus the "formal" and "informal" components of this network are resources that clients can utilize to meet their own needs.

The lack of contact between paid and unpaid caregivers suggests that formal and informal services each comprise a separate source of care, which can be mixed and matched. An individual with care needs can select a package of care—a mix of formal and informal care, to match his or her needs and circumstances—assuming that resources are available. A consumer orientation to home care is expressed most explicitly by working-age clients, who tend to see themselves as their own care managers. The younger clients in our sample were less likely to receive help from relatives and were more likely to say that they—and not someone else—made all the decisions about and arrangements for their home care. They also were more likely to train and supervise their home care workers (which is, in part, because they are more likely to hire workers directly, rather than through home care agencies).

To the extent that paid workers and family helpers are part of separate or parallel service systems the relationships *between* family and worker may *not* necessarily be important. What may be more significant is *access* to both paid and unpaid service providers. Both paid caregiving and family caregiving are resources. People with care needs but without monetary resources (or without access to public stipends) can obtain caregiving if they have family members who are willing to care for them without monetary compensation. Conversely, people who need care but who lack family caregivers can purchase care at home if they can afford the cost of paid care. To the extent that both family caregiving and paid care resources are limited or unavailable, an individual may have to do without needed care.

THE SYMBOLIC INTEGRATION OF HOME CARE WORKERS IN FAMILY LIFE

Even if home care workers rarely see or interact with their clients' relatives, the home setting and the nature of the work mean that there is often a symbolic integration of workers into the family lives of their clients. Paid caregivers are brought into family life, in part, through family talk. Most home care workers who provide personal care engage in conversations about their clients' families. Much of this talk may be superficial. Nonetheless, about three quarters of the clients in our sample say they discuss personal problems with their workers, and it is likely that much of this "confiding" involves discussion of family matters. A number of workers in our sample had virtually no contact with their clients' family members but knew a great deal about these families and had formed opinions about their behaviors, both positive and negative.

Another form of symbolic integration occurs when clients or workers view each other in quasi-family terms. Some clients and workers used family roles metaphorically in their home care relationships. One worker, in her late 20s, said some of her clients are like "grandparents" to her. Several workers noted that they were the age of their clients' adult children and sometimes seemed to be viewed in that role (see Chichin, 1991). In our sample, about a fifth of the clients said that, at least to some degree, they consider their workers "like family." Viewing home care workers as "like family" de-emphasizes the contractual framework for the relationship and implies a more enduring commitment. Saying that a worker is "like family" is a measure of affection and attachment between client and worker. This definition of the relationship, however, does not necessarily create any direct ties between the worker and other members of the client's family.

There is, finally, one other symbolic, family role for home care workers: as an advisor or intercessor in the client's family life. The advisor/intercessor role entails the worker's offering commentary on specific family actions, advice to the client about how to respond to his or her family, and/or intervention with family members. Because they do their work in the home and have frequent and close contact with their clients, home care workers sometimes become witnesses to family behavior. When they begin to talk about this behavior and offer their own perspectives, their role shifts from observation to involvement.

The advisor/intercessor role usually involves indirect relationships with the clients' families—that is, advice is given to the client about his or her family. One worker, for example, said her client was upset about the client's daughter's "fixing up her [the client's] house. I tried to comfort her about that." Another worker said: "We argued about Elaine's [client's] aunt. Elaine thought her aunt wasn't doing enough for her and could be more helpful. I tried to get her to see her aunt's point of view."

Occasionally, home care workers directly try to intercede in family behavior. A worker whose client has young children talked about her difficulties in defining her role vis-à-vis the children and commented:

> It is obvious that Virginia has lost a lot of control with her kids because of her MS. I try not to tell her kids what to do but I give them an example to go by. One time when Steve's room was a disaster, I told him at my house if my girls can't pick up, I bag everything until they learn. . . . so Steve and I went in and cleaned up his room together.

We noted above that it appears to be common for workers to view family members as neglecting their clients. In fact, more than a quarter of the workers in our sample made statements to that effect. Some of these workers also commented that they understood that "everyone is busy" or "they have their own problems."

One worker decided to do something about the lack of family involvement. She wrote a newsletter that she sent to all of the 10 children of one of her elderly clients. And she told a number of these children, personally, "loud and clear" that they were "not involved enough." Even so, at her interview she said that "Yesterday was Albert's birthday, and there was not one card from any of his children!"

One rather unusual case illustrates the awkwardness of the family intercessor role. In this case an aide, a young woman from a home health agency, was appalled by what she saw in the household. The client was an 83-year-old comatose woman who was being kept alive with tubes down her throat and who was cared for by her husband. The worker noted that the husband was almost always alone, except for three visits a week by home care workers. Early in their relationship, she suggested to the client's husband that he should "let her [the client] go." The husband, who was dependent on the paid workers and who developed a personal relationship with this aide, as well as with others (he called them at home and gave them food and flowers from his garden), was offended by her comment. He said she had no business saying that to him, and he "almost could not forgive" her for telling him to let his wife die. What happened, in effect, was that the spouse caregiver defined the paid worker as an outsider and as overstepping family boundaries.

INTERLOCKING ROLES

Although we have described family caregivers and paid home care workers as parallel service providers, what we find illustrated in a number of our cases is an *interlocking* of family caregiver and paid worker roles. These interlocking roles do not necessarily require much, if any, face-to-face contact. Rather, the family and worker roles interlock in the sense that *each provides what the other does not.*

The situation of Mrs. Malibund provides an illustration of how the roles of family caregiver and paid worker are interrelated, despite the fact that the worker and the family member have never met and have not directly coordinated their services. Mrs. Malibund is 77 and suffers from congestive heart failure. She lives in the home of her adult daughter in a working-class neighborhood. She has no energy, cannot make her own meals, cannot clean, and has difficulty remembering to take her medications. Her daughter, who works during the day, leaves food in the refrigerator and medications by her mother's bed. Her home health aide arrives several hours after the daughter has left for work, does some light housework, heats up the lunch left by the daughter, administers the medications on the nightstand, and also provides some companionship to Mrs. Malibund, who otherwise would be alone all day. This arrangement was set up by a hospital social worker as part of the discharge plan when Mrs. Malibund was hospitalized for her heart problem. A nurse from the home care agency made one visit and set up the care plan, which essentially is being implemented jointly by the worker and the daughter—who have never met or even talked on the telephone! Their activities are interlocked specifically in that the aide completes procedures begun by the daughter (lunch and administering medications). The arrangement ensures that the client's needs are covered, with the paid worker providing a set of services during the daytime and the daughter available during the evening and night hours.

In these interlocking roles the responsibilities of family caregivers and paid workers differ in a significant sense: With few exceptions, the worker role is circumscribed by time, tasks, and arrangement for compensation; the family caregiving role generally has no such framework. Although we noted earlier in this chapter that home care work often is diffuse, nonetheless workers usually are hired for a set number of hours, and their domain includes a finite number of tasks. Although it is true that most workers do some "extra" tasks, a number of clients implied that requests for extra services should be modest and/or that workers should be compensated for extra time spent. In contrast, with family caregivers, though there are certainly limits on what services can be expected, the boundaries around responsibilities tend to be substantially more diffuse and there is really no way to define or compensate for "extra" work, when the caregiving has no monetary and no time framework.

In our sample there appeared to be a few exceptions to this distinction between family care and paid care; that is, there were cases in which paid caregivers had diffuse responsibilities while family members had little direct involvement in providing care. The case of the woman whose paid caregiver had been appointed as her guardian *ad litem* was described above. In addition, there were a few disabled clients who hired live-in personal care attendants (PCAs). Work hours and responsibilities are far more diffuse for live-in PCAs than for home health aides who are hired for two- or three-hour shifts. In fact, there were several examples of conflict in relationships between clients and live-in PCAs, in which the diffuseness of responsibilities was the underlying problem. Nonetheless, virtually all PCAs have some time off, whereas family caregivers do not necessarily have any break in their "on-call" duties.

The effect is that family caregiving is woven around access to paid care. This is illustrated in a number of our cases. Family caregivers provide meals on weekends when "Meals-on-Wheels" are unavailable; they fill in when paid workers cannot come; and they shop, clean, provide personal care, and so on—whatever paid workers do *not* provide. Furthermore, family caregivers, even when paid care is used, tend to retain an on-call role—that is, they are available when or if needed (for example, if a worker does not show up).

SUMMARY AND IMPLICATIONS

Our study has examined the interrelationships of formal and informal care in microcosm. We have observed how family caregivers and paid home care workers are part of care systems that are both parallel (or separate) and also linked together. These "informal" and "formal" care systems seem to represent separate systems of care in that there is often little or no contact between families and workers. We were surprised to find that the families in our sample had limited involvement in case management and in arrangements for home care. On the other hand, our study also revealed linkages, both symbolic and practical, between family care and paid home care. Given the home setting, home care workers become part of their clients' family worlds. Moreover, for those clients with involved families, the responsibilities of family caregivers and paid home care workers are overlapping and interlocking, even when there are no explicit or direct efforts at coordinating services.

Our case data have provided ample illustrations of the differences in structure between family care and paid home care, as described by Litwak and colleagues (see Chapter 4)—most specifically, that families offer long-term commitment; paid workers do not. Even so, we would argue that family care and paid home care by paraprofessional workers are more similar than different, and both are problematic. The needs for care are defined idiosyncratically, so the care must be individually tailored. The tasks have no clear boundaries or limits. The responsibilities are diffuse and are social rather than medical; the purpose is to help the recipient of care to get on with his or her life. The rewards are, largely, intangible and personal.

Our microcosmic analysis of the interpersonal dynamics of the client-worker-caregiver triad needs to be understood within the larger context of long-term care policy—that is, *the lack of access to paid home care.*

Care at home is expensive—in time and/or money. In this country, most individuals with long-term care needs and most family caregivers cannot afford much or any paid home care. Judith Heumann, in testimony to the Senate Committee on Labor and Human Resources, asserted that access to personal assistance services is "a major civil rights issue." She described her personal anguish at having to ask for assistance that was voluntary because she had no resources for paid care. She also asserted that she has been denied jobs because potential employers fear that she might need personal assistance. She stated:

> I was raised to live the American dream of equal opportunity. I always thought that meant getting a well-paying job, getting married, owning a nice house and car, and going on vacations. But how can I reach that dream of equal opportunity without the assistance I need? . . . I am not unique. Millions of people with disabilities require some sort of personal assistance. Most exhaust personal and family resources, both financial and emotional. Some are forced into dehumanizing institutions at great expense to the taxpayer. (Heumann, 1991)

Horowitz (1985) cautions that "those who advocate additional service supports for older people and their families are pitted against those who would like to increase family care in order to reduce public expenditures" (p. 200). In a recently published longitudinal study of care networks for the elderly, Stoller and Pugliesi (1991, p. 188) report that networks do *not* tend to expand when persons become more disabled and in need of care. The implication is that a small number of caregivers provide more services as needs increase. The authors conclude that the burdens on informal care providers increase as the older person's health diminishes and that formal services are an essential supplement to the care provided by networks when the networks' capacity is exceeded.

As noted in the introduction, there has been limited research on the linkages between formal and informal care. Clearly, more research is needed on the complementary and overlapping roles of paid care and family care and the implications for quality and cost. Of particular interest would be studies on the relationships between paid and family caregivers for persons with cognitive impairments. The finding in this sample, that paid home care workers often seem to have minimal interaction with the families of their clients, may suggest that the clienteles for paid home care and for family care are somehow different—that is, that family caregivers and paid home care workers tend to serve persons with differing medical, economic, or social needs. Various studies have shown that older persons with family caregivers tend not to use formal services. It is not clear, however, why this is so. It is possible that, in the United States, with our limited paid home care and our assumptions about family responsibilities, persons with family resources are subtly and systematically discouraged from entering the formal care system.

The sample in this study is *not* representative of people with long-term care needs, in part because it is comprised exclusively of people who *do* receive paid home care (at least twice a week). But even in our sample we find that care recipients tend to be underserviced. Clients often "make do"—that is, they manage in their daily lives while having important needs unmet (such as regular toileting, bathing, and getting outdoors). One implication of the lack of public funding for paid home care is that people with care needs do not receive much care.

Lack of access to paid home care also has implications for family caregivers. Our analysis of the interlocking roles of family and paid workers suggests that family caregiving is organized around paid care and is defined in relation to the availability of other services. A major policy concern has been to encourage and increase family care in order to place limits on public expenditures for long-term care. But how much should families be "squeezed"? Even when family caregivers benefit from some home care, as our study shows, paid care is almost always a very expensive and a very limited commodity. It seems clear that family caregivers also are underserviced.

NOTES

1. A distinction ought to be made, however, between commitment to the person and commitment to the tasks of caregiving. A close relative (spouse, daughter, son, etc.) may always care (have an emotional attachment) but may not always be a caregiver. Even spouses may give up the caregiver role if the work becomes too burdensome, physically or emotionally.

2. In a previous paper (Fischer et al., 1990) we described caregiving for familyless elderly by non-kin (neighbors and friends) as "care without commitment." Informal non-kin caregivers and paid home care workers are similar in that neither has a long-term obligation to provide care.

3. We are referring to paraprofessional workers: home health aides and personal care attendants. There are other "formal" providers of home care—physicians, nurses, pharmacists, and so on—for whom the home care tasks are much more clearly circumscribed.

4. The sample may have a "positive bias"—that is, there is likely to be an underestimate of problems in home care relationships, for two reasons. First, the home care agency directors, who selected the clients for the study, may have been reluctant to reveal problem

cases. Second, the sample includes only long-term home care clients; it is possible that there are more difficulties in short-term arrangements, and/or that clients with long-term needs do not continue using home care if they have too many difficulties.

REFERENCES

Archbold, P. G. (1990). The impact of caring for an ill elderly parent on the middle-aged off-spring. *Journal of Gerontological Nursing, 6,* 78-85.

Callahan, J. J. (1989). Play it again, Sam: There is no impact. *The Gerontologist, 29,* 5-6.

Cantor, M., & Little, V. (1985). Aging and social care. In R. H. Binstock & E. Shanas (Eds.), *Handbook of aging and the social sciences* (2nd ed., pp. 745-782). New York: Van Nostrand Reinhold.

Chichin, E. R. (1991). The treatment of paraprofessional workers in the home. *Pride Institute Journal of Long-term Home Health Care, 10*(1, Winter), 26-27.

Christianson, J. (1988). The evaluation of the national long term care demonstration: The effect of channeling on informal caregiving. *HSR: Health Services Research, 23*(1), 99-117.

Daatland, S. O. (1983). Use of public services for the aged and the role of the family. *The Gerontologist, 23,* 650-656.

Eustis, N. N., & Fischer, L. R. (1991). Relationships between home care workers and their clients: Implications for quality of care. *The Gerontologist, 31,* 447-456.

Fischer, L. R. (1986). *Linked lives: Adult daughters and their mothers.* New York: Harper & Row.

Fischer, L. R., & Eustis, N. N. (1988a). DRGs and family care for the elderly: A case study. *The Gerontologist, 28,* 383-389.

Fischer, L. R., & Eustis, N. N. (1988b). *Relationships between home care workers and their clients: A report for the Blandin Foundation.* St. Paul, MN: Blandin Foundation Fellowship Program.

Fischer, L. R., & Eustis, N. N. (1990). Quicker and sicker: How changes in Medicare affect the elderly and their families. *Journal of Geriatric Psychiatry, 22*(2), 163-191.

Fischer, L. R., Rogne, L., & Eustis, N. N. (1990). Support systems for the familyless elderly: Care without commitment. In J. Gubrium & A. Sankar (Eds.), *The home care experience* (pp. 129-144). Newbury Park, CA: Sage.

Heumann, J. (1991, July 25). Presentation before the Senate Committee on Labor and Human Resources.

Horowitz, A. (1985). Family caregiving to the frail elderly. *Annual Review of Gerontology and Geriatrics, 5,* 194-246.

Kemper, P. (1988). The evaluation of the national long term care demonstration. *HSR: Health Services Research, 23*(1), 161-173.

Litwak, E. (1985). Complementary roles for formal and informal support groups: A study of nursing homes and mortality rates. *The Journal of Applied Behavioral Science, 21*(4), 407-425.

Litwak, E., & Szelenyi, I. (1969). Primary group structures and their functions: Kin, neighbors and friends. *American Sociological Review, 34,* 465-481.

McAuley, W. J., & Arling, G. (1984). Use of in-home care by very old people. *Journal of Health and Social Behavior, 23,* 54-64.

McAuley, W. J., & Blieszner, R. (1985). Selection of long-term care arrangements by older community residents. *The Gerontologist, 25,* 188-193.

Montgomery, J. E. (1982). The economics of supportive services for families with disabled and aging members. *Family Relations, 31*(1), 19-28.

Mundinger, M. O. (1983). *Home care controversy: Too little, too late, too costly.* London: Aspen Publications.

Newhouse, J., & McAuley, W. J. (1987). Use of informal in-home care by rural elders. *Family Relations, 36*(4), 456-460.

Newman, S. J., & Stuyk, R., with Wright, P., & Rice, M. (1990). Overwhelming odds: Caregiving and the risk of institutionalization. *Journal of Gerontology, 45*(5), S173-S183.

Simon-Rusinowitz, L., & Hofland, B. (1989, October). *The impact of varying perspectives on client autonomy in long term care: Home care for the elderly vs. attendant services for the disabled.* Paper presented at the Annual Meetings of the Gerontological Society of America, Minneapolis, MN.

Stoller, E. P., & Pugliesi, K. L. (1991). Size and effectiveness of informal helping networks: A panel study of older people in the community. *Journal of Health and Social Behavior, 32,* 180-191.

Stone, R., Cafferata, G. L., & Sangl, J. (1987). Caregivers of the frail elderly: A national profile. *The Gerontologist, 27,* 616-626.

Surpin, R., & Grumm, F. (1990, April). Building the home care triangle: Clients and families, paraprofessionals and agencies. *Caring,* pp. 6-15.

Sussman, M. B. (1985). The family life of old people. In R. H. Binstock & E. Shanas (Eds.), *Handbook of aging and the social sciences* (2nd ed., pp. 415-449). New York: Van Nostrand Reinhold.

12

The Caregiver as
the Hidden Patient

Challenges for Medical Practice

JACK H. MEDALIE

Medical practitioners have long been trained to do everything possible for their patients (part of the Hippocratic oath taken upon graduation from medical school) and usually regard the people around the patient—family and friends—as allies in the management of the identified patient. In some cases, however, these "helping" people become unwilling participants or even antagonists in respect to the care.

Whether family and friends become allies or unwilling participants, family practitioners who take care of other family members often witness symptoms, illnesses, and even fatal diseases developing in the caregiver and/or other members of the patient's intimate group (Dody, 1986; Hasselkus, 1988; Rabins, Mace, & Lucas, 1982). These conditions usually are associated with, or are the result of, increased stress due to altered roles, relationships, and functions brought about by the presence of a serious and long-term illness in a close family member.

The objectives of this chapter are threefold. The first is to illustrate how the effect of caring for patients with serious diseases, who are in different stages of their life cycle, can sometimes lead to illness in the caregiver or in the whole family constellation. The caregivers or families in these situations need to be regarded as "hidden patients" who covertly or overtly can develop serious illnesses. The second objective is to discuss the models of care used in family practice and how the caregivers fit into a suggested comprehensive model. Finally, guidelines are developed regarding the management or intervention techniques clinicians can use in the challenging situation of dealing with a seriously ill patient, the caregiver, and the intimate primary group.

My first experience of the hidden patient phenomenon occurred when I was a young physician practicing in a rural area. A middle-aged couple with no children, Mr. and Mrs. N. Y., had moved into one of the villages under my care four weeks after he had suffered a myocardial infarction. His convalescence at home was extremely difficult due to his inconsiderate demands and refusal to leave his bed, except to go to the bathroom. His wife attended to his every need day and night and although her neighbors helped with some household chores, she had no real support system in their new neighborhood. This went on for several months and although I visited their home approximately twice a week, I, as I had been trained, concentrated on the patient and did not pay special attention to his wife. Finally, the burden of his care and their disturbed relationship became too much for her, and she committed suicide. Adding to my shock, her husband, whom I had been unable to motivate to leave his bed, not only got up, but within two weeks of her funeral was working a full day in the fields on a nearby farm!

In many ways this was an eye-opening experience for me as a young physician. It not only made me doubt my own ability but also made me question whether the well-trained biomedical clinician that my medical school and residency training had produced was adequate for the tasks of primary care medicine. The answer was obviously no. It also raised the question: Who was the patient and what was the physician's responsibility in regard to the patient's helpers?

During the ensuing years my additional experiences, as well as those of my colleagues, made me realize that our biomedical training had to be extended in a number of different directions. The first and major lesson to be learned was the concept that I called the *hidden patient* (Medalie, 1975), a term also used a few years later by Fengler and Goodrich (1979). In most cases the caregiver of a seriously ill, long-term patient adjusts to both the pleasant and unpleasant periods and manages to cope with the extra burdens. If, however, this caregiver's self-sufficiency and/or social support is inadequate, she or he may overtly or covertly develop some pathology, and thus the hidden patient becomes a real patient. At times the whole family system adjusts dysfunctionally and produces a scapegoat, or some other pathology, in which case the whole family can be regarded as the hidden patient. The pathology that the hidden patient develops often occurs during the course of the patient's illness, but sometimes only develops or becomes apparent after the death of the identified patient.

The previous clinical vignette of the caregiver's suicide illustrates the hidden patient effect when the patient is an adult. This effect also can be seen at every stage of the individual or family life cycle. Families in the early stages of the life cycle are involved in caregiving as part of their normal development. Every mother is a caregiver to her children and similarly her coping ability will depend on her children's health and behavior, her own health and self-sufficiency, and the support she receives from her husband (or companion) and others, of whom the physician can play a key role (Wasserman, Inui, & Barriatua, 1984).

The mood alterations and other stress-related symptoms seen in mothers and sometimes fathers may be accentuated and aggravated when a child has a serious congenital condition (Down's syndrome, severe spina bifida, Fallots' tetralogy, cystic fibrosis) or an acquired one such as acute leukemia. All these childhood conditions increase the family's financial problems, decrease their social participation, and often lead to marital and family distress. The hidden patient is the family system, which might choose or identify any member as the patient brought to the physician. It might be the overly protective mother who keeps going despite a helpless and hopeless feeling and an underlying depression; the frustrated father with muscular and joint pains or headaches; or one of the other children who has been neglected and develops symptoms such as eneuresis, abdominal pains, or unusual behavior. Sometimes dysfunction becomes chronic and irreversible and leads to separation and divorce. Most families, however, seem to obtain sufficient support so that the child's chronic illness brings them together in a more meaningful bonding relationship. A feature of these adjusted families is the increased sensitivity and understanding of other people's disabilities displayed by the normal siblings when they reach adulthood.

FAMILY VIGNETTES

Family M. P. T.

The following vignette shows a young couple dealing with their congenitally retarded child. Despite an improved and good relationship between them, their own health deteriorated.

A young married couple gave birth to their first child after an uneventful pregnancy. The birth was a normal vaginal delivery but the infant soon exhibited evidence of multiple abnormalities, the main one being Down's syndrome, which was confirmed by chromosomal analysis. In addition to the usual mental retardation and external physical signs, the infant also had esophageal atresia, which led to difficulty in swallowing. This was surgically repaired, but the infant continued to be in poor health until further cardiological investigations revealed a septal defect between the two sides of the heart. Despite the parents' feelings that the child should be left alone, they consented to the open heart operation after very strong pressure from the surgeons and hospital. The operation was successful and the child was partially able to function but needed full-time attention.

After trying for nearly 18 months to care for the infant at home, the parents had her admitted to a very good home for retarded children. It was expensive but with both parents working they managed to support themselves and their institutionalized child. During the course of the next five years (the child had at least one serious complication each year but survived them all), both parents developed serious illnesses. The mother developed signs of irritable bowel syndrome, which necessitated hospitalization on two occasions, and the father developed a bleeding duodenal ulcer. Because they decided not to have any more children, the father had a vasectomy.

The hidden patient is often the main caregiver (Mrs. N. Y.), but families usually respond like a system (Family M. P. T.) in that every individual in the system and the system as a whole are affected by any serious condition that descends upon one member. Thus every member of the family is affected in some way, but usually not as badly as the main caregiver, who bears the brunt of the stressful situation. This is further complicated in dysfunctional families, in which sometimes, with or without serious illness of the caregiver, the family develops pathology of its own, as shown in the following vignette.

Y. M.'s Family

Y. M., a 12-year-old boy, was referred by a school counselor to a psychiatrist due to aggressive behavior in school. He was the youngest of five siblings (see Figure 12.1), with three much older brothers and a sister 3 years his senior.

A number of individual and family sessions brought this story to light. Twelve years earlier, his father, Mr. R. M. (an overweight salesman), was

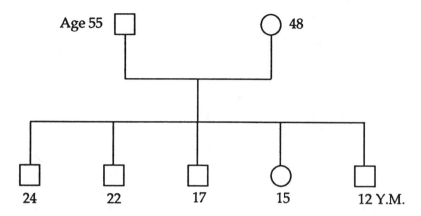

Figure 12.1. Y. M.'s Family Tree

admitted to a hospital for a transient cerebral ischemic attack with a blood pressure of 250/130. He responded well to treatment and has been under close medical supervision since, with his blood pressure under reasonable control. At the time of hospital discharge he and his wife were warned by the attending physician that he should not overexert himself physically or become too upset because either of these things could cause his blood pressure to rise and he would be a candidate for a stroke. As both Mr. and Mrs. R. M. had had members of their family die from strokes, they took this warning very seriously. Mr. R. M., who previously had played football and baseball with his children, stopped all physical activities and withdrew from all family arguments or conflicts. Mrs. R. M., the mother of five children, found herself the caregiver of her husband ("my sixth child"), who became very dependent on her. She tried to take over the roles of both father and mother but found it very difficult, especially when the three eldest boys quarreled with each other or teased and sometimes hit the two youngest children. She also tried to stop the children's fighting and noise by warning them of the effect it had on their father. Both Mr. and Mrs. R. M. learned that when the children got out of hand, the father's complaint of a headache brought peace very quickly.

This stifling atmosphere went on for years with a negative effect on everyone, especially the two younger adolescent children. The frustrations of the older boys and even the mother were taken out on the youngest boy, who was picked on, blamed, and frequently punished for many incidents in the home. The result of this scapegoating of Y. M. led to a great deal of negative behavior at home, while at school he became very aggressive to his peers and very disturbing to his teachers.

During the course of family therapy a more realistic approach was taken to Mr. R. M.'s hypertension. After his eldest sons told him they "had no father," he gradually took back some of his previous roles and became a participant in their family life again. This took a great burden off his wife (the caregiver) and allowed the sibling relationships to become more normal. All this had a very positive effect on Y. M. at home and school.

The R. M. family exemplifies what can happen when a key family member suddenly becomes dependent and the main caregiver cannot adequately cope with his or her new roles. The atmosphere created by this upsets the functioning of the whole family system. One of the ways this system reacts is to create a scapegoat, who suffers greatly but who in a sense allows the rest of the family to more or less keep functioning. The family sessions allowed each member to speak freely and it was apparent how much each had been affected. An interesting feature to mention is that Y. M.'s aggressive behavior was in a way a healthier sign than if he had reacted by becoming quiet and even depressed. The mother, who previously was barely coping with the tasks of bringing up five children *with* the help of her husband, found herself inadequate to cope with her dependent husband, the new fathering role she was expected to fulfill, plus the mothering of her five children (Mattlin, Wethington, & Kessler, 1990). Something had to break but instead of an explosion, such as divorce or serious illness of the mother, the family unconsciously found the scapegoat phenomenon to be their solution (Vogel & Bell, 1968).

Family S.

As most studies of caregivers have been done on families in which an old person is the patient, here is a vignette illustrating an old person being looked after by an adult couple whose cultural values and beliefs kept them from fully utilizing available community resources, despite the severe stress they endured.

This Afro-American family consisted of the mother, age 78 (Mrs. G. S.), her only son, and his wife. The mother's husband died from a stroke 10 years previously, 6 months after their other son, age 45, died suddenly. The mother, who lived alone in an apartment, had shown signs of memory deterioration over the years and had developed a paranoid fear that people were stealing her money and other valuable items. This, plus her evening wanderings, caused the neighbors to complain, so her son made her move in with him and his wife (Mr. and Mrs. S. S.). He had a full-time job as a mechanic and was somewhat overweight but otherwise enjoyed good health. His wife, a charming woman, had insulin-dependent diabetes mellitus that was under good control. Despite the wife having been pregnant twice, they had no live children. She sometimes did part-time clerical work, but her main occupation centered around church activities.

From the time Mrs. G. S. came to live with her son, the burden of her care fell on his wife, her daughter-in-law. She accepted this role intellectually and spiritually, but gradually the burden of the 24-hour watchfulness began to take its toll. Particularly upsetting were Mrs. G. S.'s evening wanderings and her insistence on preparing her own meals to prevent others from poisoning her. The latter always involved the possibility of a fire in the kitchen. Despite available assistance from neighbors and the church congregation, the care of Mrs. G. S., who had Alzheimer's dementia, began to take its toll on her daughter-in-law, who insisted on doing the bulk of the care herself. The younger woman's diabetes periodically went out of control and on two occasions this necessitated brief hospitalization. These incidents usually were preceded by signs of depression.

Mr. S. S. found himself in the difficult position of peace-keeper between his mother and his wife. His coping mechanisms included increasing his alcohol intake, and gradually his blood pressure rose to hypertensive levels. Despite family conferences with their family physician and a social worker that led to short periods of respite care (accepted reluctantly), the couple continued to care for Mrs. G. S. at home for nearly four years. They would not accept the solution of a nursing home because it ran counter to their cultural and religious beliefs, and they could not afford sustained help in their home. The turning point came when Mrs. G. S. fractured her hip and during her hospitalization completely lost control of her urinary and bowel systems. At that stage the couple allowed the social worker to place the mother in a nursing home, where Mrs. G. S. died within a few weeks. The couple felt very guilty about Mrs. G. S.'s death and only after numerous contacts and counseling with their physician did the daughter-in-law's diabetes and the son's hypertension gradually stabilize, and his drinking binges decreased and then ceased.

In this vignette of an Alzheimer's patient, there was gradual deterioration of health of the middle-aged caregivers. The main caregiver, the daughter-in-law, had insulin-dependent diabetes and her husband had a tendency to drink too much before they accepted the caregiving burden. This new role caused the previous health problems of these hidden patients to become aggravated and in addition, new conditions developed: depression in the wife and hypertension in the husband. In this family, emotional and material support were available and forthcoming from their church, friends, neighbors, and medical care personnel. Despite all this, however, the 24-hour on-duty burden was not sufficiently eased.

The health effects on the caregivers of Mrs. G. S. occurred during the caregiving period. In some cases, however, the major effects occur after the death of the patient, as the next vignette illustrates.

Mrs. E. B.

Mrs. E. B. was a 46-year-old white married woman with three children. Her husband was an executive of a chain of department stores and was noted for his efficiency and management skills. Despite annual health examinations, she presented with carcinoma of the ovary with metastases in many parts of her abdominal cavity. She underwent surgery followed by chemotherapy, with alleviation of all signs and symptoms, for 18 months. She then had a recurrence and despite additional chemotherapy, succumbed to her disease a little more than a year later.

Her husband, with the assistance of their children, a cleaning woman, and friends, took responsibility for the care of the patient, household duties, and the children's needs, as well as continuing with his business activities. Whenever he was asked how things were going, he always replied, "We're managing alright, if only E. would be healthy." During the period of her illness Mrs. E. B. always kept up a happy exterior and was very supportive of her husband's efforts even though she told her physician that she was worried about her husband because he was working too hard. Her husband never complained of his own health, but approximately three weeks after her death he vomited a great deal of blood and was hospitalized and treated for a severe bleeding duodenal ulcer.

Interestingly, the husband had been treated for ulcer symptoms 25 years earlier, but had had no recurrence of symptoms until after his wife's death. Another interesting feature of this family was the source of support for the caregiver. We usually look at the people surrounding the patient and the caregiver for the necessary social support. In this instance, the major support for the caregiver was the patient herself, despite her terminal illness. The fact that the patient, despite severe illness, can be and often is the main support of the family is something practitioners tend to overlook. When this scenario occurs, the death of the patient removes the main support from the caregiver, often with serious consequences.

RISK FACTORS IN CAREGIVING

The increased death rate of spouses during the first or second year following the death of the first spouse has been documented in numerous studies since Rees and Lutkins reported their initial observations from their general practice in Wales (Rees & Lutkins, 1967). Males are generally more susceptible to this phenomenon than females, especially those elderly males who do not remarry (Osterweis, Solomon, & Green, 1984a). The factors related to this bereavement mortality are believed to include:

1. Shared risk factors. There is a high degree of spouse concordance for hypertension, hypercholesterolemia, obesity, smoking, and so on due to the phenomenon of associative mating (likes marry likes) and of couples gradually adopting similar lifestyle habits (Sackett, Anderson, Milner, Feinleib, & Kannel, 1975).
2. Shared exposure to environmental hazards.
3. Loss of social support system brought about by bereavement.
4. Effects of bereavement on the body's immune system. The stress of bereavement renders the surviving spouse more susceptible to illness, including behavior such as substance abuse, and illnesses including infections and cancer (Kiecolt-Glaser, Dura, Speicher, Trask, & Glaser, 1991; Osterweis, Solomon, & Green, 1984b).

It is not uncommon to see the surviving spouse die from the same disease, such as coronary heart disease or cerebrovascular disease. On the other hand, I have witnessed a number of surviving spouses who have died from cancer that only became clinically apparent after the death of the first spouse from a chronic condition other than cancer.

MODELS OF PRIMARY CARE

Consciously or not, clinical practice is carried out on the basis of a conceptual model(s) that has been accepted by the practitioner and integrated into his or her practice. A *model* is an integrated description of a belief system to explain natural phenomena or to visualize something that cannot be observed (Medalie, 1990). Illness is defined as the patient's complaints that bring him or her to the physician. Disease is the classification of the patient's symptoms and signs into medically accepted categories. In family practice and other primary care activities, a number of care models are used, depending on the circumstances of the patient and the illness or disease.

The models used in primary care clinical practice include the following:

1. The *biomedical model* regards disease as a derangement of underlying bodily physiochemical mechanisms. Molecular biology is the basic scientific discipline used in this model. The corollary of this is that if a condition cannot be explained on a molecular-physiochemical basis, then it should not be regarded as a disease. Some go further and question whether such a condition even should be included in the province of medicine or physicians. The remarkable advances in molecular biology have maintained the biomedical model as the dominant one in medical practice.

2. The *biopsychosocial model,* a term coined by George Engel (Engel, 1977, 1980), is "a framework for understanding the integration and interaction of the biological, psychological and social dimensions of health, disease and health care" (Doherty, Baird, & Becker, 1986). This model adds psychological and sociocultural dimensions to the basic biomedical model and serves as the foundation for the systems and epidemiological concepts of health and disease.

3. *Developmental models* are based on the work of Erikson (1950), Hill (1970), and Duvall (1977) and take into consideration the psychological developmental changes that occur over time, through sequential phases and transitions of the individual and family life cycle.

4. *Systems models* state that "all levels of organization are linked to each other in a hierarchial relationship, so that change in one affects change in the others" (Von Bertalanffy, 1952). Anything that seriously affects one unit (or individual) of a system will affect the whole system, and anything that affects the system as a whole will affect each individual

within the system. This principle has been adapted in work with families by both family therapists (Doherty & Baird, 1983) and family medicine (Christie-Seely, 1984).

5. *Epidemiological models* look beyond the individual and family to include the environment, stating that "health or disease is the result of complex interactions between the host, environment, and the agent or other stressors" (Fletcher, Fletcher, & Wagner, 1982). Epidemiological and statistical techniques have been adapted at different levels, from the individual patient all the way to community and population research (Cassel, 1974; Medalie, Kitson, & Zyzanski, 1981).

THE COMPREHENSIVE MODEL OF PATIENT-CAREGIVER-PHYSICIAN INTERACTION

The challenge for medical practitioners is multifaceted. We have to accept the fact that although our primary responsibility is to the identified patient, the patient with an acute serious illness or a chronic condition is rarely, if ever, an isolated person but rather is part of a relationship complex. The awareness of this relationship complex brings together two paradigms. The first is the circular systemic process whereby the stress of caregiving might be parlayed into a state of health or illness for the caregiver as well as the patient. The second is the "beyond-the-patient orientation" in which the traditional doctor-patient clinical relationship is extended to include the caregiver and the rest of the family within the context of their life-cycle stage and their environment. To consider the total picture of this interaction, I use an epidemiologic approach to define the areas that might need attention when practitioners try to understand or manage the situation in a comprehensive manner.

This *comprehensive model* of the patient-caregiver-physician interaction is depicted in Figure 12.2 as five overlapping circles contained within a larger one. These circles represent the patient, the caregiver, the family, the physician, and the illness interacting within the environment. This dynamic interaction is a complex process involving multiple factors. An important element of this interaction is the stage of the life cycle that each constituent has reached and how the developmental tasks have been met (Medalie & Cole-Kelly, 1992). In brief, some of the factors related to each constituent in the model are described below.

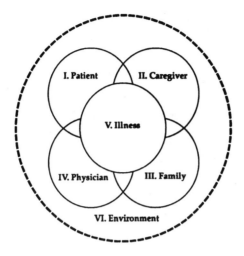

Figure 12.2. The "Patient-Caregiver-Physician" Interaction Model

The Patient

The demographic characteristics of the patient, including age, sex, marital status, and socioeconomic background, provide the important social context of interactions with formal and informal caregivers. The patient's health status, including current and past health conditions; ability to transact activities of daily living; and knowledge and understanding of health conditions represent key health-related factors. Support networks and quality of support from persons other than the designated caregiver also are considered important.

The Caregiver

Demographic characteristics of the caregiver, such as age and sex, and personal characteristics, such as education and personality, are also important factors in the model. The caregiver's relationship to the patient (spouse, daughter, friend, etc.) as well as the attitude of the caregiver toward the patient and the patient's illness must be considered. Furthermore, the effect of caregiving on the caregiver's lifestyle, health status, and the caregiver's support system are concepts that factor into the comprehensive model. Finally, adequacy and efficiency in the caregiving role and the caregiver's relationship with the physician warrant consideration.

The Family

As previously stated, the family as a unit may become a hidden patient; therefore, factors such as family structure (component of the family and members available on a daily basis or in crisis situations) and household structure (those living with the patient and caregiver) are significant to the interaction. Issues pertaining to the family functioning include previous roles of the patient and the caregiver and who has taken over or is currently helping with these roles. The family's life-cycle stage and how the present situation will affect developmental tasks of this stage are important factors in the model. Knowledge of the family's previous experience and current relationship with the physician, the family's understanding of the patient's illness, and their desire to help the caregiver round out the considerations regarding the family role in this interactive context.

The Physician

Personal characteristics of the physician—such as age and sex; stage in individual, family, and professional life cycle; and years of personal experience with the patient's illness—represent important factors relevant to the comprehensive model. The relationship between the physician and both the patient and the caregiver will shape the success of patient care. The physician's willingness to make the caregiver an integral part of the health-care team contributes to positive outcomes. It is also important to consider the physician's knowledge base regarding community referral and support services.

The Illness

The *type* of illness is a key factor because demands posed by different illnesses vary greatly. Examples of illnesses with varied demands are a mentally intact but physically disabled adult, a congenitally retarded child, or a congenitally impaired old person who is incontinent. The *stage* of illness is also important. Is it in the early, advanced, or terminal stage? Is the patient partially independent, needing intermittent help for specific purposes only, or completely dependent, needing 24-hour vigil for assistance with all bodily activities?

The Environment

Resources for basic needs, such as food, water, and heating, as well as the physical structure of the home and nature of facilities for patient and caregiver (e.g., stairs, carpets, cooking facilities, bathing, safety, etc.), are important factors in understanding patient and caregiver needs. It is also very important to be aware of the availability and accessibility of physicians 24 hours a day, emergency services, community support services, and home help. Last, the type of coverage of medical insurance is of primary concern for patient, caregiver, and family members.

The relevance of the model is that it directs the physician's attention to the multitude of factors that should be taken into consideration in situations in which a caregiver is managing a disabled individual who is either homebound or bedridden. The physician very quickly, systematically, or over the course of time, makes an assessment of the patient, the patient's illness, the caregiver, the family functioning, and the resources available in the environment, so the patient can receive the best care available. In every situation only a few factors are found to be the key ones so the physician's emphasis is specifically directed to these only.

The physician's main concern is and will be the patient, but the key to the patient's care is the caregiver (Maletta & Hepburn, 1986). Thus a primary function of the physician is to develop and maintain a good working relationship with the caregiver in order to make him or her an integral part of the health-care team. In this context it is important that the physician be aware of the common problems that may develop in the caregiver and the family. This knowledge can be used in anticipatory guidance as well as in the early diagnosis and treatment (primary and secondary prevention) of the caregiver and family.

Based on my clinical experience, particular health problems often are associated with the burden of caregiving. Caregiver symptoms include mood swings (short temper, irritable, less tolerant). This type of stress often brings forward less pleasant aspects of the caregiver's personality, especially if the caretaking task was accepted unwillingly. Other symptoms include headaches (tension or migraine are very common); fatigue; exhaustion; migratory muscular and joint pains; aggravation of previous symptoms; behavioral changes (especially in young adults or adolescent caregivers, this might be reflected in work- or school-related problems); and increase in marital and family conflicts around new roles, extra burdens, precarious finances, and lack of shared caregiving responsibilities.

Some illnesses or diseases that can develop during the first years of caregiving, or sometimes even after the stress is over (a kind of post-stress syndrome), include hypertension, low back pain, irritable bowel syndrome, migraines, myocardial infarction, duodenal ulcer, increased infections, cancer, depression, and family dysfunction, sometimes leading to separation and divorce.

GUIDELINES FOR PHYSICIANS AND OTHER HEALTH-CARE PROVIDERS

Despite the fact that each patient and caregiver differs in many respects, the above illustrates that there are enough common themes and processes to be able to devise flexible guidelines for physicians dealing with disabled patients and their caregivers. These guidelines can be divided into two interrelated areas: direct care of the patient, which indirectly helps the caregiver, and direct help to the caregiver and family.

Direct Care of Patient

1. Manage the patient efficiently and empathetically. This involves the following factors:
   - Up-to-date knowledge of the patient's medical condition
   - Knowledge of and early referral to appropriate specialists and/or other community services
   - Early diagnosis and treatment of changing conditions or complications
2. Ensure that you or your associates can be reached easily and quickly.
3. Ensure that arrangements are in place to deal with medical crises or emergencies.
4. Maximize the independence of the patient with respect to functioning, medication, and decision making.
5. Encourage both the patient and the family to make appropriate arrangements for health benefits, durable power of attorney for health care, living will, and legal and financial estate planning matters.

6. Inspect the home facilities for safety and suitability for the patient. This includes toilet facilities, hand rails, stairs, carpets, beds, chairs, wheelchairs, walkers, canes, night lights, and so on. A physical therapist would be an excellent resource for this.

7. Encourage the patient, if he or she is able, to participate in former social activities (support network) and/or encourage him or her to start new ones.

8. Despite the difficulties, periodic home visits to the patient and the caregiver in their own environment are a very positive aspect of continuing care.

Direct Help to Caregiver

1. Ensure that the caregiver is an integral part of the health team. This involves the following factors:
   - Listen carefully to the caregiver's progress report on the patient.
   - Have the caregiver present in the room when you examine the patient.
   - Involve the caregiver in all aspects of management of the patient: medications, diet, activities, and so on.
   - Ensure your (or your associates') availability to the caregiver at all times.
   - If the caregiver can, have him or her record basic daily data on the patient that can be reviewed at each visit.

2. Following an assessment of the caregiver's knowledge of the patient's illness and ability to cope with management and coordination of all activities, the physician should educate the caregiver as much as possible for the multiple chores. Roles that need to be learned include:
   - Observer of clinical changes in the patient
   - Provider of direct care (medication, food, etc.)
   - Liaison with family and friends
   - Liaison with physician and other therapists
   - Liaison with community resources

3. Acknowledge the caregiver's efforts at every contact.

4. Inquire directly about the caregiver's feelings and state of health.
   - How does he or she feel about the job? What are the difficulties and frustrations? What solutions can you offer?
   - Discuss the relationship between caregiver and patient and between caregiver and family.
   - Encourage the caregiver to talk about feelings, especially any resentment, guilt, or anger, so he or she can understand that these are normal and expected feelings.

- Is the caregiver receiving the support he or she thinks is necessary?
- Is the caregiver looking after him- or herself? Is the caregiver taking time for his or her own activities?

5. Watch for signs of excessive stress, and when observed intervene directly, if necessary, using any of the following approaches:
   - Direct medical examination and treatment
   - Helping the caregiver learn how to deal with stress, specifically by relaxing, talking to others, taking time off, or joining support groups
   - Referring the caregiver to formal counseling if needed

6. Encourage the caregiver's participation in his or her own social groups, despite fatigue.

7. It is very important to arrange periodic "respite care" for the patient so the caregiver can have a break. This can be done through other members of the family, friends, religious support groups, or community agencies that provide temporary services in the home or in their institutions.

It is also relevant to mention the problem of the patient's caring *relatives* (siblings or children) *who live far away from the patient's home.* The hassles and stress of daily caregiving often lead to frustration and even conflicts between the caregiver and the distant, well-meaning, caring relatives. The caregiver may become angry and frustrated because he or she does not think these relatives are doing enough or that they appreciate his or her efforts. The distant relatives may feel guilty about not being able to help more and may overcompensate by frequent phone calls to the caregiver and physician, offering well-meaning but often disruptive criticism and suggestions. When this occurs the physician often finds him- or herself triangulated in a conflict between the caregiver and the distant relatives. A solution to this problem is not easy, but I have found two methods very useful.

The first method is to ask all the distant relatives to designate one person as the liaison between the caregiver and the physician and the rest of the family. This makes life much easier for everyone concerned. The second method, which can be complementary to the first, is the family conference. This is a meeting of all relevant family members with the caregiver and the physician (and the patient, if he or she is cognitively able to do so). At this face-to-face conference, the problems (medical and otherwise) are discussed until there is a joint solution. Following the initial family conference, periodic review conferences (either face-to-face or via telephone) for updates are much easier for everyone.

The challenge of dealing simultaneously with a seriously ill patient and the surrounding hidden patients, especially the caregiver, can be complicated and arduous, but it usually is a small investment that brings large dividends in terms of improved health and satisfaction for all concerned—including the physician. It is hoped that the medical care and social systems will allow and encourage such an approach through appropriate incentives and rewards.

REFERENCES

Cassel, J. (1974). An epidemiological perspective on psychosocial factors in disease etiology. *American Journal of Public Health, 64,* 1040-1043.

Christie-Seely, J. (1984). *Working with the family in primary care.* New York: Praeger.

Dody, P. (1986). Family care of the elderly. *The Milbank Memorial Fund Quarterly, 64,* 34-75.

Doherty, W. J., & Baird, M. A. (1983). *Family therapy and family medicine.* New York: Guilford.

Doherty, W. J., Baird, M. A., & Becker, L. A. (1986). Family medicine and the biopsychosocial model. *Advances, 3,* 17-28.

Duvall, E. M. (1977). *Marriage and family development* (5th ed.). Philadelphia: J. B. Lippincott.

Engel, G. L. (1977). The need for a new medical model: A challenge for biomedicine. *Science, 196,* 129-136.

Engel, G. L. (1980). The clinical application of the biopsychosocial model. *American Journal of Psychiatry, 137,* 535-544.

Erikson, E. H. (1950). *Childhood in society.* New York: Norton.

Fengler, A. P., & Goodrich, N. (1979). Wives of elderly disabled men: The hidden patients. *The Gerontologist, 19,* 175-183.

Fletcher, R. H., Fletcher, S. W., & Wagner, E. H. (1982). *Clinical epidemiology.* Baltimore, MD: Williams & Wilkins.

Hasselkus, B. R. (1988). Meaning in family caregiving: Perspectives on caregiver/professional relationships. *The Gerontologist, 28,* 686-691.

Hill, R. (1970). *Family development in three generations.* Cambridge, MA: Schenkman.

Kiecolt-Glaser, J. K., Dura, J. R., Speicher, C. E., Trask, J., & Glaser, R. (1991). Spousal care-givers of dementia victims: Longitudinal changes in immunity and health. *Psychosomatic Medicine, 53,* 345-362.

Maletta, G. J., & Hepburn, K. (1986). Helping families cope with Alzheimer's: The physician's role. *Geriatrics, 41,* 81-90.

Mattlin, J. A., Wethington, E., & Kessler, R. C. (1990). Situational determinants of coping and coping effectiveness. *Journal of Health & Social Behavior, 31,* 103-122.

Medalie, J. H. (1975, December). *The hidden patient.* Presentation to the School of Medicine Faculty Retreat, Case Western Reserve University, Painesville, OH.

Medalie, J. H. (1990). Angina pectoris: A validation of the biopsychosocial model. *Journal of Family Practice, 30,* 273-280.

Medalie, J. H., & Cole-Kelly, K. (1992, March). *A dynamic life-cycle model of the doctor-patient relationship.* Paper presented at Amelia Island Conference on Empowerment, Amelia Island, FL.

Medalie, J. H., Kitson, G. C., & Zyzanski, S. J. (1981). A family epidemiological model: A practice and research concept for family medicine. *Journal of Family Practice, 12,* 79-87.

Osterweis, M., Solomon, F., & Green, M. (Eds.). (1984a). *Bereavement: Reactions, consequences and care.* Washington, DC: National Academy of Sciences.

Osterweis, M., Solomon, F., & Green, M. (1984b). Toward a biology of grieving. In M. Osterweis, F. Solomon, & M. Green (Eds.), *Bereavement: Reactions, consequences and care* (pp. 145-175). Washington, DC: National Academy of Sciences.

Rabins, P. V., Mace, N. L., & Lucas, M. J. (1982). Impact of dementia on the family. *Journal of the American Medical Association, 248*(3), 333-335.

Rees, W., & Lutkins, S. G. (1967). Mortality and bereavement. *British Medical Journal, 4,* 13-16.

Sackett, D. L., Anderson, G. D., Milner, R., Feinleib, M., & Kannel, W. B. (1975). Concordance for coronary risk factors among spouses. *Circulation, 52,* 589-595.

Vogel, E. F., & Bell, N. W. (1968). The emotionally disturbed child as the family scape-goat. In N. W. Bell & E. F. Vogel (Eds.), *A modern introduction to the family* (pp. 412-427). New York: Free Press.

Von Bertalanffy, L. (1952). *Problems of life.* New York: John Wiley.

Wasserman, R. C., Inui, T. S., & Barriatua, R. D. (1984). Pediatric clinicians' support for parents makes a difference: An outcome-based analysis of clinician-parent interaction. *Pediatrics, 74*(6), 1047-1053.

13

Caregiving Issues
in Families of Children
With Chronic Medical Conditions

ANNE E. KAZAK
DIMITRI A. CHRISTAKIS

It's upsetting that they [autistic adults] must live with strangers. . . . Where are their families?

Mother of a 5-year-old with severe Pervasive Developmental Disorder after reading a newspaper article on group homes for autistic adults

This chapter presents a theoretical framework for understanding issues related to parenting and caregiving when a child has a serious, chronic medical condition. Building upon a social-ecological and systems model, this framework emphasizes individuals, and systems (e.g., parents, families, siblings, schools, hospitals) at multiple levels of analysis as they relate to caregiving demands. We organize empirical research, theoretical papers, and clinical examples related to caregiving in families with a disabled or chronically ill child to illustrate this theoretical orientation. The family is considered as embedded within broader caregiving systems. Some of these systems are well known (e.g., hospitals, schools); others reflect the broader culture (e.g., impact of gender). Consistent with the lifespan orientation of this book, we delineate issues developmentally. The growing utilization of home medical care also is addressed, specifically with respect to the impact on caregiving for children. We conclude with recommendations for future research and intervention on caregiving systems for these children and their families.

BACKGROUND

The impact of serious childhood illness on families is well known in terms of general family stress and the family reorganization necessary for successful adaptation. However, with respect to the breadth and diversity of the population of children with chronic health problems, existing research often has not clarified the nature of specific caregiving demands, nor has it adequately explored the interrelationships between the child, illness, caregivers, and others.

Estimates indicate that 10-12% of school-age children in the United States have a chronic health problem (Hobbs, Perrin, & Ireys, 1985). We discuss children with a range of medical conditions, including those typically considered chronic illnesses (e.g., cystic fibrosis), physical disability (e.g., spina bifida, cerebral palsy), and mental retardation. The problems such varied chronic pediatric conditions pose are diverse; the impact of these problems on caregivers and the specific caregiving demands are equally diverse.

For example, the demands of some conditions, such as childhood cancers, have changed with the advent of new therapies and resulting improved survival rates. Prior to the mid-1970s, pediatric cancer was almost inevitably fatal. Although the loss of a child is traumatic, the relatively short course of the illness minimized prolonged caregiving responsibilities. Today, with more intense and successful treatments, additional parental caregiving for extended periods of time is necessary. Similarly high levels of caregiving demands also are incurred by the growing number of infants and young children receiving highly technical, specialized medical care at home, including the medically fragile children discussed in Chapter 5 of this volume.

Although caregiving is necessary across all serious pediatric conditions, the role that particular illnesses and conditions play in affecting caregiving demands is unclear. Conceptually, the ways in which different illnesses may impact upon family functioning have been approached both noncategorically and specifically. A noncategorical approach emphasizes commonalities across conditions in coping with childhood chronic illness (Stein & Jessop, 1982). Although clarification of these commonalities is important, much of the literature on childhood chronic illness has been based upon studies that mix illness groups with no clear rationale. Without identification of possible illness parameters that may affect caregiving, it may be premature to conclude that such parameters may not have different psychological effects on both caregivers and their children.

Rolland (1984, 1987) has proposed a model for understanding psychosocial characteristics of illnesses that may impact upon families and caregiving. The four dimensions outlined are *onset, course, outcome,* and *degree of incapacitation.* Each of these characteristics has implications specifically related to caregiving for ill children. For example, in a family with a terminally ill child, caregiving responsibilities may intensify with time. During this period, caregivers must cope with their grief and loss while providing more intense care for the dying child. In contrast, a disease with a stable course may demand a steadier level of caregiving and necessitate family reorganization, but major changes and emotional upheaval are not anticipated.

SOCIAL ECOLOGY, SYSTEMS THEORY, AND CHILDHOOD CHRONIC ILLNESS

Social ecology (Bronfenbrenner, 1979) provides a useful model for understanding the ways in which childhood chronic illness reciprocally impacts upon individuals and systems internal and external to the family (Kazak, 1986, 1987, 1989). Emanating from the work of developmental psychologists, social ecology typically considers the child as the center of nested concentric spheres of influence (Figure 13.1). At its inception this contextual approach to understanding children represented a shift from laboratory-based research and provided a model that could guide field-based studies of children's behavior at different levels of analysis.

The first such level is the *microsystem,* or patterns of activities, roles, and interpersonal relations experienced by the developing person, including the immediate family. Within the microsystem one can examine parent-child interactions and the development of sibling bonds. These are areas of inherent interest in the case of families with ill children. Understanding the nature of parent-child or sibling interactions in such families elucidates ways in which they are like other families but also provides insight into substantive differences associated with having children with special needs.

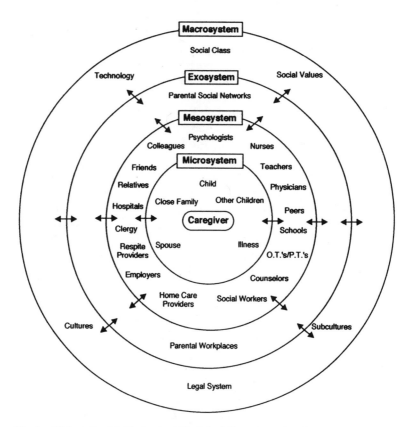

Figure 13.1. A Social-Ecological Model of Caregivers for Children With Chronic Medical Conditions

Mesosystems are interrelated microsystems. For children, the meso-systemic level of analysis explores the relationships between families and schools or families and hospitals. Although these relationships are important for any child or family, families with a chronically ill child often have particular learning and/or school needs that accentuate the importance of family/school relationships. Moreover, there is an additional long-term relationship with members of the health-care team that changes as the nature and demands of treatment change.

The *exosystem* is an environment that does not affect the child directly, but that nevertheless has profound indirect effects. Typically exosystemic work has considered the impact of parental social networks and employment on children. Given the importance of caregiving for chronically ill children and the fact that the vast majority of caregiving is provided by parents, understanding the social context in which parents function is critical. For example, the extent to which family and friends are supportive of caregiving demands can impact on the child and family. Similarly, health-care needs of chronically ill children can necessitate parental absences from work. The extent to which parental employers are flexible in this respect may affect the child indirectly through increased or decreased parental stress associated with work.

Finally, at the outermost level is the *macrosystem,* which is the impact of subculture, culture, and general belief patterns on the entire system. The values of our society and the attitudes toward persons with disabilities, particularly as they are manifested in laws and policies affecting families caring for children with chronic health-care needs, must be considered in a thorough and thoughtful understanding of caregivers. The ways in which caregiving is valued or devalued may affect caregivers' self-concept and the nature of the care that ultimately is provided. At a more tangible level, a lack of supportive local, state, and federal policies and services (e.g., education, transportation) can have direct effects on caregiving styles and the level of stress caregivers face.

Other important components of social-ecological theory include reciprocity and the importance of change in the natural progression of development. Emphasizing the interactive rather than the linear nature of development and relationships, reciprocity is a cornerstone of contextual theory. Children's temperament and the nature of their illness impact on their caregivers just as caregivers' style and resources impact on their interactions with their children. Transitions are critical as well and can be either expected or unexpected. Developmentally expected transitions (e.g., starting school, leaving school) as well as unexpected (e.g., accidents, recurrence of illness) affect families and warrant further attention.

A systems perspective on caregiving in families with pediatric illness emphasizes the interrelatedness of all components of the family and the wide range of variables that may contribute to caregiver adjustment. Systems theory posits complex interrelationships among these variables and argues against simple linear causal explanations. The need for identifying research methodologies and data to understand the gestalt of caregiving for ill children remains.

THE SOCIAL-ECOLOGICAL
FRAMEWORK OF CAREGIVERS

In this chapter we make a major shift in the social-ecological model to emphasize caregivers. A framework that emphasizes the interrelatedness of individuals and systems that affect the process of caregiving, Figure 13.1 shows this social-ecological model, putting the caregiver at the center. Our focus here is on the two innermost spheres of influence: the *microsystem,* which for our purposes consists of all immediate family members and the illness, and the *mesosystem,* which includes parental social support networks (family and friends), the educational system, and all members of the complex health-care system. Although at least equally important, the exosystem and macrosystem are not discussed in detail in this chapter. We have chosen to emphasize those levels of the model for which the most research evidence exists. We explore below the influences the microsystem and mesosystem exert on caregivers for chronically ill or medically disabled children, but first we address more general issues related to caregiving.

Caregiving and Parenting

With respect to children, *caregiving* and *parenting* are two closely related, often overlapping, but not necessarily identical roles. In a broad sense parenting can be viewed as accepting substantial responsibility for a child. It can include socialization, guidance, discipline, and financial and emotional support. Parenting is a lifelong process that changes with phases of a child's development. Caregiving may be viewed as the hands-on aspects of raising a child. Whereas a *parent* can be removed from the day-to-day details of child care, a *caregiver* is directly involved with them. Among other things, caregiving includes changing diapers, applying bandages, bathing and clothing, teaching, playing with, supervising, and transporting the child. Chronically ill or disabled children may have additional demands, such as flushing intravenous lines, attaching and removing ventilators, or suctioning endotracheal tubes. In general, children with chronic conditions may require caregiving for a longer period of their lives than healthy children typically do. Although our emphasis in this section has been on concrete demands, caregiving is a process that also involves psychological involvement and impacts that are very important, although more difficult to articulate. Within Figure 13.1, the caregiving responsibilities define many but not all important aspects of the relationships that the caregiver has with persons in the microsystem.

Parenting can be provided by many persons: biological parents, custodial and noncustodial parents, stepparents, other adults both within and outside the nuclear family unit, extended family, respite care workers, and teachers. In this chapter we focus on *parents* (usually mothers) who do the majority of *caregiving* for children with chronic health-care needs. In addition to direct parenting and caregiving for the children, they also must negotiate other systems (e.g., health care, schools, community agencies) intimately involved in their child's short- and long-term well-being. Thus parental caregivers share caregiving with members of both their microsystem and their mesosystem.

Developmental (Lifespan) Issues

Several important developmental issues often are neglected in the literature on caregiving and children. The most obvious is the developmental level of the child. Caregiving demands for infants, active preschoolers, and adolescents differ. The developmental level of the child may be a more pertinent concern in understanding the impact of caregiver burden than illness type and warrants further consideration. For example, adolescents with any chronic medical condition must struggle with the transition to young adulthood and must make educational and vocational decisions and choices about living arrangements that are somewhat different from their nonaffected peers. The caregiving demands on parents and siblings may intensify at a time when all family members may desire more autonomy. These issues are more directly related to adolescence than to a particular illness.

Related to the child's developmental level is the developmental level of the family itself. General schema of family development are available (Carter & McGoldrick, 1980) but tend to focus on normal, or normative, sequences of family development. The implications of family transitions (such as the birth of a second or third child, separation or divorce, children leaving home, or grandparent illness) may be quite complicated for a family with a child with a chronic health problem and often are related to the manner in which a developmentally unexpected event (serious, potentially life-threatening illness in a child) is integrated into one's understanding of being a parent. A child's illness can affect a parent's own development and that of the family in other more tangible ways as well. A parent (often a mother) who may have anticipated not working outside the home for a few years while raising young children may revise that timetable in light of an ill child, or a family may pass up a transfer or promotion in order that a parent (often a father) will not have to change job demands, relocate self or family, or move the child to a potentially less optimal school system.

Intergenerational experiences impact on family caregiving as well. Previous family legacies and encounters with illness and caretaking become incorporated into the family's style. For example, the mother quoted at the outset of the chapter expects that her other children will care for her daughter when they are adults. Her experiences are based upon her own supportive, extended family and her husband's experiences as a successful survivor of a much more chaotic family system. Thorough family evaluations, including an understanding of intergenerational experiences with illness and caregiving, are integral to helping the family plan long-term care.

Links With Care of the Elderly

Despite obvious similarities, research on kin caregiving for the elderly and for disabled children has not been linked. This is unfortunate because a great deal of useful information could be exchanged.

Among other topics, work on caregiving for the elderly has addressed the interfacing of formal and informal help systems (Noelker & Bass, 1989), caregiver burden (Stephens, Kinney, & Ogrocki, 1991), and gender effects of caregiving (Young & Kahana, 1989). All of these issues have clear parallels with caregiving for disabled children. Often, the endpoint evaluated in home care of the elderly is institutionalization, that is, when and why a family opts for nursing home placement. Insofar as families resort to institutionalization of an elder when the burden of care becomes too great, it can serve as a marker of family systems that have been overwhelmed. For caregivers of disabled children, institutionalization is seldom an option, but the risk of burnout is as present. One of the goals of studying kin caregivers of elderly is to identify which caregivers are at risk for burnout and to learn how to know when they are near the edge. The findings of studies of caregivers for elderly, especially those designed to predict or alleviate burnout, could be meaningfully applied to families caring for disabled children. For example, Mohide and colleagues (1990) conducted a randomized trial of caregiver support in the home care treatment of elderly patients with dementia. Included were caregiver-focused health care, education about dementia and caregiving, regularly scheduled in-home respite, and a self-help caregiver support group. Their intervention produced a clinically important improvement in quality of life, a slightly longer mean time to long-term institutionalization, and a greater sense of satisfaction with the role as caregiver. A program with similar goals and means might very well be effective for families with medically disabled children.

Moreover, many of the methodologies employed in the study of the home care for the elderly could be modified and used for the disabled or chronically ill child paradigm. For example, Birkel (1987) has a particularly interesting and useful model for assessing caregiver and elder well-being. His is one that examines what he calls the home care household, which includes the physical context of the home, the patterns of its residents, and the interaction between the two. Of note, he pays due attention to allocations of space within the household—sick rooms, play areas, common living areas—and investigates how varied access impacts on the dynamics of the family. We now turn to address the caregiver's microsystem and its components.

MICROSYSTEM: THE FAMILY AND
CAREGIVING FOR A PEDIATRIC CONDITION

The family, or microsystem, of the disabled child has been the subject of much attention in the literature. Early studies, following an intuitive line of reasoning, posited that the increased stress of having a handicapped child at home would have negative repercussions throughout the immediate family, affecting the child, the siblings, the parents, and their marital relationship. Those studies and their conclusions recently have been revisited and revised. The results of this literature have important implications for caregivers and caregiving systems.

Most prominent, some research indicates no differences with respect to global family outcome (adjustment) variables between families with and without children with a range of conditions (Cadman, Rosenbaum, Boyle, & Offord, 1991; Kazak & Marvin, 1984; Kazak & Meadows, 1989; Kazak, Reber, & Snitzer, 1988). Importantly, these samples reflect large representative samples and are not biased with respect to clinical problems.

The acceptance of the broad range of family functioning seen in families with chronically ill children and the abandonment of a deficit orientation toward these families is contingent, in part, on understanding the implications of some widely utilized research designs. As an example, employing a null hypothesis model allows researchers to accept (and hence present and publish) only data in which group differences were determined. Findings of no difference cannot be accepted as being of scientific merit under this model. Several studies have proposed reconsideration of the null hypothesis model. A similar research design that may promote a model of expecting deviance in families with chronically ill children is the use of comparison (or control) groups. Securing appropriate control groups is difficult and wrought with many problems. Studies that examine differences between more and less successful coping with childhood chronic illness may help clarify why some families do better than others who also have chronically ill children.

It is also important that researchers accept and consider the wide diversity in family structures, racial and ethnic backgrounds, and styles. Given the high rate of divorce and the prevalence of single-parent households in the United States, family research on caregiving must approach these issues with a broad frame of reference, and without the expectation of two married adults in the household. Similarly, racial and ethnic variability need to be explored more systematically. Studies of black and Hispanic families of children with cancer show potentially adaptive patterns (i.e., extreme closeness, mother-child alliances, different types of responses to childhood pain) that differ from those often associated with positive adaptation (Baskin, Forehand, & Saylor, 1986; de Parra, de Cortazar, & Covarrubias-Espinoza, 1983; Pfefferbaum, Adams, & Aceves, 1990).

Fundamentally, families who have children with special needs can cope successfully and look much like other families despite the additional caregiving demands. They can be viewed as normal families coping with an abnormal situation in that most families do not have a child with a chronic health problem. A social-ecological framework may help identify those factors that can contribute to more or less successful coping and to understand the ways in which caregivers and caregiving systems function in this regard. For example, what qualities of spousal and/or friendship relationships relate to positive adaptation to caregiving demands? How can health-care teams interact effectively with parents to ameliorate caregiving problems?

The Affected Child

Children with chronic physical problems have long been noted to be at higher risk for psychopathology than unaffected children. Friedrich (1977) noted that secondary psychological problems often can become the primary handicap for a physically disabled child. A large survey of more than 3,000 children ages 4-16 and residing at home in Ontario, Canada, found children with chronic illness and associated disability to have a threefold risk of psychiatric disorder. Children with chronic medical conditions without an associated disability were found to have a twofold increased risk (Cadman, Boyle, Szatmari, & Offord, 1987). Other investigators, however, found lower rates of psychopathology and provide some clarification of the types of factors that may affect the development of psychological problems. Wallander, Varni, Babani, Banis, and Wilcox (1988) found on average more behavioral problems in their study of 270 children with 6 chronic physical disorders, but they concluded that only a small portion could be considered clinically maladjusted. In most cases maladjustment appears to be related to neurological impairments, which are widely accepted as more stressful for both the child and the caregiver. This raises the question of what role the illness type itself plays in caregiver demands.

The Illness

How do characteristics of disabled children, their medical condition, and the demands of their treatment affect parenting and caregiving? Is it unquestionably more difficult to parent a child with a severe disability than a child with a milder difficulty? Are caregivers a variable that accounts for the diversity in adjustment seen among medically disabled or chronically ill children?

One school of thought has maintained that a disability and its attendant limitations place an added burden on children and thereby put them at increased risk for psychiatric or adjustment problems. From this hypothesis would follow the expectation that the more severe the disability, the more severe the burden and, hence, the greater the frequency and extent of adjustment problems. Indeed, some investigators have found an association between the degree of children's disabilities and their psychiatric problems (Cadman et al., 1987; Daniels,

Miller, Billings, & Moos, 1987; Steinhausen, Schindler, & Stephan, 1983), whereas others have found none (Breslau, 1985; Wallander, Feldman, & Varni, 1989). That there is no incontrovertible evidence for a direct, linear, cause-and-effect relationship between illness burden and maladjustment implies that mediating variables must exist. Parental coping styles and abilities may be those variables. Children with a moderately serious health problem may do worse than those with a more severe one if the former do not have caregivers who can adequately help them cope, or whose coping styles for themselves are ineffective. Assuming that medically disabled children are no less diverse in their intrinsic disposition than abled children, it follows that their adjustment should be equally environmentally influenced.

Parents and Other Adults in the Family as Caregivers

As defined in this chapter, caregiving for disabled children is parenting with additional demands related to having a child with chronic medical concerns. Nonetheless, "parent" is a role assumed by an adult in a family. It is important (for parents and professionals alike) to place parenting in perspective as one role played by adults in families. In our discussion we separate the caregiver's role as a parent from his or her role as a spouse.

In theory the similarities between parenting a disabled child and a nondisabled one may be overlooked. In either case a caregiver must be sensitive and responsive to the child's needs. But in practice there is a salient difference. Our society is centered on caring for the needs of what it deems normative children. Parents have their own parents to use as positive or negative role models in caring for a normal child. They usually can talk with family or friends about experiences that, on the most fundamental level, should not be largely different from their own. Such is often not the case for parents of disabled children. For example, discussions about when children walked or talked or how they were toilet trained are common, helpful, and invigorating for most new parents but can be quite alienating for parents of disabled children.

Furthermore, the mechanics of child rearing are established for healthy children. The *machinery* is in place, and consequently a substantial part of parenting is almost rote. As an example, a parent can enroll his or her normal 5-year-old in school, go to an open house to learn of the child's progress, attend annual Parent-Teacher Association (PTA) meetings, and read report cards. For a disabled child, however, parents must take a decidedly more active role in an uncharted territory without a guide. Formal education often begins earlier. They may have no personal or familial experiences on which to base their actions. Friends and relatives, though they can provide tremendous and invaluable emotional support, cannot readily relate to the differences of living with a handicapped or chronically ill child. Caregivers often must engage their child's school or school board, or they may have to seek legal counsel to ensure that their child's needs are met. The process of obtaining and ensuring an appropriate, quality education for a medically disabled child is much more time-consuming than it is for normal children, and it often demands advocacy skills and assertiveness that individual parents may not possess.

These differences in caregiving requirements for medically disabled children exist within the home, the extended family, and the community. For example, almost any child can accompany a parent or grandparent on a shopping trip. The child must be supervised and engaged in a developmentally relevant manner in the tasks at hand. For disabled and abled children alike, the rules and expectations for behavior in public must be communicated. For the disabled child, other caregiving demands also must be negotiated: the wheelchair that may not fit in narrow aisles; the behaviorally unpredictable children who may damage themselves or property and may need a lengthy time-out period; or the children with cancer who may become fatigued and unable to keep up with others. There are numerous ways in which any of these stressful circumstances can be handled. The personality, experiences, resourcefulness, and characteristics of caregivers can mediate the outcomes for both parent and child.

All of the demands and differences that having a handicapped or medically disabled child pose are not without their cost. Olshansky (1962) may have been the first to give the pervasive negative feeling that parents with disabled children sometimes experience a name. Chronic sorrow succeeds the acute grief they feel at having a child who is not normal. It remains in the background of their subconscious, insidiously informing day-to-day activities but largely kept in check until it is readily brought to the foreground at what would be developmental milestones in a normal child's life. For example, many researchers (Gath, 1978) have commented that the care of a newborn handicapped child, excepting extreme cases, is not all that different from the care of any newborn. With the commencement of school and the inevitable tracking of a handicapped child to a program that is different from that of a parents' neighbors' or friends' children, one such milestone is reached and chronic sorrow can become a flare-up of an acute grief reaction.

Caregiver burden is complicated not only by such psychological stressors but also by economic ones. Ensuring prompt and adequate reimbursement for medical services remains a source of stress (Leonard, Brust, Janny, & Patterson, 1991). Respite care is often not funded. Physical therapy, speech therapy, occupational therapy, and nutrition service coverage can be limited and infrequent (Fox & Newacheck, 1990). These macrosystemic issues and frustrations underlie daily life and can contribute to increased caregiver distress.

Marital Relationships

The once common notion that having a handicapped child will *inevitably* have an adverse effect on a marriage and likely result in divorce is no longer accepted as valid (Sabbeth & Levethal, 1984). Kazak and Marvin (1984) report no difference in marital satisfaction between parents of handicapped children and controls. They distinguish between the *parenting* role, in which differences were found, and the marital role. Cadman and colleagues (1991), analyzing the Ontario Child Health Study data, found no increase in familial dysfunction. Darling (1987) notes that many parents comment on an increased family cohesiveness brought on by a need to rally together for the handicapped child's benefit.

In the past, anecdotal accounts of closeness, normality, or even happiness often have been dismissed or interpreted as denial on the part of parents. There is now a clearer understanding of the range of marital reactions to having a chronically ill or disabled child and a more reasonable acknowledgment that some of the research methods we have relied upon actually may have biased our understanding.

Nevertheless, from a systems perspective the vulnerability of the marital relationship is evident. The birth of any child changes the nature of the marital dyad. Parental expectations of what a child will be like begin long before birth. This, too, at least in Western culture, is part of the process of becoming a parent. It is common for would-be parents to fantasize about their unborn child's appearance, demeanor, or future accomplishments. Expectant parents do not spend time or energy planning what to do or how to act if their newborn is somehow medically disabled. Indeed, they spend time and energy repressing their fears of such an outcome.

When a child is born with special health-care needs or diagnosed with a serious health problem in childhood, uncertainty, increased involvement with medical systems, and a higher level of caregiving demands intertwine with and impact on the marriage. It may be more difficult for the marriage to stabilize and reorganize to accommodate the needs of the child. A closer focus upon the ways in which spouses negotiate critical events over the course of a disabled child's life is needed to identify personal and systemic characteristics associated with positive adaptation.

Siblings

In many instances the chronically ill child is not the only child in the family system and caregiving needs extend to other children in addition to the disabled child. How caregivers relate to other children in their families is an important area of family research. In a study of 25 preschool siblings of children with cancer and a matched group of comparison families, Horwitz and Kazak (1990) examined the ways in which mothers viewed siblings as alike or different from the ill child. Mothers of children with cancer were more likely to view the sibling as being like the child with cancer than were comparison mothers who rated their two well children. In light of the generally high level of family and sibling outcome found, it is suggested that this tendency to view siblings as being like the ill child may have been an adaptive way to minimize the impact of the illness and maintain a view of both children being relatively normal and alike.

The relatively small body of literature that examines the impact of childhood chronic illness on siblings has yielded conflicting results. Some studies show few if any differences in the behavior of siblings of handicapped or chronically ill children (Breslau, Weitzman, & Messenger, 1981). Others (Breslau & Prabucki, 1987; McAndrew, 1976) found negative behavior that could be attributed by maternal report to the presence of the handicapped child. Whatever effects siblings do show also have not been correlated with the degree of disease or disability of their brother or sister (Breslau et al., 1981; Wood et al., 1988), suggesting again that it is the impact of a given disease on a *family* and not directly on the sibling that has consequences.

Inasmuch as siblings of handicapped or chronically ill children are at risk for psychiatric problems, however, a greater stress is added to the microsystem of caregivers. They must both be attentive to the needs of their disabled child and be wary of the effects that added attention and the illness itself may be having on their other children. Relying primarily on outcome measures for siblings, the research literature pays virtually no attention to how parents and family members balance the needs of all children with respect to caregiving.

From a systems standpoint, what protects or endangers a sibling may be the role he or she is asked to play vis-à-vis an ill brother or sister. That is, how the caregiver chooses or neglects to integrate the child into the caregiving context of the family may be the determining factor. It may be that too much involvement with caregiving responsibilities puts the siblings at risk (McHale & Gamble, 1989), or perhaps it is that too little involvement does so. Ultimately, parents, by deciding how much and what kinds of interactions children will have with their disabled siblings, play a decisive role in the psychological adjustment outcome of the well children.

Gender and Caregiving
for Chronically Ill Children

Traditionally the majority of caregiving responsibilities have been the mother's. The role of gender in understanding the differential roles and impact of childhood chronic illness on women and men in families often is ignored. The majority of literature on parenting describes mothering. The need to clarify mothering and fathering is important, as is the effort necessary to engage fathers in meaningful research on both parenting and caregiving for a disabled child.

Gender itself only recently has been getting the consideration it warrants. Much work of late has focused on the differing roles men and women play in caring for the disabled or sick child. Early studies often noted that fathers assumed increased financial burdens secondary to the increased costs of the disabled child and, hence, spent more time at work, whereas mothers spent more labor-intensive time caring for their child and, hence, spent more time in social isolation. Changing demographics and societal attitudes have allowed—often demanded—that more women enter the workforce. That, coupled with more open-minded assessments of gender roles and coping strategies, has led to some interesting changes in the literature.

What once was viewed as an amplification of standard family roles— mother as homemaker/nurturer, father as breadwinner—brought on by the added caretaking and economic necessities of having a handicapped child might, in fact, have had an additional impetus. Parks and Pilisuk (1991), in a study of gender-based differences in coping with the stress of caring for a parent with Alzheimer's disease, explore what they identify as four styles of coping. One of their subscales, withdrawal, describes a "business-as-usual" facade. It was characterized by an unwillingness to let other people know how bad things really are or how the subject feels about a situation and a reluctance to be around people or to talk to anyone about the distressing situation. Withdrawal was found to be more common in men than women.

Spending more time out of the house then, ostensibly solely to shoulder the increased financial burden, in fact may have served a twofold purpose. Men may have been practicing withdrawal in the old family schema by working harder as an excuse to avoid interacting with their disabled child or having to talk about their feelings regarding the child, and simultaneously to project an even more convincing business-as-usual picture. Presently, these differences in coping styles may be being manifested with women doing a larger "second shift," working outside the home and then assuming the lion's share of caretaking responsibilities at home. What emerges is a chicken-and-egg paradox of sorts. Do gender-based coping differences lead to gender-based roles in caregiving for the disabled child or vice versa? An exploration of coping strategies used in this population of families, with attention as well focused on any associations between the type of burden experienced and the means of coping utilized, would be extremely interesting.

Bristol, Gallagher, and Schopler (1988) studied the effect of a young developmentally disabled and nondisabled male child on adaptation and family roles of both parents. They note that fathers of disabled children assumed less responsibility for child care than comparison fathers, even in mother-employed families, and, more important, that this decrease in child involvement was specific to the disabled children and not their siblings.

The disparity in gender roles has led to a disparity in gender tolls. Maternal stress in caring for a disabled child is noted to be the only stress higher than comparison parents (Kazak, 1987). Several studies have found that mothers of disabled children suffer significantly higher levels of depression/anxiety than control mothers of healthy children (Breslau, Staruch, & Mortimer, 1982; Jessop, Riessman, & Stein, 1988). A depressed mother, particularly when her depression is attributable in large part to her caregiving responsibilities, clearly functions suboptimally as a caretaker and can bias assessments of child adaptation (Brody

& Forehand, 1986), thus further confounding attempts to assess a disabled child's functioning.

THE MESOSYSTEM: HEALTH-CARE SYSTEMS, SCHOOLS, AND PARENTAL SOCIAL NETWORKS

The mesosystem of any caregiver includes formal and informal support systems for the caregiver and institutions with which the caregiver interacts. With respect to formal support, caregivers of children with chronic illness must interact with a large number of diverse professionals. As Figure 13.1 shows, these include physicians, nurses, therapists (physical, occupational, speech), teachers and school administrators, and psychologists and social workers. All of these professionals are a part of the systems in which they work. Understanding the systemic characteristics, of families and other microsystems, is important. A further complication exists in the case of home care, in which traditional boundaries are rearranged and professionals entering the home need to negotiate a partnership with the parental caregivers. Informal supports include nuclear and extended family members, friends, and others available to caregivers.

Hospitals and Health-Care Systems

The ways in which health-care systems (formal caregiving systems) interface with family systems and support parental caregiving in childhood chronic illness are largely unexplored. In general the medical model of health care is seen as being in opposition to family-centered care, and the models for meaningful parental involvement in health care and health-care policies of hospitals are limited.

Arguing cogently for a systemic view of chronic illness that includes medical staff, family, and patient, Reiss and De-Nour (1989) discuss roles for each member of the illness caregiving system over the developmental course of the illness. Applying their adult-focused model to childhood chronic illness necessitates consideration of the role of the patient's individual development. Changing developmental abilities alter the pediatric patient's role in participation in medical decisions and in terms of understanding the need for relationships with formal and informal caregivers. Pertinent as well are the ways in which parents or caregivers work collaboratively, with each other and with formal caregivers at a family level.

Home Care

Some of the traditional boundaries between care provided in a hospital or clinic setting and that provided at home have changed with the rapid growth of pediatric home care. Many families with ill children provide some degree of care, in conjunction with professional home care providers, once delivered only in a hospital setting. Nutritional support, intravenous antibiotics, chemotherapy, and home ventilators are examples of high-technology medical care now possibly provided at home.

The presence of professionals in the home can itself be a source of stress. Particularly stressful for parents are difficulties collaborating with and arranging for services (Weiss, 1991) and integrating themselves into the treatment plan (Crutcher, 1991). For home care, parents and professionals may differ with respect to responsibility and control. Parental caregivers may feel that professionals should comply with certain (sometimes unspoken) expectations and priorities. The effectiveness of home care is associated with the degree to which parents' and professionals' priorities are similar (Mueller & Leviton, 1986). Physical and occupational therapists recognize that parents must be considered as equals in the development and implementation of a treatment plan (Bazyk, 1989).

A safe and well-orchestrated home care plan involves close collaboration among family, hospital, and home care providers. Parents must be trained and participate in assessments and plans for home services. The physical modifications necessary (e.g., keeping medications and supplies away from young children) must be made, as well as establishment of schedules for nursing assistance in the home. Effective communication channels for assistance with routine and emergency medical needs must be established. In a study of home versus hospital chemotherapy and antibiotics for children with cancer, families were found to prefer home care, in terms of the impact on the entire family and upon the child's quality of life during the period of home care (Lange, 1991). Understanding how caregivers, who prefer home care, cope with the different levels of demands home care poses might enable health providers to extend this option to more families.

The growth of the home medical care system exemplifies the interconnectedness of the mesosystem and broader systems. The home care movement has been spurred by two potentially divergent goals: cost containment and beneficence. Ideally, as is often stated, home care can be both cheaper and better than hospitalization. But inasmuch as the impetus for it is economic, problems arise. A cost-containment strategy leads to a triage system in which resources are allocated according to assessed need in an effort to maximize benefit at a fixed level of expenditure. This is not without its problems. Jessop and Stein (1991), in a provocative study designed to understand who benefits most from a pediatric home care program, found that maximal benefit was derived from those whose illness burden was small and whose coping resources (social, educational, financial, personal) were low. Prior to their study, home care was principally directed at families with the least coping resources and the greatest illness burden. Practicing in a climate of scarce resources might mean that those who are worse off, who more desperately need help, should not get it if the goal is solely to maximize benefit.

If the commitment to home care was based entirely on the idea that it is preferable to both child and family (caregivers), then a commitment to pay for whatever services are necessary—education, respite, counseling—would follow. Costs, of course, must be contained, as they always should maximize efficiency. However, it is conceivable that home care ultimately may not be a tremendous cost saver, but rather a more humane alternative to repeated routine hospitalization. Balancing these societal issues will require involvement and advocacy from all caregivers involved with children, including parents, teachers, and health-care professionals.

School Systems

Two important federal laws (P.L. 94-142, The Education for All Handicapped Children Act, in 1975, and an amendment to that law, P.L. 99-457, in 1986) have mandated educational services to children with special health-care needs, including preschool children and their families. These laws mandate parental involvement in the determination of educational goals and methods and provide channels for interaction between school systems and families of children with serious health-care needs.

As important as schools are in the lives of all children, and particularly for children with chronic health-care needs and possible learning problems, little attention has been paid to the ways in which educational systems and family systems interact around caregiving issues. Given the lack of interrater agreement often found between parent and teacher report measures, it is not surprising to find that teachers and parents show differences with respect to what they feel predicts adjustment of chronically ill children (Ayoub, Perrin, & Willett, 1991). Power and Bartholomew (1987) propose interesting theoretical styles of interaction between schools and families (e.g., avoidant, competitive, collaborative) that are ripe for research to operationalize these concepts and examine the impact of different styles and goodness of fit. Of interest, as well, is the process by which both family and school react to a perceived problem and how beliefs, problem-solving styles, and flexibility of all systems involved respond to crisis situations.

Parental Social Support Networks

Social support represents an important alternative to examining social isolation in families with chronically ill children. Whereas isolation is associated with health risk and psychopathology, social support is a strong protective factor (Cassel, 1976; Cobb, 1976). A striking statement in support of social support comes from House, Landis, and Umberson (1988), who state, "The evidence regarding social relationships and health increasingly approximates the evidence in the 1964 Surgeon General's report that established cigarette smoking as a cause or risk factor for mortality and morbidity from a range of diseases."

Size and other characteristics of parental social networks emerge as consistent differences between families with and without impaired children. Social networks of families with handicapped children have been found to be smaller, more dominated by family members, and more closely knit than others, with associations between these characteristics and parental distress (Kazak, 1987; Kazak & Wilcox, 1984; Kazak et al., 1988; Quitner, Gluekauf, & Jackson, 1990). Social support and its meanings may vary with age of the child or demands of the illness. Florian and Krulik (1991) present evidence of no relationship between social support and loneliness in mothers of children with life-threatening conditions, whereas a relationship between the two did exist for mothers of chronically ill children.

CONCLUSIONS

A social-ecological systems model provides a framework by which contextual factors affecting caregiving for chronically ill children can be understood. By examining family, school, and health-care system variables, issues that impact on caregiving can be identified for further research. A social-ecological approach also can incorporate the many changes in pediatric health care that have taken place in a relatively short period of time and have impacted upon children with serious health needs and their families. The ways in which seriously ill children are cared for by their families, the school system, the community, and the health-care system are in transition. The increase in home care, the survival of children once considered fatally ill, and the upsurge of technology-dependent children all have produced changes in the social-ecological systems of families with ill children. Many of these changes have ramifications that are not yet fully understood.

Our focus here has been specifically on the caregivers, elements of the social-ecological framework that often are overlooked in a child-centered model. Future research is needed to examine the impact on caregivers of having a seriously ill child and on the ways in which all caregiving systems interact. From a social-ecological perspective, identification of caregivers' characteristics that facilitate adaptive coping is needed. Similarly, the ways in which effective partnerships (with spouses, teachers, health-care providers) are established and the process by which they work effectively are in need of further research.

More research on gender issues related to caregiving is clearly warranted. A better understanding of what precisely puts female caregivers at increased risk for depression would be the first step toward helping them. Research on male caregivers' roles, with attention to why they often avoid caretaking responsibilities, might illuminate ways to help get them more involved.

As our analysis has emphasized, the family system is only one (albeit a critically important) system involved in the care of seriously ill children. Understanding other systems (e.g., schools and medical systems) and how they interact with families is critical. Serious childhood health problems necessitate long-term relationships among children, caregivers, and professionals. Clarification of the processes by which these relationships develop should be helpful in designing services and in providing policy recommendations.

REFERENCES

Ayoub, C., Perrin, E., & Willett, J. (1991, April). *Adjustment of children with a chronic illness: Child, parent, and teacher perspectives on the characteristics of the child.*

Paper presented at the biannual meeting of the Society for Research in Child Development, Seattle, WA.

Baskin, C., Forehand, R., & Saylor, C. (1986). Predictors of psychological adjustment in mothers of children with cancer. *Journal of Psychosocial Oncology, 3,* 43-54.

Bazyk, S. (1989). Changes in attitudes and beliefs regarding parent participation and home programs: An update. *American Journal of Occupational Therapy, 43*(11), 723-728.

Birkel, R. (1987). Toward a social ecology of the home-care household. *Psychology and Aging, 2*(3), 294-301.

Breslau, N. (1985). Psychiatric disorders in children with physical disabilities. *Journal of the American Academy of Child Psychiatry, 24,* 87-94.

Breslau, N., & Prabucki, K. (1987). Siblings of disabled children. *Archives of General Psychiatry, 44,* 1040-1046.

Breslau, N., Staruch, K. S., & Mortimer, E. A. (1982). Psychological distress in mothers of disabled children. *American Journal of Diseases of Childhood, 136,* 682-686.

Breslau, N., Weitzman, M., & Messenger, K. (1981). Psychologic functioning of siblings of disabled children. *Pediatrics, 67*(3), 344-353.

Bristol, M., Gallagher, J., & Schopler, E. (1988). Mothers and fathers of young developmentally disabled and nondisabled boys: Adaptation and spousal support. *Developmental Psychology, 24*(3), 444-451.

Brody, G., & Forehand, R. (1986). Maternal perceptions of child maladjustment as a function of the combined influence of child behavior and maternal depression. *Journal of Consulting and Clinical Psychology, 54*(2), 237-240.

Bronfenbrenner, U. (1979). *The ecology of human development.* Cambridge, MA: Harvard University Press.

Cadman, D., Boyle, M., Szatmari, P., & Offord, D. R. (1987). Chronic illness, disability, and mental and social well-being: Findings of the Ontario Child Health Study. *Pediatrics, 79*(5), 805-813.

Cadman, D., Rosenbaum, P., Boyle, M., & Offord, D. (1991). Children with chronic illness: Family and parent demographic characteristics and psychosocial adjustment. *Pediatrics, 87,* 884-889.

Carter, E., & McGoldrick, M. (1980). *The family life cycle: A framework for family therapy.* New York: Gardner.

Cassel, J. (1976). The contribution of the social environment to host resistance. *American Journal of Epidemiology, 104,* 107-123.

Cobb, S. (1976). Social support as a mediator of life stress. *Psychosomatic Medicine, 38,* 300-314.

Crutcher, D. (1991). Family support in the home: Home visiting and Public Law 99-457: A parent's perspective. *American Psychologist, 46*(2), 138-140.

Daniels, D., Miller, J. J., Billings, A. G., & Moos, R. H. (1987). Psychosocial functioning of siblings of children with rheumatic disease. *Journal of Pediatrics, 109*(2), 379-383.

Darling, R. B. (1987). The economic and psychosocial consequences of disability: Family-society relationships. In M. Ferrari & M. Sussman (Eds.), *Childhood disability and family systems* (pp. 45-61). New York: Haworth.

de Parra, M., de Cortazar, S., & Covarrubias-Espinoza, G. (1983). The adaptive pattern of families with a leukemic child. *Family Systems Medicine, 1,* 30-35.

Florian, V., & Krulik, T. (1991). Loneliness and social support of mothers of chronically ill children. *Social Science Medicine, 32*(11), 1291-1296.

Fox, H., & Newacheck, P. (1990). Private health insurance of chronically ill children. *Pediatrics, 85*(1), 50-57.

Friedrich, W. (1977). Ameliorating the psychological impact of chronic physical disease on the child and family. *Journal of Pediatric Psychology, 2,* 26-31.

Gath, A. (1978). *Down's syndrome and the family: The early years.* New York: Academic Press.

Hobbs, N., Perrin, J., & Ireys, H. (1985). *Chronically ill children and their families.* San Francisco: Jossey-Bass.

Horwitz, W., & Kazak, A. (1990). Family adaptation to childhood cancer: Sibling and family systems variables. *Journal of Clinical Child Psychology, 19,* 221-228.

House, J., Landis, K., & Umberson, D. (1988). Social relationships and health. *Science, 241,* 540-545.

Jessop, D., Riessman, C. K., & Stein, R. (1988). Chronic childhood illness and maternal mental health. *Developmental and Behavioral Pediatrics, 9*(3), 147-156.

Jessop, D., & Stein, R. (1991). Who benefits from a pediatric home care program? *Pediatrics, 88*(3), 497-505.

Kazak, A. E. (1986). Families with physically handicapped children: Social ecology and family systems. *Family Process, 25,* 265-281.

Kazak, A. E. (1987). Families with disabled children: Stress and social networks in three samples. *Journal of Abnormal Child Psychology, 15*(1), 137-146.

Kazak, A. E. (1989). Families of chronically ill children: A systems and social-ecological model of adaptation and challenge. *Journal of Consulting and Clinical Psychology, 57*(1), 25-30.

Kazak, A. E., & Marvin, R. S. (1984). Differences, difficulties and adaptation: Stress and social networks in families with a handicapped child. *Family Relations, 33,* 67-77.

Kazak, A. E., & Meadows, A. (1989). Families of young adolescents who have survived cancer: Social-emotional adjustment, adaptability, and social support. *Journal of Pediatric Psychology, 14,* 175-191.

Kazak, A. E., Reber, M., & Snitzer, L. (1988). Chronic childhood disease and family functioning: A study of phenylketonuria. *Pediatrics, 81,* 224-230.

Kazak, A. E., & Wilcox, B. (1984). The structure and function of social networks in families with handicapped children. *American Journal of Community Psychology, 12,* 645-661.

Lange, B. (1991). Unpublished raw data collected from Family Centered Community-based Services for Children with Cancer. Project funded by the Bureau of Maternal and Child Health.

Leonard, B. J., Brust, J. D., Janny, D., & Patterson, J. (1991). Home care reimbursement for technology-dependent children: Its impact on parental distress. *Alternative Lifestyles, 12*(1), 63-76.

McAndrew, I. (1976). Children with a handicap and their families. *Child: Care, Health and Development, 2,* 213-237.

McHale, S., & Gamble, W. (1989). Sibling relationships of children with disabled and nondisabled brothers and sisters. *Developmental Psychology, 25*(3), 421-429.

Mohide, E. A., Pringle, D. M., Streiner, D. L., Gilbert, J. R., Muir, G., & Tew, M. (1990). A randomized trial of family caregiver support in the home management of dementia. *Journal of the American Geriatrics Society, 38,* 446-454.

Mueller, M., & Leviton, A. (1986). In-home versus clinic-based services for the developmentally disabled child: Who is the primary client—Parent or child? *Social Work in Health Care, 11*(3), 75-88.

Noelker, L., & Bass, D. (1989). Home care for elderly persons: Linkages between formal and informal caregivers. *Journal of Gerontology, 44*(2), 563-570.

Olshansky, S. (1962). Chronic sorrow: A response to having a mentally defective child. *Social Casework, 43*, 190-193.

Parks, S. H., & Pilisuk, M. (1991). Caregiver burden: Gender and psychological costs of caregiving. *American Journal of Orthopsychiatry, 61*(4), 501-509.

Pfefferbaum, B., Adams, J., & Aceves, J. (1990). The influence of culture on pain in Anglo and Hispanic children with cancer. *Journal of the American Academy of Child and Adolescent Psychiatry, 29*, 642-647.

Power, T., & Bartholomew, K. (1987). Family-school relationship patterns: An ecological assessment. *School Psychology Review, 16*, 498-512.

Quitner, A., Gluekauf, R., & Jackson, D. (1990). Chronic parenting stress: Moderating versus mediating effects of social support. *Journal of Personality and Social Psychology, 59*, 1266-1278.

Reiss, D., & De-Nour, A. (1989). The family and medical team in chronic illness: A transactional and developmental perspective. In C. N. Ramsey, Jr. (Ed.), *Family systems in medicine* (pp. 435-444). New York: Guilford.

Rolland, J. (1984). Towards a psychosocial typology of chronic and life threatening illness. *Family Systems Medicine, 2*, 245-262.

Rolland, J. (1987). Chronic illness and the life cycle: A conceptual framework. *Family Process, 26*, 203-221.

Sabbeth, B., & Levethal, J. (1984). Marital adjustment to chronic childhood illness. *Pediatrics, 73*, 762-768.

Stein, R., & Jessop, D. (1982). A noncategorical approach to childhood chronic illness. *Public Health Reports, 97*, 354-362.

Steinhausen, H., Schindler, H., & Stephan, H. (1983). Correlates of psychopathology in sick children: An empirical model. *Journal of the American Academy of Child Psychiatry, 22*, 559-564.

Stephens, M., Kinney, J., & Ogrocki, P. (1991). Stressors and well-being among caregivers to older adults with dementia: The in-home versus nursing home experience. *The Gerontologist, 31*(2), 217-223.

Wallander, J., Feldman, W., & Varni, J. (1989). Physical status of psychosocial adjustment in children with spina bifida. *Journal of Pediatric Psychology, 14*(1), 89-102.

Wallander, J., Varni, J. W., Babani, L., Banis, H. T., & Wilcox, K. T. (1988). Children with chronic physical disorders: Maternal reports of their psychological adjustment. *Journal of Pediatric Psychology, 13*(2), 197-212.

Weiss, S. (1991). Stressors experienced by family caregivers of children with pervasive developmental disorders. *Child Psychiatry and Human Development, 21*(3), 203-216.

Wood, B., Boyle, J. T., Watkins, J. B., Nogueira, J., Zimand, E., & Carroll, L. (1988). Sibling psychological status and style as related to the disease of their chronically ill brothers and sisters: Implications for models of biopsychosocial interaction. *Developmental and Behavioral Pediatrics, 9*(2), 66-72.

Young, R., & Kahana, E. (1989). Specifying caregiver outcomes: Gender and relationship aspects of caregiving strain. *The Gerontologist, 29*(5), 660-666.

14

Relationships Between
the Frail Elderly's Informal
and Formal Helpers

LINDA S. NOELKER
DAVID M. BASS

Gerontologists have had a long-standing interest in the elderly's social relationships and social support, particularly their integration in the family system and intergenerational exchanges. With the increasing number of chronically disabled aged, a substantial amount of recent gerontological research has focused on vulnerable or frail elderly and their use of assistance. Much of this research is confined to care by immediate family members (spouses and adult children), leading some to argue that caregiving research is characterized by an "ideology of intimacy" (Krause, 1990; Lee, 1985). This restricted focus detracts from the importance of other informal helpers, such as siblings, friends, and neighbors, and of formal service providers as the frail elderly's caregivers (Krause, 1990; Penning, 1990).

The emphasis on immediate family caregivers also takes attention away from developing models of the relationship *between* informal and formal helpers as partners in the caregiving process. Conceptual advances in this area have been further limited by an overwhelming reliance on cross-sectional research designs that prohibit investigation

---

AUTHORS' NOTE: This chapter was prepared with support from the National Institute of Mental Health (MH 45918-02). The authors thank their colleague Gary Deimling for his helpful comments on the manuscript.

of changes in the mix of informal-formal helpers over the course of long-term caregiving (Jette, Tennstedt, & Branch, 1992).

To promote more conceptual and empirical attention to the relationship between informal and formal helpers, this chapter reviews three existing conceptualizations of this relationship. The basic tenets of each approach are outlined along with its underlying assumptions and empirical support. The chapter also reviews findings from the authors' research on the frail elderly's informal and formal helpers, which led to the development of an integrated model that draws on the strengths of prior conceptual work.

EXISTING MODELS OF INFORMAL-FORMAL RELATIONSHIPS

The Hierarchical Compensatory Model

A widely recognized conceptual approach linking informal and formal helpers is Cantor's hierarchical compensatory model (1979). It posits that the source of assistance follows a pattern based on the primacy or closeness of social relationships. A key element in the model is the notion of succession, meaning that societal norms about the primacy of relationships govern the elderly's preferences for help. These norms make the frail elder's spouse the first choice as caregiver, followed by children, and then other kin. Thus caregiving activities are expected to be performed by the closest family member who is available and capable of helping. If kin are unavailable, friends and neighbors are the next choices for assistance, followed by formal service providers. When the involvement of formal helpers is necessary, their assistance typically is confined to a relatively narrow range of tasks, in contrast to the informal support network, which provides a far broader base of assistance.

More recently Cantor (1989, 1991) has enlarged the hierarchical compensatory model to the "social care system." This expansion of the model maintains its emphasis on assistance source and hierarchy; however, it gives greater attention to the interrelatedness of the informal and formal systems. The social care system allows for more fluidity or overlap among the hierarchical levels and acknowledges that the elder's functional status and the availability of informal care influence assistance use. Yet the basic principle that family and then other informal helpers are the first choice for assistance is at the foundation of the broader reformulated model.

Implicit in the hierarchical compensatory model are several assumptions. One is that there is societal consensus on norms of filial obligation dictating the primacy of helpers. However, in a pluralistic society comprised of many racial and ethnic groups, both the content and strength of filial norms are likely to vary across population groups. Empirical evidence supports this view by showing that intergenerational family exchanges vary in relation to available resources as well as cultural norms (Akiyama, Antonucci, & Campbell, 1990). When there is cultural divergence on filial norms, the influence of individual preferences for care and other factors are likely to play a more important role than the hierarchical model indicates.

The model also gives a secondary role to the specific types of help needed in relation to the resources of available helpers. The dimensions of a task, such as frequency and amount of time required and skill level, are seen as having some effect on the choice of helpers. However, in this model the type of task is of less importance in helper choice than the nature of support preferences, in which immediate kin predominate.

The hierarchical model as well as other conceptualizations of family care implicitly regard it as the preferable care arrangement as it appears to be the first choice of older people and their kin. Yet research shows that informal caregivers, namely spouses and adult children, often continue functioning as the sole care provider even when the type and amount of help needed by the frail older relative exceed the caregiver's capacity (Frankfather, Smith, & Caro, 1981; Gerace & Noelker, 1990; Hess & Soldo, 1985). In these situations the negative effects of informal care are conceptualized chiefly in terms of caregiver stress and burden rather than care-receiver health and well-being or quality of care. This approach stands in sharp contrast to outcomes of interest in formal care settings for frail elderly, in which negative effects are centered on patient outcomes such as nutritional status, depression, and mismanaged medications.

Empirical Support for the Model

Support for the hierarchical compensatory model derives from studies of older persons' informal support systems that consistently identify the prominent place of primary kin caregivers. Cantor's initial research (1979) on the model was designed to test the relative importance of task and helper relationship in the support choices of inner-city elderly. Findings showed that when respondents were asked to choose to whom other than a spouse they would turn if 10 types of instrumental and affective support were needed, children were the overwhelming choice. This pattern persisted even when controls for the proximity and frequency of contact with children were introduced. Formal sources of help rarely were selected regardless of task. Cantor's subsequent research (1983), guided by the hierarchical model, investigated various types of informal caregivers (spouse, child, other relative, friend, or neighbor) in relation to the nature and extent of caregiving strain they reported.

More recent research has offered less support for the hierarchical compensatory model. Auslander and Litwin (1990) compared Israeli elderly who did and did not apply for public social services in order to test the premise that older persons use formal services when informal helpers are unavailable or unable to provide sufficient help. Based on the hierarchical model, it was expected that those who applied for formal assistance more often would lack informal supports. Results did show that applicants for formal services had smaller networks, had fewer immediate and proximate kin, and perceived the network as less emotionally supportive. However, the only significant difference in network composition was that applicants less often had a spouse. No differences were found in the presence of children, other family members, friends, and neighbors. Thus available children and other informal helpers did not uniformly provide assistance in the absence of a spouse. Moreover, structural and qualitative characteristics of the informal network, such as composition, size, and perceived quality, were shown to have important influences on the source of assistance.

In a study of Manitoba elderly, Penning (1990) found limited support for the hierarchical model. There was evidence for a hierarchical ordering of informal helpers; when spouses were present, they were named most often as helping with tasks, followed by children for spouseless elderly. However, support was not found for the compensatory premise of the model, meaning that elderly without a spouse were more likely to make do without help than to receive help from children. There also was no evidence indicating that the availability or sufficiency of informal help affected the use of formal help.

The Task-Specific Model

A second conceptual approach to the relationship between informal and formal support is Litwak's task-specific model (1985). In this model, sources of help are governed by the types of tasks for which assistance is needed. The model maintains that the structural characteristics of informal and formal groups differ, making each group more suitable for providing certain types of help.

The informal system, by virtue of its primary group structure, is most appropriate for unpredictable, nonuniform, and nontechnical tasks. The formal system's group structure makes it the best for handling specialized and predictable tasks. Hence a chief premise of the model is that assistance patterns are governed by the goodness of fit between group and task characteristics.

Because informal and formal groups are structurally suited to different types of tasks, dual specialization or task segregation occurs. This means that certain tasks fall within the domain of informal helpers, whereas others are in the purview of formal helpers. The clear division of labor between formal and informal helpers promotes efficiency in task performance and inhibits intergroup conflict stemming from differences in the structural characteristics of each group.

The model's focus on the fit between characteristics of tasks and groups assumes positive outcomes for appropriate matches; however, these outcomes have not been well explicated or widely investigated. For example, the model posits that dual specialization minimizes conflict between informal networks and formal systems, yet the prevalence, nature, and manifestations of this conflict are unclear. Apart from intergroup conflict, other outcomes of interest, such as burden and strain among informal caregivers and formal helpers' job satisfaction, are not an integral part of the model. Similarly, the outcomes for frail elderly, such as improved functioning, lessened emotional strain, and satisfaction with the care arrangement, are not an explicit focus of the model.

The model's more macro orientation toward group structures also takes attention away from the diversity that is found within primary groups and formal systems. Although informal groups share certain characteristics, such as an affective orientation, they vary considerably in their structural features (size, composition, density of ties) and in the sociodemographic, attitudinal, and other personal characteristics of their members. The relative impact of these factors, in contrast to the goodness of fit between group and task characteristics, on caregiving outcomes has not been established.

Empirical Support for the Model

Findings from Litwak's (1985) research on a sample of persons over 65 years of age from New York and Florida lend empirical support to the task-specific model. His application of the model included a variety of other constructs, such as ethnicity, age, and family size, that modified assistance patterns but did not change the fundamental principle of linking task characteristics and group structure.

Recent research using a national sample of unmarried elderly women offered some support for the task-specific model (Soldo, Wolf, & Agree, 1990). Results from this investigation indicated that adult children are better suited to help with personal care and instrumental activities of daily living when compared to other informal caregivers. Also, as previously reviewed, some support was found for Litwak's task-specific model in Penning's (1990) study. Different types of helpers, particularly spouses and adult children, assisted with different activities. This study, however, as in many empirical investigations of the task-specific model, examined only a narrow range of tasks rather than the full continuum of assistance needed by frail older persons. Furthermore, studies testing the task-specific model often use hypothetical support situations to elicit helper choices because respondents have relatively few, if any, impairments and assistance needs. To adequately test this model, research should be designed to determine the contributions made by all helpers across a broad range of tasks with which frail elderly actually receive assistance.

Supplementation

A third conceptualization of the informal-formal relationship is supplementation (Edelman, 1986). Although this concept has not been incorporated into a broader model or framework of the informal-formal relationship, it does offer an alternative perspective to the hierarchical and task-specific models. Supplementation posits that formal support buttresses the informal network by sharing in the impaired aged's care. The concept of "task sharing" between the informal and formal systems distinguishes supplementation from the hierarchical compensatory model, in which formal service use is associated with unavailable or insufficient informal help. Supplementation differs from the task-specific model because formal and informal helpers can assist with the same tasks without negative outcomes such as intergroup conflict.

Supplementation generally refers to routine rather than highly skilled or technical care. In fact, the model asserts that most care needed by chronically ill and disabled older persons is ongoing routine assistance with personal care and activities of daily living. It emphasizes that routine care can be time-consuming and exhausting for informal caregivers, particularly elderly spouses, who can benefit from relief or respite service. Hence, in this conceptual approach, a primary purpose of formal help is to share the care with informal helpers rather than to substitute for them or solely provide specialized types of help.

The concept of supplementation countermands the policy position that increasing the availability of formal services will encourage families to relinquish their caregiving role, thereby increasing the public costs of caring for frail elderly (Greene, 1983). Although supplementation acknowledges that in some instances services are used as a replacement for kin care when families are unable or unwilling to accept caregiving responsibilities, it maintains that formal services mainly are used by family caregivers who require support and periodic, not permanent, relief from their responsibilities. In these situations formal service use can forestall caregiver stress or burnout, thus enabling family caregiving to continue over a longer period.

Supplementation assumes that the frail elderly's increasing dependency and the consequent strain on informal helpers govern the type and volume of both informal and formal assistance use. As the elderly's care needs grow, the efforts of informal helpers increase, along with their burdens, and the formal system responds with supportive services. Similar to the hierarchical compensatory and task-specific models, supplementation assumes a rationality or orderliness to the informal and formal systems that some conflict theorists may view more as the exception than the rule. Formal systems do not always allocate services in response to caregiver burden and, in fact, may be prohibited from doing so (Carrilio & Eisenberg, 1983; Noelker, 1984). Also, as was previously noted, informal caregivers frequently resist service use despite the jeopardy to their own health and well-being.

Empirical Findings

In a sample of homebound elderly persons in Chicago, supplemental help from formal providers was more frequently observed than substitution of formal for informal help (Edelman & Hughes, 1990). Findings from this panel study showed that informal caregiving patterns were stable even four years after formal services were introduced. Moreover, an increase in formal service use was associated with increased informal care. The increase in both formal and informal help was interpreted as an indicator of escalating care needs and caregiver strain. A more conclusive explanation of the findings could not be given because no measures of caregiver strain or service goals, such as respite for the caregiver, were included in this research. At the same time the results are seen as supporting the concept of supplementation because informal helpers maintained their role even when formal assistance was used, thus contradicting the premise that formal services will be used to substitute for informal care.

The authors' research also supports the concept of supplementation (Noelker & Bass, 1989). Our study of 519 spouse and adult-child primary caregivers who lived with their frail older relative showed that in 37% of the cases help with at least one type of task was given by both the primary caregiver and a formal service provider. Similarly, when the elder's care needs and caregiver burden were greater, more intense service use occurred.

TOWARD AN INTEGRATED MODEL OF INFORMAL-FORMAL ASSISTANCE

Each conceptualization outlined above provides a plausible description of the relationship between informal and formal helpers. The literatures on family caregiving and formal service use, however, suggest that these models and their application have several limitations. One is that research on help provided by informal caregivers has tended to investigate only a limited number of tasks or task categories with which chronically impaired elderly receive assistance. These studies have tended to focus on a particular type of help, such as personal care, or on broad categories of help, such as emotional support and activities of daily living.

Within any one category, tasks are likely to vary in difficulty, skill level, and time required. For example, in the personal care category, activities such as bathing or transferring from bed to chair require lifting and thus demand strength and stamina on the caregiver's part. Helping with these tasks is likely to be especially problematic for older caregivers, who frequently have chronic illnesses and related functional impairments of their own. In contrast, providing assistance with eating by cutting meat, buttering bread, or feeding the impaired person is less physically demanding. With this in mind, subsequent research on caregiving and service use should give more attention to the variety of tasks within assistance categories as well as to help provided with a wider variety of tasks.

A second limitation hampering refinement of caregiving models is that research studies often have investigated the elderly's choice of helpers in relation to *hypothetical* tasks with which assistance may be required at some later point. These models cannot be adequately tested to determine variability in informal-formal relationships until all persons actually involved in helping are investigated. Moreover, every helper's contribution in relation to all tasks with which he or she provides assistance should be investigated.

A third limitation of the caregiving models is their relatively static orientation, reflected in the focus on a single factor seen as exerting the primary influence on informal-formal helper relationships across time. It is more likely that changes occur in the nature of informal-formal helper relationships during the course of caregiving and that a number of factors, apart from task characteristics or helper preferences, have important influences on these changes. The fact that each model has received some empirical support suggests that no one approach adequately represents the dynamic features of frail elderly's helping networks over the different phases or stages of long-term caregiving.

A fourth limitation of existing conceptualizations is that they do not incorporate the wide range of contingencies influencing help-seeking behavior. Research on predictors of service use by older persons has delineated a number of these contingencies, some of which include personal characteristics of the impaired person and informal helpers, characteristics of the service environment such as the availability of services in a community, and beliefs about the efficacy of formal assistance. Contingencies that account for differences in contact with a service and service use patterns, such as adequate insurance coverage, also affect the interface between formal and informal helpers.

Another limitation of existing conceptual approaches is that their application has tended to include a narrow range of informal helpers. For example, a disproportionate amount of attention has been given to the primary or nuclear kin caregiver (Krause, 1990; Lee, 1985). This limitation is further compounded by the fact that definitions of "primary" have varied across investigations, which prohibits cross-study comparisons of results (Barer & Johnson, 1990). Based on recent evidence underscoring the active role of secondary informal caregivers (Tennstedt, McKinlay, & Sullivan, 1989), subsequent investigations should reflect a more comprehensive view of informal helpers that moves beyond the primary caregiver to the total helping network.

Research on the elderly's use of formal services also has adopted a narrow view of the formal network, often because of methodological or design limitations. For example, in a number of studies of community-residing elderly, the samples were categorized as service users and nonusers, regardless of type of service used or the number of service providers. This approach was necessary because the low incidence of service use precluded examination of specific services (see Bass & Noelker, 1987, for a review of these studies). Other studies have attempted to compensate for the small number of users by grouping services under a broader rubric, such as home health care, that encompasses different services such as nursing, speech and physical therapies, and home health aide service.

Last, little systematic attention has been given to informal helpers' use of services designed for caregivers, such as support groups, respite care, and education programs. The availability of caregiver services has grown during the past decade, and several of these services provide education and counseling for caregivers about how to access community services on behalf of their impaired relative. Consequently, future studies should give attention to the nature and extent of service use by caregivers and how their use of services affects patterns of service use by the frail elderly.

Empirical Grounding of the Integrated Model

Our development of an integrated conceptual model began with the assumption that each conceptual approach reviewed here accurately depicted the informal-formal relationship in some caregiving circumstances. The model's development emanated from an empirical investigation that examined the predictors of the frail elder's use of formal help with 13 personal care and home health tasks using cross-sectional data from 586 caregiving families (Bass & Noelker, 1987).

This study was premised on the assumption that both the frail elder's and primary kin caregivers' characteristics are important determinants of service use. When primary caregivers are spouses or adult children living with a frail older relative, they can have a direct influence on formal service use by arranging for the service. They also can exert an indirect influence by altering the older person's perceptions of service need, imparting knowledge about service availability, or affecting service providers' assessments of need to include caregiver burden and strain. Findings from this research sensitized us to the following: the importance of including both elder and caregiver variables as predictors of service use, the greater involvement of both informal and formal helpers when the elder is more disabled, and the differences in predictors of *contact* with the service and *volume* of use.

Our subsequent research gave more detailed attention to the nature of task sharing and task segregation by primary kin caregivers and service providers around the same personal care and home health tasks (Noelker & Bass, 1989). This investigation sought to develop a typology of informal-formal helper relationships that was not based on any one conceptual approach, but defined the relationships as they emerged from study data.

Findings offered some support for each of the three conceptual approaches. Specifically, results showed that 42% of the families relied exclusively on informal helpers, a type that we defined as "kin independence" from the service sector. In these cases the spouse or adult child primary caregiver provided the personal and home health care with which the impaired elder needed help. This type is consistent with the *hierarchical compensatory model* because nuclear kin gave the needed assistance.

Another 21% of the primary caregivers reported that formal service providers helped with different personal and home health tasks than those performed by the spouse or adult child caregiver. This group of families represented the *task-specific model* and its concept of dual specialization.

In 9% of the cases, service providers assisted with the same personal and home health tasks as primary kin caregivers, thus representing the *supplementation model*. Primary kin caregivers and service providers in the remaining 28% of families shared in the performance of some personal and home health tasks, but at least one additional task was performed exclusively by a formal helper. This relationship combined *task specialization and supplementation* to form an unanticipated type defined as supplementation/specialization.

Subsequent analyses sought to explain why this variation existed in informal-formal relationships by identifying the factors or contingencies that accounted for them. The Andersen model, widely employed in research designed to predict service use (Andersen & Aday, 1978), provides a framework for conceptualizing these explanatory factors into categories related to characteristics of the service users. As noted earlier, this framework was expanded in our first study to include characteristics of the primary kin caregiver as well as the frail older person (Bass & Noelker, 1987).

The expanded Andersen framework includes predisposing, enabling, and need characteristics of the care recipient and primary caregiver. Predisposing factors refer to sociodemographic characteristics and health-related attitudes. Enabling factors include economic and social resources that promote or inhibit service use. Some enabling characteristics are common to both members of the caregiving dyad when they share a household, such as income and proximity to service sites. Other enabling characteristics, such as education or knowledge about service availability and access, may differ for the frail elder and the caregiver.

Need characteristics of the care receiver represent the illness or disability that necessitates assistance use. Some studies indicate these factors are the strongest predictors of service use (Miller & McFall, 1991). Caregiver need characteristics encompass stress effects resulting from caregiving, such as restricted activities, health deterioration, and financial losses. In family care research these effects frequently have been assessed using measures of caregiver burden or strain (Deimling & Bass, 1986; Kinney & Stephens, 1989; Lawton, Kleban, Moss, Rovine, & Glicksman, 1989; Zarit, Reever, & Bach-Peterson, 1980).

Results from multivariate analyses showed that family care situations in which no formal services were used, representing the hierarchical compensatory model, typically had elderly care receivers with fewer physical impairments and kin caregivers who were less burdened. In contrast, high levels of impairment and burden were predictive of the supplementation/specialization type, in which formal providers and caregivers helped with some of the same tasks but formal helpers also provided specialized assistance with others. The supplementation model was more typical of women caregivers who reported more social isolation because of caregiving. The task-specific or dual-specialization type was more common to caregiving husbands who reported higher levels of burden and to less impaired care receivers.

Overall, study findings showed that some types of informal-formal relationships were related to stable characteristics such as the primary caregiver's gender. Other types were related to dynamic characteristics such as the care receiver's functional status and caregiver burden. The importance of these dynamic characteristics in distinguishing informal-formal helper relationships suggests that relationships observed at one point in time will be altered as impairment, caregiver strain, and other factors in the care situation change.

Research on the Integrated Model: Study Design

Our previous work was limited by its focus on a narrow range of informal and formal helpers (the primary spouse or adult child caregiver and home health providers) and on only 13 personal care and home health tasks. It was further limited by an inability to represent all the important predisposing, enabling, and need characteristics suggested by the expanded Andersen framework. Consequently, a larger study currently underway utilizes an expansion of the Andersen framework to examine helping patterns around a broad range of tasks. The study's first objective is to determine the factors that differentiate among various types of informal-formal relationships based on the helpers' involvement with specific tasks and task areas. Its second objective is to identify predictors of the different types of community-based services used by frail elderly and predictors of the caregiver services used by their informal helpers.

The study design is a cross-sectional survey involving in-person interviews with approximately 500 elderly clients who currently receive case management and other services from five nonprofit agencies in the greater Cleveland, Ohio, area. Interviews also are conducted with the person identified by each client as the primary informal caregiver. In addition, the clients' case managers complete a questionnaire for each client-caregiver dyad on dimensions of service use (type, units provided, reimbursement source) and service goals. The study's cross-sectional design was selected over a panel design for two reasons: Prior research has not yielded sufficient information to specify relationships between predictor variables and study outcomes, and the study's focus is on predictors of outcomes rather than changes in those outcomes.

Clients of multiservice agencies were seen as the optimal population from which to draw the study sample because these agencies make an array of services available to impaired older persons. Hence samples from this source contain active service users, thereby avoiding the problem of limited service use commonly encountered in investigations relying on general samples of community-residing elderly.

Moreover, the case managers at multiservice agencies typically can access their own agency's services on a client's behalf as well as services from other agencies (Austin, 1988; Capitman, Haskins, & Bernstein, 1986; Secord, 1987). Frail elderly with a variety of assistance needs thus benefit from the service-coordination function of case management and the "package" of services tailored to their needs. Because multiple services are commonly used by this client population, it lends itself to studies seeking to identify the predictors of different service types such as telephone reassurance, home-delivered meals, and day programs.

An additional reason that the study sample is drawn from case-managed elderly client populations is that case-management practice principles mandate full utilization of informal helpers to meet the clients' assistance needs, with formal services used to fill in the gaps. As a result clients receiving case management are likely to have varied combinations of informal and formal helpers in their support networks, making this population well suited to research on the diversity in relationships between informal and formal helpers around care tasks.

A second case-management practice principle relevant to research on informal-formal helper relationships is that the informal helpers of elderly clients should be given the support and assistance they need to function effectively in the caregiver role (Gwyther, 1988; Gwyther, Gold, & Hinman-Smith, 1988; Schneider, 1988; Seltzer, Ivry, & Litchfield, 1987). As a result of this practice principle, multiservice agencies increasingly have made caregiver counseling, support groups, respite care, and other services available to clients' informal helpers. The advantage for this research study is that case-managed client populations lend themselves to investigations of service use by both elderly clients and informal caregivers and to the relationship between their patterns of service use.

Another advantage to drawing the study sample from clients of multiservice agencies is that agency staff can provide more rigorous data than client and caregiver respondents on specific dimensions of service use such as units provided and reimbursement sources. When derived from agency accounting and billing records, the data is likely to be more timely and accurate than information reported by service consumers because the information is used for service reimbursement purposes and is audited.

The Study's Conceptual Approach

To link informal and formal helpers around a variety of care tasks and task areas, a list of tasks with which frail elderly need assistance was compiled. This list was based on our survey research data on the types of help provided to frail elderly, information from care plans for the Benjamin Rose Institute's community-based clients, and a review of data collection instruments from other studies of informal caregiving and formal service use. As Table 14.1 shows, 44 tasks were identified and were grouped into 9 task areas. The purpose of grouping the tasks into areas was to simplify and shorten the interview process. More specifically, information on each helper's identity and characteristics is obtained for all task areas; however, categorical information about helpers is collected for each task (primary caregiver, other informal helper, formal helper).

The task areas and tasks are linked with corresponding services that provide assistance with the different tasks. As Table 14.1 shows, the 44 tasks correspond to 28 health and social services designed for community-residing frail older persons. This approach enables us to identify both the nature and extent of formal service use and the various combinations of informal and formal helpers around specific tasks, because the characteristics of each formal helper (e.g., day-care worker, home health aide) are ascertained in relation to each task area and the categories of helper types are determined for each task.

The study's conceptual framework was expanded to include a wider array of predisposing, enabling, and need factors for frail elderly and their informal helpers as shown in Table 14.2. The predisposing factors that were added to gender, age, race, and caregiver-receiver relationship were service-use beliefs and beliefs about filial obligation. Service beliefs were included based on research showing that beliefs about the availability, accessibility, acceptability, and affordability of services influence service seeking and use (Collins, Stommel, King, & Given, 1991; McKinlay, 1972; Mechanic, 1979; Petchers & Milligan, 1988). Moreover, these beliefs are likely to derive from an individual's cultural background, and thus they can help to clarify black-white differences found in both informal and formal assistance use (Gerace & Noelker, 1990; Gibson, 1982; Soldo et al., 1990).

Beliefs about family responsibility were conceptualized as perceived obligations to provide care to ill or impaired family members, to share this responsibility with other persons from outside the family, and to monitor or manage formal services used by older relatives (Teresi, Toner, Bennett, & Wilder, 1988). Previous studies suggest that beliefs about filial obligations also account for black-white differences in the size and composition of the elderly's helping networks, the duration and intensity of informal caregiving, and the use of nursing home care (see Antonucci & Cantor, 1991, for an overview).

The category of enabling factors also was expanded to include qualitative features of the helping network, conceptualized as appraisals of the adequacy, promptness, and supportiveness of help given by network members. This addition results from recent research findings on social support indicating that these qualitative features are conceptually and empirically distinct from the structural and functional features of helping networks (Seeman & Berkman, 1988; Vaux & Athanassopulou, 1987; Vaux et al., 1986).

Additional enabling factors in the expanded framework include income sources, insurance for health and social services, and perceived adequacy of finances. Because our preliminary studies demonstrated the importance of household income as a predictor of the volume of home health service use, greater attention is being given in this research to aspects of income that can more directly affect service use, such as health insurance coverage. In addition, subjective and objective features of financial resources are included based on prior investigations showing that some elderly and informal caregivers, regardless of actual income level, are reluctant to accept service in order to conserve their savings in anticipation of future care needs, namely, nursing home care (George, 1987; Saperstein, 1988).

As Table 14.2 shows, relatively more emphasis is being given in our current study to the need characteristics of both care receivers and caregivers because the importance of these characteristics has been demonstrated in prior studies of the elderly's service utilization (Bass & Noelker, 1987; McAuley & Arling, 1984; Miller & McFall, 1991). Although our original conceptualization of care-receiver need factors was multidimensional, covering physical, cognitive, and behavioral impairments, this category was broadened in the expanded model. Additional care-receiver need characteristics include diagnosed health conditions, health symptoms, sensory limitations, and mental status. The last is of particular importance as recent research has shown that the use of formal and informal help differs for frail elderly who are either cognitively intact or impaired (Birkel & Jones, 1989; Soldo et al., 1990).

TABLE 14.1 Task Areas and Corresponding Service Types

Task Areas and Tasks	Corresponding Service Types
Socioemotional Support	
Counseling	Therapeutic or mental health counseling service
Problem solving	Friendly visiting service
Information/advice	Companion service
Emotional support	Senior centers
Temporary relief/respite	Adult day care
Socializing	Support groups/peer counseling
	Hospice
Care Management	
Getting service information/referral	Care management service
Planning for services	Information and referral service
Locating services	Advocacy
Coordinating assistance use	Relocation and placement
Monitoring services	
Advocacy	
Personal Care	
Bathing	Home health aide service
Grooming	Adult day care
Toileting	Short-stay residential care
Dressing	Hospice
Feeding	
Transferring bed or chair	
Ambulation in house	
Health Care	
Blood pressure monitoring	Home health aide service
Giving injections	In-home nursing service
Catheter care	Occupational, physical, or speech therapy
Colostomy care	Short-stay residential care
Tube feeding	Adult day care
Cleaning or dressing wounds	Hospice
Monitoring medications	
Checking pulse/respiration	
Instruction about care	
Special exercise/therapy	

TABLE 14.1 Continued

Task Areas and Tasks	Corresponding Service Types
Checking and Monitoring	
Continuous supervision	Telephone reassurance
Regular checking	Friendly visiting service
Telephone monitoring	Emergency monitoring service
	→ Adult day care
	Short-stay residential care
	Hospice
Household	
Washing dishes	Homemaker service
Laundry	Chore service
Light cleaning	→ Home-delivered or congregate meals
Preparing meals	Hospice
Heavy housework	
Finances	
Paying bills	→ Money management service
Banking	
Outside Household	
Shopping/errands	Case aide service
Yard maintenance	→ Chore service
Home maintenance	
Transport and Escort	
	→ Transportation/escort service
	Adult day care

Informal caregivers' subjective reports about the care receivers' cognitive status also are included as need characteristics, along with more objective assessments of cognitive status. The relative influence of these two types of mental status measures on caregiver burden and service use is of substantive interest, as is the relationship between them because a large portion of family care studies rely only on caregivers' reports. Last, recent advances in the conceptualization and measurement of caregiver burden and caregiving's effects on informal helpers indicate that

TABLE 14.2 Predictor Characteristics and Service Use Outcomes

	Pertains to:	
Predictor Characteristics	*Care Receiver*	*Primary Caregiver*
Predisposing Characteristics		
A. Family and Household Structure	✓	✓
B. Occupation and Employment Status		✓
C. Beliefs About Service Use	✓	✓
Acceptability		
Availability		
Accessibility		
D. Beliefs About Family Responsibility	✓	✓
Enabling Characteristics		
A. Financial Resources		
Income and income sources	✓	✓
Perceived adequacy	✓	✓
Insurance coverage	✓	✓
B. Education	✓	✓
C. Structure of Informal Helping Network	✓	✓
D. Appraisal of Network Quality	✓	✓
Need Characteristics		
A. Health Status	✓	✓
Perceived health	✓	✓
Health conditions	✓	✓
Reported health symptoms	✓	✓
Reported sick days	✓	
B. Physical Functioning		
Activities of daily living (ADL)	✓	
Instrumental activities of daily living (IADL)		✓
Incontinence		✓
Sensory limitations	✓	
Disability	✓	
C. Symptoms of Care Receiver's Mental Impairment		
Assessed cognitive status	✓	
Subjective memory problems		✓
Reported cognitive incapacity		✓
Disruptive behaviors		✓
Social functioning		✓

TABLE 14.2 Continued

Predictor Characteristics	Pertains to:	
	Care Receiver	Primary Caregiver
D. General Well-being		
Depression	✓	✓
Life satisfaction	✓	✓
E. Positive and Negative Caregiving Effects		
Caregiving satisfaction		✓
Caregiving mastery		✓
Physical health change		✓
Emotional health change		✓
Relationship strain		✓
Social activity restriction		✓
Work and financial care-related strain		✓
Service Use Outcomes		
A. Care Receivers' Assistance Use	✓	
Task areas and service or help	✓	
Supplemental service data		✓
B. Caregiver Service Use		✓
Service types		✓
Volume of service use		
Auspice, provider type, location, cost		

improvements are required in this need category to enhance the predictive power of the caregiver need characteristics (Lawton et al., 1989).

The expanded conceptualization shown in Table 14.2 suggests a broader view and more diverse measures of the service-use outcomes because these measures are likely to have different predictors (Bass & Noelker, 1987). The service-use dimensions of interest include the provider organization or auspice, reimbursement source, and volume and duration of use. These dimensions contrast with a single dimension, service contact in a prior period, often the past 6 months, that is widely used in other studies. However, 6 months is considered too lengthy for reliable recall and a 2- to 3-month time period has been recommended (George, 1989).

CONCLUSIONS AND IMPLICATIONS

Conceptual and empirical interest in the relationship between the frail elderly's informal and formal helpers is driven by policy and program development issues as well as theoretical concerns. At the policy level a cautionary stance has been taken toward supporting increased services for chronically disabled elderly and family caregivers, ostensibly based on the fear that families will withdraw their help and come to rely on formal services to meet the care needs of older relatives. The fear of formal service substitution also stems from the less explicitly articulated policy consideration that family volunteerism is less expensive than government support for comprehensive health and social services.

To date, research findings consistently suggest that the fear of service substitution is groundless in the majority of family care situations. Informal care is not supplanted by formal support even when the latter is available and affordable. The belief that family care is less expensive also may be erroneous because it ignores the indirect social costs of caregiving. These costs are evidenced by changes in caregivers' labor-force participation and by various types of care-related strain that can undermine caregivers' emotional and physical health.

Service program planners and practitioners also have an interest in conceptual models for informal-formal helper relationships, because these models and related research findings influence the development of services for frail elderly and their families. For example, conceptual approaches emphasizing the primacy of the informal network and the importance of filial responsibility point to services that enlarge, undergird, and coordinate the activities of informal helpers. In accordance with this approach, formal services are indicated when informal helpers are absent or when care receivers require highly skilled care that informal helpers cannot provide. Formal services are contraindicated when their provision would disrupt or displace informal caregiving.

An alternative conceptual model focused on enhancing the elderly's autonomy and independence points to services that foster rehabilitation, health promotion, environmental adaptation, and the use of assistive devices to avoid or minimize the elderly's functional dependence on others. The importance of these service programs is supported by empirical research showing that older persons with greater autonomy demonstrate better morale and higher levels of life satisfaction (Krause, 1990; Lee, 1985). Additional support comes from studies showing that some older persons with financial resources prefer to purchase services rather than rely on family members (Archbold, 1982; Bass & Noelker, 1987). Guided by this conceptual approach and related research findings, formal services should be made available as an alternative to informal care in order to keep the elderly person from feeling beholden to or dependent on family members.

Policy and practice considerations related to the frail elderly's care also are affected by factors that distinguish long-term care of the aged population from younger age groups with chronic impairments. One factor is the lack of certainty about which informal caregiver takes primary responsibility for the older person's care. Although the aged's informal network often includes multiple individuals, the primary caregiver plays the central role in direct care and how informal services are used (Bass & Noelker, 1987).

The lack of clarity about who fills the primary caregiver role for frail elderly stands in contrast to the care of chronically ill children, where the primacy of the parent is nearly universal. When illness or accident occurs for middle-aged adults, a spouse typically is available to become the primary informal helper. In later life, however, the majority of elderly requiring long-term care are widowed women. Although most of these women have children, the question is which child, if any, will accept primary responsibility for the parent's care. Taking on the primary caregiver role can pose a major dilemma for adult children when they do not live near the parent or have other family and work obligations. The lack of an adult child primary caregiver increases the likelihood that the parent's care network will be more heavily weighted toward formal services, including nursing home care.

Our research indicates that accurate identification of the primary caregiver is less problematic when the elder and caregiver live together regardless of how they are related. These situations may be more similar to caregiving for younger populations. When the impaired elder lives alone, however, it is not uncommon to receive conflicting reports from family members and case managers about who has primary responsibility. A solution adopted by some researchers is to avoid directly asking for the primary caregiver's identity, determining it from a series of questions that indicate who helps most frequently with a list of specific tasks (Barer & Johnson, 1990).

A second factor that distinguishes later life caregiving from care for other age groups relates to the onset of the need for care and the nature of the precipitating condition. At earlier life stages it is more typical for a single disease of acute onset or traumatic injury to necessitate caregiving.

In contrast, chronically impaired older persons frequently have multiple health conditions, such as diabetes, hypertension, and arthritis, that disable them over many years. In these situations informal care can begin almost imperceptibly and evolve over a decade or more in scope and intensity. As a result of the gradual onset the elderly's informal helpers often have difficulty when asked to specify exactly when they began giving assistance.

The gradual onset of impairment also suggests that informal helpers slowly increase their caregiving responsibilities without considering the relevance of formal services. However, a dramatic downward turn or crisis that interrupts the gradual decline in functioning and rapidly escalates care needs can induce families to turn to the formal system. This "crisis orientation" may help explain the consistent finding that formal service use by impaired elderly is linked with increased informal assistance.

The multiplicity of disease conditions in later life also complicates the frail elderly's use of formal care. When multiple conditions are present the patient typically is confronted with a wider array of formal care providers and organizations. There are more physicians and other specialists, more medications prescribed, more clinics to attend, and other support organizations to contact for information (e.g., stroke club, lung association, cancer society). In contrast, at earlier life stages the chronically ill person and family often can identify with a single disease condition and participate in one service arena.

Last, caregiving in later life as opposed to earlier ages is influenced by societal values and expectations about the "normalcy" of decreased abilities in later life and the elderly's closer proximity to death. This contrasts with expectations for younger disabled persons, in which the orientation tends to be more futuristic with an objective of maximizing activity and social integration. For younger persons these expectations increase the aggressiveness of interventions and a service orientation toward family as well as patient. For the frail elderly there is less certainty about the frail elder's role in the family and family members' roles in the care process. These factors, along with a concern for maintaining the autonomy of the older person, complicate the development of informal-formal helper relationships around the care of frail elderly.

REFERENCES

Akiyama, H., Antonucci, T. C., & Campbell, R. (1990). Rules of support exchange among two generations of Japanese and American women. In J. Sokolovsky (Ed.), *Growing old in different societies* (pp. 127-138). Belmont, CA: Wadsworth.

Andersen, R., & Aday, L. (1978). Access to medical care in the U.S.: Realized and potential. *Medical Care, 4,* 533-546.

Antonucci, T. C., & Cantor, M. H. (1991). Strengthening the family support system for older minority persons. In *Minority elders: Longevity, economics, and health* (pp. 32-37). Washington, DC: Gerontological Society of America.

Archbold, P. G. (1982). All-consuming activity: The family as caregiver. *Generations, 7,* 12-13.

Auslander, G. H., & Litwin, H. (1990). Social support networks and formal help seeking: Differences between applicants to social services and a nonapplicant sample. *Journals of Gerontology: Social Sciences, 45,* S112-S119.

Austin, C. D. (1988). History and politics of case management. *Generations, 12*(5), 7-10.

Barer, B. M., & Johnson, C. L. (1990). A critique of the caregiving literature. *The Gerontologist, 30,* 26-29.

Bass, D. M., & Noelker, L. S. (1987). The influence of family caregivers on elders' use of in-home services. *Journal of Health and Social Behavior, 28,* 184-196.

Birkel, R. C., & Jones, C. J. (1989). A comparison of the caregiving networks of dependent elderly individuals who are lucid and those who are demented. *The Gerontologist, 29,* 114-119.

Cantor, M. H. (1979). The informal support system in New York's inner city elderly: Is ethnicity a factor? In D. E. Gelfand & A. J. Kutznik (Eds.), *Ethnicity and aging* (pp. 153-174). New York: Springer.

Cantor, M. H. (1983). Strain among caregivers: A study of experience in the United States. *The Gerontologist, 23,* 597-604.

Cantor, M. H. (1989). Social care: Family and community support systems. *Annals of the American Academy of Political and Social Sciences, 503,* 99-112.

Cantor, M. H. (1991). Family and community: Changing roles in an aging society. *The Gerontologist, 31,* 337-346.

Capitman, J. A., Haskins, B., & Bernstein, J. (1986). Case management approaches in coordinated community-oriented long-term care demonstrations. *The Gerontologist, 26,* 398-404.

Carrilio, T. E., & Eisenberg, D. M. (1983). Informal resources for the elderly: Panacea or empty promises? *Journal of Gerontological Social Work, 6,* 39-47.

Collins, C., Stommel, M., King, S., & Given, C. W. (1991). Assessment of the attitudes of family caregivers toward community services. *The Gerontologist, 31,* 756-761.

Deimling, G. T., & Bass, D. M. (1986). Symptoms of mental impairment among elderly adults and their effects on family caregivers. *Journal of Gerontology, 41,* 778-784.

Edelman, P. (1986). The impact of community care to the home-bound elderly on provision of informal care [Special issue]. *The Gerontologist, 26,* 234A.

Edelman, P., & Hughes, S. (1990). The impact of community care on provision of informal care to homebound elderly persons. *Journals of Gerontology: Social Sciences, 45,* S874-S884.

Frankfather, D. L., Smith, M. J., & Caro, F. G. (1981). *Family care of the elderly.* Lexington, MA: D. C. Heath.

George, L. K. (1987, July). *Respite care and support groups: Benefits for caregivers and barriers to use.* Paper presented at the conference Caring for Frail Elderly: A Partnership of Family and Community, Cleveland, OH.

George, L. K. (1989). Services research: Research problems and possibilities. In E. Light & B. Lebowitz (Eds.), *Alzheimer's disease treatment and family stress: Directions for research* (pp. 401-433). Washington, DC: Government Printing Office.

Gerace, C. S., & Noelker, L. S. (1990). Clinical social work practice with black elderly and their family caregivers. In Z. Harel, E. McKinney, & M. Williams (Eds.), *Black aged: Understanding diversity and service needs* (pp. 236-258). Newbury Park, CA: Sage.

Gibson, R. (1982). Blacks at middle and late life: Resources and coping. *Annals of the American Academy of Political and Social Sciences, 464,* 79-90.

Greene, V. L. (1983). Substitution between formally and informally provided care for the impaired elderly in the community. *Medical Care, 21,* 609-619.

Gwyther, L. (1988). Assessment: Content, purpose, outcomes. *Generations, 12*(5), 11-15.

Gwyther, L., Gold, D., & Hinman-Smith, E. (1988). *Older people and their families: Coping with stress and conflict.* Durham, NC: Duke University Center for the Study of Aging and Human Development.

Hess, B., & Soldo, B. (1985). Husband and wife networks. In W. J. Saur & R. T. Coward (Eds.), *Social support networks and the care of the elderly: Theory, research and practice* (pp. 67-92). New York: Springer.

Jette, A. M., Tennstedt, S. L., & Branch, L. G. (1992). Stability of informal long-term care. *Journal of Aging and Health, 4,* 193-211.

Kinney, J. M., & Stephens, M. P. (1989). Caregiving hassles scale: Assessing the daily hassles of caring for a family member with dementia. *The Gerontologist, 29,* 328-335.

Krause, N. (1990). Perceived health problems, formal/informal support, and life satisfaction among older adults. *Journals of Gerontology: Social Sciences, 45,* S193-S205.

Lawton, M., Kleban, M., Moss, M., Rovine, J., & Glicksman, A. (1989). Measuring caregiving appraisal. *Journals of Gerontology: Psychological Sciences, 44,* P61-P71.

Lee, G. (1985). Kinship and social support among the elderly: The case of the United States. *Aging and Society, 5,* 19-38.

Litwak, E. (1985). *Helping the elderly: The complementary roles of informal networks and formal systems.* New York: Guilford.

McAuley, W., & Arling, G. (1984). Use of in-home care by very old people. *Journal of Health and Social Behavior, 25,* 54-64.

McKinlay, J. B. (1972). Some approaches and problems in the study of the use of services—An overview. *Journal of Health and Social Behavior, 13,* 115-152.

Mechanic, D. (1979). Correlates of physician utilization: Why do major multivariate studies of physician utilization find trivial psychosocial and organizational effects? *Journal of Health and Social Behavior, 20,* 387-396.

Miller, B., & McFall, S. (1991). The effect of caregiver's burden on change in frail older persons' use of formal helpers. *Journal of Health and Social Behavior, 32,* 165-179.

Noelker, L. S. (1984). Family care of elder relatives: The impact of policy and programs. In *Conference proceedings on family support and long term care* (pp. 52-85). Excelsior, MN: InterStudy.

Noelker, L. S., & Bass, D. M. (1989). Home care for elderly persons: Linkages between formal and informal caregivers. *Journals of Gerontology: Social Sciences, 44,* S63-S70.

Penning, M. (1990). Receipt of assistance by elderly people: Hierarchical selection and task specificity. *The Gerontologist, 30,* 220-227.

Petchers, M. K., & Milligan, S. E. (1988). Access to health care in a black urban elderly population. *The Gerontologist, 28,* 213-217.

Saperstein, A. (1988, October). *Clinical issues in respite care.* Paper presented at the conference Respite for Family Caregivers: Advances in Program Design and Evaluation, Cleveland, OH.

Schneider, B. (1988). Care planning: The core of case management. *Generations, 12*(5), 16-18.

Secord, L. (1987). *Private case management for older persons and their families: Practice, policy, potential.* Excelsior, MN: InterStudy.

Seeman, T. E., & Berkman, L. F. (1988). Structural characteristics of social networks and their relationship with social support in the elderly: Who provides support. *Social Science and Medicine, 26,* 737-749.

Seltzer, M. M., Ivry, J., & Litchfield, L. C. (1987). Family members as case managers: Partnership between the formal and informal support networks. *The Gerontologist, 27,* 722-728.

Soldo, B. J., Wolf, D. A., & Agree, E. M. (1990). Family, households, and care arrangements of frail older women: A structural analysis. *Journals of Gerontology: Social Sciences, 45,* S238-S249.

Tennstedt, S., McKinlay, J., & Sullivan, L. (1989). Informal care for frail older persons: The role of secondary caregivers. *The Gerontologist, 29,* 677-683.

Teresi, J., Toner, J., Bennett, R., & Wilder, D. (1988). Caregiver burden and long-term planning. *Journal of Applied Social Sciences, 13,* 215-256.

Vaux, A., & Athanassopulou, M. (1987). Social support appraisals and network resources. *Journal of Community Psychology, 15,* 537-556.

Vaux, A., Phillips, J., Holly, L., Thomson, B., Williams, D., & Stewart, D. (1986). The Social Support Appraisals Scale (SS-A): Studies of reliability and validity. *American Journal of Community Psychology, 14,* 195-219.

Zarit, S., Reever, K., & Bach-Peterson, J. (1980). Relatives of the impaired elderly: Correlates of feelings of burden. *The Gerontologist, 20,* 649-655.

Conclusion

This volume has focused on expanding the caregiving paradigm and enhancing conceptual understandings through greater appreciation of context. What have we learned through this exploration and what future directions do we need to look toward?

It may be fair to argue that caregiving research has had an uneven course of development with some areas of research receiving a great deal of attention and others being relatively neglected (Zarit, 1989). At the same time it is important to note that those areas that have received the most research attention, such as caring for aged patients with Alzheimer's disease, also have made the most strides in conceptual and methodological development. They can thus inform newer and developing areas of interest. In time, new research areas also tend to generate their own characteristic research traditions, in terms of both conceptual and methodological orientations.

The present volume has sampled alternative conceptual and research traditions that characterize caregiving research focusing on different points in the life course. The diverse orientations represented in the contributions to this volume suggest a need for greater communication among the diverse constituencies of caregiving. Our understanding can be enriched by perspectives of those involved in the caregiving process at different points during the life course and in different illness situations. In addition, the field can be enriched by perspectives of researchers and practitioners from different disciplines.

There are multiple benefits to expansion of the caregiving paradigm. Articulation of a broader paradigm results in moving beyond unidimensional and molecular approaches to caregiving. More comprehensive and holistic approaches to caregiving are likely to enhance the heuristic value of research in this area. Thus where the care receiver suffers from a designated illness, such as mental illness, other conditions such as physical illness also would be taken into account. Furthermore, the comprehensive paradigm moves toward recognizing that in many cases the care receiver "gives" or the caregiver "receives" in a family relationship. In some situations such as those of an elderly couple, in which both spouses suffer from chronic illness, it may be misleading to designate only one party as caregiver and the other as care receiver. Research may more profitably focus on reciprocal caregiving transactions.

Consideration of the temporal dimensions of caregiving, and particularly a life-span oriented approach to caregiving, opens up diverse new content areas for research. Thus, for example, a useful new temporal direction for the study of caregiving relates to understanding caregiving careers. Recent efforts have begun to evaluate the cumulative effects of caregiving throughout the lifespan on caregiver career, starting with the "in home care" stage, proceeding to the "institutionalization" stage, and terminating in the "bereaved" stage (Pearlin, Mullen, Semple, & Skaff, 1990).

The impact of time on social role performance has been the subject of growing attention by social scientists concerned with life-course perspectives (Clausen, 1986; Elder, 1985). The life-course trajectory of caregiving responsibilities also differs based on the type of illness considered. On one extreme are parents of children with developmental disabilities such as autism or Down's syndrome. These parents face predictable lifelong caregiving responsibilities. On the other extreme are illnesses such as cancer that may go into remission and from which recovery is possible but where recurrence of the illness looms as a threat to survival of the care receiver. Each trajectory of illness and life-course stage may call for different research strategies in considering processes and outcomes of caregiving. Thus, for example, cross-sectional studies of older adults confronting the care of adult children with Down's syndrome may be useful. In contrast, understanding of caregiving to children with cancer may require longitudinal studies that follow parents from diagnosis to alternative trajectories of recovery, remission, or intensification of illness.

The contributions to this volume move in the direction of recognizing the important practice and policy implications of research in the field of caregiving. Interventions can benefit from expansion of the caregiving paradigm by noting differential objectives of intervention involving different actors in both the family and formal systems and interventions at different points in the illness and life course. For example, the expanded paradigm recognizes needs of both members of the caregiver-care receiver dyad. Integrated models of service delivery call for addressing needs of both caregivers and care receivers and for recognizing that such needs and desires may not always be symmetrical (Gonyea, Seltzer, Gerstein, & Young, 1988). Thus research is needed to test the appropriateness and effectiveness of intervention models for caregiving families that vary systematically with stages of the life cycle.

Directives for policy also may be enriched by considering contextual influences of culture, ethnicity, and social class. Filial obligations and attitudes toward caregiving are powerfully shaped by culture and ethnicity (Yu et al., 1993). Thus service options such as respite care in a nursing home may be wholly acceptable to one group whereas they are totally unacceptable to another. Accordingly, policies that foster such services may meet with varying success.

The expanded caregiving paradigm, illustrated in contributions to this volume, also provides some direction for bridging the gap between conceptualization and empirical work in the area of caregiving research. To the extent that we can identify salient processes of caregiving, research can be undertaken to examine the mechanisms by which caregiving demands or behaviors impact on well-being of both caregivers and care receivers. We can then go beyond answering only questions about the impact of caregiving on psychological well-being of those providing care and move toward addressing the questions of how or why favorable outcomes might be generated and adverse outcomes avoided.

The journey toward such progress is likely to benefit from a diversity of methodological approaches. There is need for further work to identify processes or mechanisms involved in caregiving. Qualitative and observational studies that could prove to be particularly useful in identifying such processes can focus on the phenomenology of both caregivers and care receivers along with eliciting biographical narratives that can place caregiving in a temporal and life-span developmental context. Such studies also can shed light on previously unrecognized issues that may shape attitudes, behaviors, and feelings of those giving and receiving care.

Critical dimensions of caregiver-care receiver transactions also may be identified through observational research in naturalistic studies in health-care settings and in private homes. Laboratory studies of social interactions between caregivers and care receivers under controlled conditions also could add to our understanding of processes such as cooperation, compliance, self-disclosure, and other social behaviors.

Where predictors of important transactions and outcomes in caregiving have been identified, the field might greatly benefit from prospective studies and macrolevel studies that permit consideration of caregiving systems rather than examinations of just individuals involved in caregiving transactions.

It is our hope that the contributions in this volume pave the way for improved conceptualization and operational approaches achieved through an extended caregiving paradigm, increased diversity in research methods, and enhanced communication among researchers and practitioners from different disciplines. We believe this volume will be useful to students, researchers, practitioners, and policy makers as they direct their imaginations toward moving the fields of practice and scholarship forward in a quest for better understanding of the caregiving paradigm.

REFERENCES

Clausen, J. A. (1986). *The life course.* Englewood Cliffs, NJ: Prentice Hall.

Elder, G. H., Jr. (1985). Perspectives on the life course. In G. H. Elder, Jr. (Ed.), *Life course dynamics, trajectories, and transitions, 1968-1980* (pp. 23-49). Ithaca, NY: Cornell University Press.

Gonyea, J. G., Seltzer, G. B., Gerstein, C., & Young, M. (1988). Acceptance of hospital-based respite by families and elders. *Health and Social Work,* 201-208.

Pearlin, L. I., Mullen, J. T., Semple, S. J., & Skaff, M. M. (1990). Caregiving and the stress process: An overview of concepts and their measures. *The Gerontologist, 30,* 583-594.

Yu, E., Liu, W. T., Wang, Z., Levy, P. S., Katzman, R., Zhang, M., Qu, G., & Chen, F. (1993). Caregivers of the cognitively impaired and the disabled in Shanghai, China. In S. H. Zarit, L. I. Pearlin, & K. W. Schaie (Eds.), *Caregiving systems: Formal and informal helpers* (pp. 3-30). Hillsdale, NJ: Lawrence Erlbaum.

Zarit, S. H. (1989). Do we need another "stress and caregiving study?" *The Gerontologist, 39,* 147-148.

Index

About the Editors

David E. Biegel, Ph.D., is the Henry L. Zucker Professor of Social Work Practice and Professor of Sociology, Mandel School of Applied Social Sciences, Case Western Reserve University. He currently also serves as Co-Director of the Center for Practice Innovations at the Mandel School. He has been involved in research, scholarship, and practice pertaining to the delivery of services to hard-to-reach population groups and the relationship between informal and formal care for the past 15 years. His recent research activities have focused on natural support systems for persons with chronic mental illness, family caregiving, and mental health and aging. His recent books include: *Family Caregiving in Chronic Illness: Alzheimer's Disease, Cancer, Heart Disease, Mental Illness, and Stroke* (co-authored with Esther Sales and Richard Schulz, Sage, 1991); *Family Preservation Services: Research and Evaluation* (co-edited with Kathleen Wells, Sage, 1991); and *Aging and Caregiving: Theory, Research, and Policy* (co-edited with Arthur Blum, Sage, 1990).

Eva Kahana, Ph.D., is Pierce T. and Elizabeth D. Robson Professor of Humanities, Chair of the Department of Sociology, and Director of the Elderly Care Research Center at Case Western Reserve University. She received her doctorate in human development from the University of Chicago and did a postdoctoral fellowship with the Midwest Council on Social Research in Aging. She has received the Gerontological Society of America Distinguished Mentorship Award. She is currently a Mary E. Switzer Distinguished Fellow of the National Institute of Disability and Rehabilitation. In the past year she has received the Heller Award from Menorah Park Center for the Aged and was named the Distinguished Gerontological Researcher in the State of Ohio. She has published extensively in the areas of stress, coping and health of aged, late-life migration, and environmental influences on older persons.

May L. Wykle, Ph.D., R.N., F.A.A.N., is the Florence Cellar Professor of Gerontological Nursing, the Director of the University Center on Aging and Health, and the Associate Dean for Community Affairs at the Frances Payne Bolton School of Nursing, Case Western Reserve University. She has received a National Institutes of Mental Health Geriatric Mental Health Academic Award and was Director of a five-year Robert Wood Johnson Teaching Nursing Home Project. Her research area is geriatric mental health, self-care, and family caregiving. She is currently the Principal Investigator of a 4-year study, "Black vs. White Caregivers' Formal/Informal Service Use." She has written many articles, chapters, and books. She received the 1993 Leadership Award for Excellence in Geriatric Care from the Midwest Alliance in Nursing.

About the Contributors

Joan Aldous, Ph.D., is the William R. Kenan, Jr., Professor of Sociology at the University of Notre Dame. She has written a paper commissioned for the United Nations titled "Families in the Development Process" and has received the Ernest W. Burgess Award in recognition of her continuous and meritorious contributions to theory and research in the family field of sociology. Her research has concerned parent-child relations with primary- and middle-school-age children and pre-retirement couples' interchanges with their adult children. Her articles have been published in numerous journals.

David M. Bass, Ph.D., is Assistant Director of Research at The Margaret Blenkner Research Center of The Benjamin Rose Institute. He has conducted numerous studies and published extensively on issues related to the effects of chronic illness on aged persons and their family members. Special areas of interest include the utilization and impact of formal services, social support, the effect of Alzheimer's disease on family members, bereavement, and the organization of long-term care. He currently is Co-Principal Investigator of a project examining the relationship between formal and informal assistance use by elderly receiving case-management services.

Patricia Flatley Brennan, Ph.D., R.N., is Associate Professor of Nursing and Systems Engineering at Case Western Reserve University. She received her master's degree in nursing from the University of Pennsylvania and her doctorate in industrial engineering at the University of Wisconsin-Madison. Following 7 years of clinical practice in critical care nursing and psychiatric nursing, she has held several academic nursing positions. She developed and directed the Computer Link, an electronic network designed to reduce isolation and improve self-care among home care patients. In 1991 she was elected as a Fellow of the American Academy of Nursing, and in 1992 she became Associate Editor for the *Journal of the American Medical Informatics Association.*

Venkatesan Chakravarthy is a Ph.D. student in the Mandel School of Applied Social Sciences, Case Western Reserve University. Besides family caregiving with the chronically ill, his research interests include infant mortality and female infanticide in India. He currently is involved in the Healthy Family Healthy Start Project as a Research Assistant. The goal of the project is to reduce infant mortality in the selected areas of the City of Cleveland and Warrensville Heights.

Dimitri A. Christakis, M.D., is a Resident in Pediatrics at the Seattle Children's Hospital and Medical Center and the University of Washington. He graduated from Yale University and the University of Pennsylvania School of Medicine. His current research interests include the impact of medical interventions on child development and the medical ethical development of physicians in training.

Nancy N. Eustis, Ph.D., is Special Assistant in Disability, Aging, and Long-Term Care Policy, Office of the Assistant Secretary for Planning and Evaluation, U.S. Department of Health and Human Services. She is on leave from her position as Professor of Public Affairs and Planning at the Humphrey Institute of Public Affairs, University of Minnesota, where she teaches courses in social policy, aging policy, and evaluation research. She is senior author of *Long-Term Care for the Elderly: A Policy Perspective* and coeditor of *Aging and Disabilities: Seeking Common Ground.*

Lucy Rose Fischer, Ph.D., is Research Investigator in Geriatrics at Group Health Foundation in Minnesota. She is the author of three books and has published numerous professional articles and research reports on intergenerational family relationships, informal caregiving, paid home care, health care, volunteering, and qualitative research methods. She has been on the faculties of the University of Minnesota and St. Olaf College and was Senior Research Scientist at the Amherst H. Wilder Foundation. She is a Fellow of the Gerontological Society of America.

Barbara A. Given, Ph.D., R.N., F.A.A.N., is Professor and Director of the Center for Nursing Research in the College of Nursing and Associate

Director for the Cancer Center at Michigan State University. She has served on the Institute of Medicine panel to advise the Department of Defense on its Breast Cancer Program. She has been actively involved in research of long-term and home care for more than 9 years. She has been awarded grants from the National Cancer Institute, the National Institute of Nursing Research, the National Institute on Aging, and the American Cancer Society. Recently, she has received a grant to examine the formal and informal costs of cancer care for patients over the age of 65 with either breast, colon, lung, or prostate cancer. She has authored and coauthored numerous articles on supportive and continuing care for families of elderly patients with cancer and other chronic diseases.

Charles W. Given, Ph.D., is Professor in the Department of Family Practice in the College of Human Medicine at Michigan State University. He has been involved in research and scholarship related to home care of the elderly and chronically ill for the past decade. The focus of this work is to understand the family and patient experience and patterns and cost of formal and informal care. He is widely published about caregiving patterns of informal and formal care. Current research activities include serving as Principal Investigator on a 5-year longitudinal intervention study of rural patients with cancer and as Co-Principal Investigator of a 4-year study on patterns and costs of cancer for elderly individuals with cancer.

Ronald J. Hammond, Ph.D., is Assistant Professor of Sociology at Utah Valley State College. He received graduate training in gerontology and sociology of the family from Brigham Young University. He recently completed a postdoctoral fellowship in gerontology with the Department of Sociology, Case Western Reserve University. His current research pertains to family and cross-cultural aspects of aging, especially concerning the divorced and separated. He has worked on the development of various grants, published articles, produced and directed an educational documentary, and is currently developing an undergraduate gerontology program at Utah Valley State College.

Dorothy Jones Jessop, Ph.D., is Director of Research and Evaluation at the Medical and Health Research Association of New York, Inc., a self-sustaining not-for-profit organization that seeks to secure funds for health services and health-services research for underserved populations in New York City. She has part-time academic appointments as an

Associate Professor in the Department of Pediatrics at Albert Einstein College of Medicine and an Associate Research Scientist in the Division of Sociomedical Sciences at Columbia University School of Public Health. She received her doctorate in sociology from New York University. She has spent more than 20 years working on applied social research projects and evaluations. Her major research interests are in the area of chronic physical illness and in disabilities, especially mental retardation, and she publishes primarily in these areas.

J. Randal Johnson, Ph.D., is Adjunct Assistant Professor of Sociology at Case Western Reserve University. He also is a Research Associate at the Geriatric Care Center at Fairhill Institute, where he acts as Research and Methodological Consultant to the Geriatric Fellows Program. His research is focused primarily on the positive and negative effects of social support networks on the mental and physical well-being of frail elderly persons. He currently is involved as Principal Investigator and Co-Principal Investigator, respectively, in two pilot studies: "Factors Associated With Negative Interactions Between Caregivers and Care-Receivers" and "A Family Intervention With Elderly Female Alcoholics" (with Dr. James Campbell). He also is Co-Investigator on the second phase of the "Adaptation to Frailty" Merit Award study.

Boaz Kahana, Ph.D., is Professor of Psychology and Director of the Center on Aging at Cleveland State University. He received his doctorate in human development and psychology from the University of Chicago in 1967. He is a Fellow of the Gerontological Society of America, the American Psychological Society, and the American Orthopsychiatric Association, where he served as Chair of the Study Group on Aging. He is a clinical and adult developmental psychologist with special interest in late-life sequelae of extreme trauma. He has been awarded research grants dealing with stress and extreme stress among the elderly in community and institutional settings. He is currently Co-Principal Investigator of a longitudinal Merit Award study of retirees who have relocated to Florida. His funded research and publications also have focused on the sequelae of external trauma among elderly survivors of the Holocaust and Pearl Harbor. He is author of numerous articles and chapters dealing with stress, coping, and adaptation among the elderly.

Catherine F. Kane, Ph.D., R.N., is Associate Professor of Nursing and Psychiatric Medicine, University of Virginia; Director of Education and

Evaluation, Western State Hospital; and Faculty Associate of the University of Virginia's Southeastern Rural Mental Health Research Center. Her career has focused on nursing care of the seriously mentally ill and their families. She has conducted research and published on issues regarding long-term care of the seriously mentally ill and programs to support families caring for this population. Her current research focuses on predicting long-term care needs of the seriously mentally ill and models of community care.

Anne E. Kazak, Ph.D., is Associate Professor of Psychology in the Departments of Pediatrics and Psychiatry at the University of Pennsylvania; Director of Psychosocial Services in the Division of Oncology at The Children's Hospital of Philadelphia; and a licensed clinical psychologist. Her research interests focus on child and family adaptation to pediatric medical conditions. She is the author of more than 45 papers in the area. She is currently the Principal Investigator on three research and service provision grants.

Kyle Kercher, Ph.D., is Associate Professor in the Department of Sociology at Case Western Reserve University. He currently also serves as Director of the Education, Epidemiology, and Health Services Research Administration of the Northeast Ohio Multipurpose Arthritis Center. He received his doctorate from the University of Washington, where he also did a postdoctoral fellowship in gerontology. He is involved in a number of longitudinal studies of the elderly and is Principal Investigator of a 5-year project analyzing buffers of the arthritis-disability cascade among old-old persons. His current research interests and publications concern adaptation to frailty among the aged, and structural equation models of physical health and psychological well-being.

Barbara J. Leonard, Ph.D., is Associate Professor of Nursing in the School of Nursing at the University of Minnesota. Her research focuses on the care of children with special health-care needs and their families. She is currently the Director of two federally funded training grants on the care of children with special health-care needs. In addition, she heads the Pediatric Nurse Practitioner area of study within the School of Nursing.

Eugene Litwak, Ph.D., is a Professor in the Department of Sociology and Head of the Division of Sociomedical Sciences at the School of

Public Health, Columbia University. His research has been on the roles of formal organizations and informal groups (such as family, friends, and neighbors) in modern industrial societies. His current research is in three fields: (a) caregiving needs and optimal forms of support for minority women who are HIV seropositive, (b) the coordination between agencies delivering mental health services to adolescents, and (c) the interaction between stages of health of older people and types of retirement communities.

Jack H. Medalie, M.D., M.P.H., F.A.A.F.P., is the Dorothy Jones Weatherhead Professor Emeritus, of Family Medicine at Case Western Reserve University. He has practiced medicine in various countries, including Africa, Israel, and the United States. He also directed a Family and Community Health Center in a low socioeconomic area of Jerusalem for 10 years and developed and chaired three new departments of family medicine in Israel and in Cleveland, Ohio. His major research interests have revolved around epidemiological investigations of chronic diseases—coronary heart disease, angina pectoris, diabetes, duodenal ulcer, and hypertension—in large population groups. A feature of this research was the interaction of psychosocial factors with biological ones in the search for risk factors relating to the development of these diseases. He has published a number of books and more than 100 articles in various medical journals. He was elected to the Institute of Medicine of the National Academy of Sciences in 1978 and is currently finalizing research projects related to physical activity and heart disease, intermittent claudication, and various new medical educational ideas.

Elizabeth Midlarsky, Ph.D., is Professor in the Department of Clinical Psychology and Director of the Center for Lifespan and Aging Studies at Teachers College, Columbia University. She is former editor of the *Academic Psychology Bulletin.* Her ongoing research interests include predictors and consequences of altruism and helping from early childhood through late life, in siblings of people with disabilities, and among non-Jewish rescuers of Jews during the Holocaust, as well as psychotherapy with diverse populations. She is coauthor of the volume *For the Sake of Others: Altruism and Helping by Older Adults,* and is currently Principal Investigator of a study on predictors and barriers to mental-health-care utilization and help seeking by older adults.

Shirley M. Moore, Ph.D., R.N., is Assistant Professor of Nursing, Case Western Reserve University. Her research has focused on interventions to support families coping with acute and chronic illness. She most recently has been a member of research projects designed to determine the effect of a computer network intervention to support home care with two groups: persons living with AIDS and caregivers of persons with Alzheimer's disease.

Heather J. Moulton, M.P.H., is the Project Coordinator for Research and Technology at Aging in America, Bronx, New York. She received her M.P.H. and M.S. degrees from Columbia University. She has had extensive long-term care experience as an occupational therapist. Her research interests focus on caregiving linkages between formal organizations and informal social support.

Linda S. Noelker, Ph.D., is Associate Director for Research at The Benjamin Rose Institute and Director of the Institute's Margaret Blenkner Research Center. For the past 20 years she has conducted applied aging research on the nature and effects of family care for frail aged and the elderly's patterns of service use. She has published widely on the aged's support networks, the well-being of family caregivers, predictors of service use, and the nature of social relationships in nursing homes. Her current research activities include serving as Principal Investigator of a project on informal and formal assistance use by elderly receiving case-management services. She is also the Principal Investigator of two studies on the quality and effects of relationships between nursing home residents and nurse assistants.

Joan M. Patterson, Ph.D., is Associate Professor of Maternal and Child Health in the School of Public Health and the Director of Research for the Center for Children With Chronic Illness and Disability, both at the University of Minnesota. Using a biopsychosocial paradigm, her research is focused on examining the reciprocal impacts of chronic illness in child and family functioning. Of particular interest is the development and evaluation of interventions for preventing psychopathology in individuals and families coping with chronic physical illness. Her current research activities include serving as Co-Principal Investigator of a longitudinal study of children with a variety of chronic illness conditions to determine the child, family, and community factors associated with psychological and social competence in the child and family. She has served as an International Rehabilitation Consultant to the government of India and has published extensively about families and stress, particularly the stress of chronic illness.

Li-yu Song, Ph.D., is Research Program Manager of the Center for Social Work Practice Innovations at Case Western Reserve University. She has extensive research experience in the mental health problems of adolescents and elderly, including working as the Research Coordinator of the Three-Year Adolescent Follow-up Study from 1988 to 1991. Her recent work has focused on factors associated with caregiver burden of persons with chronic mental illness and the relationship between violence exposure and mental health sequelae among adolescents. She has published articles in various journals.

Rosalie F. Young, Ph.D., is Associate Professor and Graduate Director of Community Medicine, Wayne State University School of Medicine. She has conducted research on health of the aged and has been Principal Investigator and Co-Principal Investigator on several studies. Her current focus is on cultural aspects of family management of Alzheimer's disease. She is the author of a book on health and aging and has published numerous articles and abstracts.